Long-Term Management of Dementia

T0199648

Long-Term Management of Dementia

Edited by
Douglas W. Scharre
Director, Division of Cognitive Neurology
Department of Neurology
The Ohio State University
Columbus, Ohio, U.S.A.

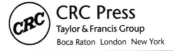

CRC Press
Taylor & Francis Group
Boca Raton   London   New York

CRC Press is an imprint of the
Taylor & Francis Group, an informa business

CRC Press
Taylor & Francis Group
6000 Broken Sound Parkway NW, Suite 300
Boca Raton, FL 33487-2742

First issued in paperback 2019

© 2011 by Taylor & Francis Group, LLC
CRC Press is an imprint of Taylor & Francis Group, an Informa business

No claim to original U.S. Government works

ISBN-13: 978-0-8493-3853-3 (hbk)
ISBN-13: 978-0-367-38339-8 (pbk)

This book contains information obtained from authentic and highly regarded sources. While all reasonable efforts have been made to publish reliable data and information, neither the author[s] nor the publisher can accept any legal responsibility or liability for any errors or omissions that may be made. The publishers wish to make clear that any views or opinions expressed in this book by individual editors, authors or contributors are personal to them and do not necessarily reflect the views/opinions of the publishers. The information or guidance contained in this book is intended for use by medical, scientific or healthcare professionals and is provided strictly as a supplement to the medical or other professional's own judgement, their knowledge of the patient's medical history, relevant manufacturer's instructions and the appropriate best practice guidelines. Because of the rapid advances in medical science, any information or advice on dosages, procedures or diagnoses should be independently verified. The reader is strongly urged to consult the relevant national drug formulary and the drug companies' and device or material manufacturers' printed instructions, and their websites, before administering or utilizing any of the drugs, devices or materials mentioned in this book. This book does not indicate whether a particular treatment is appropriate or suitable for a particular individual. Ultimately it is the sole responsibility of the medical professional to make his or her own professional judgements, so as to advise and treat patients appropriately. The authors and publishers have also attempted to trace the copyright holders of all material reproduced in this publication and apologize to copyright holders if permission to publish in this form has not been obtained. If any copyright material has not been acknowledged please write and let us know so we may rectify in any future reprint.

A CIP record for this book is available from the British Library.
ISBN-13: 978-0-8493-3853-3

Visit the Taylor & Francis Web site at
http://www.taylorandfrancis.com

and the CRC Press Web site at
http://www.crcpress.com

To my spouse, Meta Scharre, whose love and support
made this book possible.

Preface

Dementing conditions are becoming very common as the population grows older. Currently, it is estimated that 28 million people worldwide have dementia. This number will rise dramatically as the life expectancy of humans increases and as the populations in the United States and other countries age. Economic costs will also mount. Alzheimer's disease by itself is already the third most costly condition in the United States behind heart disease and cancer, when the costs of caregivers and nursing homes are taken into account. Until we find a cure, optimal long-term management is our best course of action to help alleviate the devastating costs and the impaired quality of life seen in our dementia patients.

Individuals with Alzheimer's disease will typically live 8 to 12 years after they start misplacing their keys or eyeglasses on a regular basis. After the diagnosis is made, there are many years of management decisions that lie ahead for the physician and caregivers. Every stage presents with new challenges. The patients' needs change and old issues become passé as new ones take their place. Caregiver roles must also change to keep up with the new issues. Some of these changes are predictable and others come as a surprise. Health care providers need to provide the correct timing of treatment and management direction that will optimize care. Pharmacotherapy, management of behavioral and functional problems, and appropriate referral to assist with social and legal issues are some of the important decisions that need to be made. There is a need to be proactive, efficient, cost conscious, and practical in the long-term management of dementia syndromes.

This book is intended to be a resource for solutions to common management problems that arise in caring for dementia patients over the long haul. Many monographs focus on diagnosis and treatment issues of dementia. Books that discuss long-term management are few. Our focus is more on the art than on the science of managing dementing illnesses. We wish to provide practical information and valuable insights regarding the many complex management problems that arise in dementia. Clinicians, nurses, social workers, therapists, caregivers, family members, and all that are involved in enhancing the quality of care for the dementia patient should find this book useful.

As background information, the first couple of chapters deal with the scope, risk factors, assessment, and diagnosis of the more common dementing conditions. The management issues begin with a discussion of the pharmacotherapy of cognition. Some treatments are indicated early in the course and others for later stages. There are standard, controversial, and unproven but widely used therapies. Neuropsychiatric symptoms are very common in dementia but currently there are no U.S. FDA-approved medications for treating the behavioral problems in dementia. The literature provides some suggestions regarding preferred drug approaches. Behavioral modification techniques are also very useful and may reduce the use of medications.

The rest of the book focuses on the management of specific issues in dementia. These topics range from managing instrumental and basic activities of daily living to resolving common ethical and legal dilemmas. Functional abilities are seldom regained once lost. Driving, safety, nutritional, and hygiene issues are frequent concerns for families. Maintaining patient functional abilities, being proactive regarding potential safety concerns, and knowing when to increase supervision improves the quality of life for patients. Paying for these dementia-related services requires careful planning and important tips and caveats regarding financial decision making are discussed. Physicians play an important role in monitoring patients, in follow-up care, in direction of ancillary care, in the management of the medical complications of dementia, in end-of-life care, and in medical–legal issues. Caregivers have to deal with many issues over the long course of their loved one's dementing illness and need special attention from health care providers and support groups to avoid burnout and reduce stress. Readers can look up specific topics of interest. Our hope is that this book will become a useful companion and a helpful resource of information in caring for the individual with dementia over the entire course of their disease.

—DWS

Acknowledgments

I would like to express my appreciation to Rebecca Davis, RN, LISW, Shu Ing Chang, PharmD, and the staff at Forest Hills Center in Columbus, Ohio, and the long-term dementia patients whom they serve for their support.

Contents

Preface vii
Acknowledgments ix
Contributors xiii

1. Scope of dementia: epidemiology and public health impact   1
   Patricia A. Boyle and David A. Bennett

2. Diagnosis of mild cognitive impairment and dementia   25
   Maria Kataki

3. Pharmacotherapy of cognition   56
   David S. Geldmacher

4. Behavior management in dementia   71
   Douglas W. Scharre

5. Management of function: instrumental activities of daily living   127
   Catherine Anne Bare and Martha S. Cameron

6. Management of function: basic activities of daily living   141
   Gail A. Greenley

7. Health economics and financial decision making   150
   Christopher Leibman and Trent McLaughlin

8. The primary care physician's role in the recognition, diagnosis, and management of dementia   169
   Larry W. Lawhorne

9. Ethical issues in dementia   188
   Caroline N. Harada and Greg A. Sachs

10. Legal issues in dementia   210
    Marshall B. Kapp

11. Caregiver stress and possible solutions   225
Mary D. Dodge and Janice K. Kiecolt-Glaser

12. Local and national resource listing   239
Nancy Theado-Miller

Index 245

Contributors

Catherine Anne Bare, RN, BS   Care Consultation Team, Alzheimer's Association, Central Ohio Chapter, Columbus, Ohio, USA

David A. Bennett, MD   Robert C. Borwell Professor of Neurological Sciences; Director, Rush Alzheimer's Disease Center, Rush University Medical Center, Chicago, Illinois, USA

Patricia A. Boyle, PhD   Assistant Professor, Department of Psychology, Rush Alzheimer's Disease Center, Rush University Medical Center, Chicago, Illinois, USA

Martha S. Cameron, MS, OTR/L   Care Consultation Team, Alzheimer's Association, Central Ohio Chapter, Columbus, Ohio, USA

Mary D. Dodge, FNP-BC   Center for Health and Wellbeing, University of Vermont, Burlington, Vermont, USA

David S. Geldmacher, MD, FACP   Harrison Distinguished Teaching Associate Professor of Neurology, University of Virginia Health System, Charlottesville, Virginia, USA

Gail A. Greenley, BSN, RN   Director of Nursing, Forest Hills Center, Columbus, Ohio, USA

Caroline N. Harada, MD   Assistant Professor of Medicine, Division of Gerontology, Geriatrics, and Palliative Care, University of Alabama at Birmingham, Birmingham, Alabama, USA

Marshall B. Kapp, JD, MPH   Director, Center for Innovative Collaboration in Medicine and Law, Florida State University College of Medicine; Professor, Department of Geriatrics, and Courtesy Professor, Florida State University College of Law, Tallahassee, Florida, USA

Maria Kataki, MD, PhD   Assistant Professor of Neurology, Division of Cognitive Neurology, The Ohio State University; Cluster Leader, The Independent Study Program, CNS Pathophysiology Module Leader, Consultant Regency Manor Nursing Home, Columbus, Ohio, USA

Janice Kiecolt-Glaser, PhD   Distinguished University Professor, S. Robert Davis Chair of Medicine, and Professor of Psychiatry and Psychology, Institute for Behavioral Medicine Research, The Ohio State University College of Medicine, Columbus, Ohio, USA

Larry W. Lawhorne, MD   Chair, Department of Geriatrics, Boonshoft School of Medicine, Wright State University, Dayton, Ohio, USA

Christopher Leibman, PharmD, MS   Senior Director and Head, Health Economics/Market Access, Janssen Alzheimer Immunotherapy R&D, LLC, South San Francisco, California, USA

Trent McLaughlin, PhD   Director, Health Economics, Janssen Alzheimer Immunotherapy R&D, LLC, South San Francisco, California, USA

Greg A. Sachs, MD, FACP   Chief, Division of General Internal Medicine and Geriatrics, Department of Medicine, Indiana University School of Medicine; Scientist, IU Center for Aging Research, Regenstrief Institute, Inc.; and Wishard Hospital, Indianapolis, Indiana, USA

Douglas W. Scharre, MD   Director, Division of Cognitive Neurology, Department of Neurology, The Ohio State University, Columbus, Ohio, USA

Nancy Theado-Miller, MSN, RN, CS, CNP   Nurse Practitioner, Memory Disorders Clinic, The Ohio State University Medical Center, Columbus, Ohio, USA

1 Scope of dementia: epidemiology and public health impact

Patricia A. Boyle and David A. Bennett

INTRODUCTION

Dementia is an acquired syndrome characterized by a progressive deterioration in intellectual functions, including memory, language, reasoning, and judgment. The term "dementia" does not refer to a specific disease, but rather to a cluster of symptoms that accompany certain diseases or conditions. Dementia is largely a condition of elderly persons, with more than 98% of those affected are older than 65 years. It is estimated that approximately 28 million people worldwide currently suffer from dementia, and this number is expected to double by 2020 and possibly quadruple by 2050 (1,2). Dementia poses a considerable burden to society and is recognized as one of the most significant public health challenges facing the twenty-first century. There are many causes of dementia. However, from a public health perspective, there are two main causes of interest. Alzheimer's disease, a progressive neurodegenerative disorder, is the most common cause of dementia and accounts for at least 60% to 70% of all cases and up to 90% in some studies (2–5). Cerebrovascular disease is the second most common cause of dementia (i.e., vascular dementia or vascular cognitive impairment) and accounts for about 15% to 20% of all cases, often occurring in combination with Alzheimer's disease (4,5).

Epidemiology is the study of disease occurrence in human populations. The two primary aims of epidemiologic research are to: (*i*) document the frequency and distribution of disease for determination of public health priorities and resource allocation, and (*ii*) identify risk factors associated with disease in order to inform treatment and ultimately disease prevention efforts. Epidemiology typically focuses on conditions that are common and associated with significant morbidity and mortality, and disease occurrence is often studied in relation to risk factors (6). The linking of disease occurrence to risk factors reflects the underlying assumption that the clinical expression of disease is modifiable; that is, clinical signs and symptoms of disease can be delayed, prevented, or alleviated.

In this chapter, we review the epidemiology of dementia, including its incidence and prevalence and overall public health and economic impact. Factors associated with an increased (promoting) and decreased (protective) risk of dementia are discussed. It is noteworthy that to distinguish between dementia subtypes can be difficult; however, subtypes frequently co-occur. Therefore, some epidemiologic studies focus on dementia as a general syndrome, whereas others focus on the most common subtypes of dementia, especially Alzheimer's disease and vascular dementia. Although there are other causes of dementia including the Lewy body diseases, and frontotemporal degeneration, Alzheimer's disease and vascular dementia are the primary focus of this review.

EPIDEMIOLOGY OF DEMENTIA

Incidence

Estimating the frequency of disease is an important goal of epidemiologic research. Incidence refers to the number of new cases of a condition that occur in a population over a given period of time. Because the number of new cases depends on the length of follow-up and because follow-up time varies across studies and persons, the total follow-up time is computed by summing all person-times. Incidences per year are typically provided. Incidence rates represent the number of new cases divided by the person-years at risk, and incidence rates usually refer to the number of new cases per 1000 person-years. Thus, incidence rates represent the number of new cases of a condition per every thousand persons per year.

The incidence of dementia has been examined in several different study populations (5,7–25). Recently, investigators from the Cardiovascular Health Study examined the incidence of dementia in more than 3500 persons (7). As in other U.S.-based studies, the incidence of dementia, Alzheimer's disease, and vascular dementia increased dramatically with age (9,11,12,16,24). Sex differences were not found within race, but race differences were reported. That is, scaled to age 80, the incidence of dementia in whites was about 33 per 1000 person-years, whereas that of African Americans was about 56 per 1000 person-years; notably, the racial difference was reduced considerably after adjusting for age and education. Type-specific incidence was about 19 per 1000 person-years for Alzheimer's disease and 14 for vascular dementia in whites, compared with 35 and 27 per 1000 person-years for African Americans.

In an attempt to generate reliable age-specific incidence rates for dementia, Alzheimer's disease, and vascular dementia, respectively, data from eight European population-based studies were pooled (5). More than 40,000 person-years of follow-up and more than 800 new cases of dementia were reported among persons aged 65 and older; 60% to 70% of those were classified as Alzheimer's disease and 15% to 20% were classified as vascular dementia. Dementia incidence increases dramatically with age, rising from just over 2 per 1000 person-years among those aged 65 to 69 to about 70 per 1000 person-years among those aged 90 and older. Rates were higher among women than men, particularly among those older than 80 years, and continue to increase with age, although this sex difference is at least in part due to the fact that women tend to live longer than men. Incidence rates were similar for Alzheimer's disease and increase with age from about 1 per 1000 person-years among those aged 65 to 69 to about 54 among those aged 90 and older. Rates for vascular dementia were lower than for Alzheimer's disease but showed a similar increase with advancing age. The incidence rates derived from the pooled data generally are consistent with those from other site-specific European, Canadian, and U.S.-based studies (8–25).

Taken together, the studies examining the incidence of dementia worldwide suggest several important conclusions: First, the occurrence of dementia is strongly related to age. Dementia is infrequent in persons younger than 65 years but quite frequent in those older than 65 years. The risk of developing dementia continues to increase dramatically with advancing age, with incidence rates approximately doubling with every five additional years of age after 65 (5,7,8). Second, Alzheimer's disease is by far the most frequent type of dementia worldwide. The incidence of Alzheimer's disease may be higher among women than men, particularly those older than 80 years, although this is hard to know for sure because of increased longevity among women (25). The incidence of Alzheimer's disease may also be more common among racial and ethnic minorities than whites, although this disparity is at least partially due to methodologic factors. Finally, vascular dementia is the second most frequent type of dementia. Although there are relatively few studies on the sex- and race-specific incidence of vascular dementia, and conflicting reports do exist, its incidence appears to be higher in men than women and higher among African Americans compared with whites (7,16,23).

Mortality from Dementia

Despite widespread recognition that dementia reduces life expectancy, the estimated length of survival following dementia onset varies widely from about three to nine years across studies (26–32). One of the longest estimates for median survival came from an early study of outpatients with Alzheimer's disease and was just over nine years (26). Another early study estimated the length of survival among persons with Alzheimer's disease and vascular dementia to be about five years for both (27), and a more recent study estimated survival to be about six years for persons with Alzheimer's disease as compared with three years for those with vascular dementia (31). It is noteworthy, however, that some early studies examined survival from the time persons with dementia entered the study rather than survival from the onset of disease (26,27). Such studies may not have included many severe cases and therefore may have suffered length bias, which results in an overestimation of survival. To address this issue, a team of investigators examined survival after adjustment for length bias in a cohort of more than 800 participants of the Canadian Study of Health and Aging (28). Estimated survival after the onset of dementia (all subtypes) was just over three years, in contrast to almost seven years in the unadjusted models. When findings were stratified by dementia subtype, persons with probable Alzheimer's disease and vascular dementia had an estimated survival of just over three years, as compared with almost four years for those with possible Alzheimer's disease. Notably, the duration of survival decreased as the age of dementia onset increased, and there was a shorter (though nonsignificant) duration of survival among men as compared with women.

More recently, investigators have attempted to examine the risk of mortality and length of survival in studies of incident dementia, which allow for comparisons with nondemented elderly and eliminate the concern regarding length bias. For example, one study examined the risk of mortality in more than 3500 participants of the Cardiovascular Health Cognition Study (32). After controlling for age, sex, and race, persons with vascular dementia were more than four times more likely to die during follow-up than those with normal cognition, whereas those with Alzheimer's disease were more than twice as likely to die than those with normal cognition. Median survival from dementia onset to death was about 4 years among those with vascular dementia and about 7 years among those with Alzheimer's disease, as compared with 11 years for those with normal cognition. Although the estimated length of survival did not differ between men and women in that study, sex differences were found in another study of persons with Alzheimer's disease, such that men with Alzheimer's disease had a substantially reduced life expectancy (about four years) compared with women (about six years) (30). In other studies, dementia severity, presence of neuropsychiatric symptoms, comorbid conditions, and motor dysfunction also have been reported to be associated with decreased survival times among persons with dementia.

Prevalence

Estimates of the length of survival after dementia onset and the risk of mortality from dementia are necessary for planning and distribution of resources for the care of persons with dementia and are used to determine the prevalence of dementia. Prevalence refers to the number of persons with a condition per a given unit of population at a specific point in time. Prevalence therefore reflects a combination of the number of new (incident) cases and the length of time one survives with the disease; thus, for diseases that result in death within a year of onset (e.g., glioblastoma), the incidence and prevalence are essentially the same. By contrast, prevalence is higher than incidence for diseases in which persons live for several years, as is the case with dementia. Importantly, however, prevalence estimates are more variable than incidence rates because dementia develops slowly over several years and its onset is difficult to determine precisely; thus, estimates vary across studies depending in part on the extent to which persons with mild disease are included (33).

The prevalence of dementia has been examined in several different study populations (1–4,34–36). Like its incidence, the prevalence of dementia increases substantially with age. For example, the Cardiovascular Health Study recently reported a prevalence of about 9% in those younger than 75, compared with about 33% in those aged 80 to 84 and about 45% among persons aged 85 and older (7). The prevalence of Alzheimer's disease was higher than that of vascular dementia, although vascular dementia was higher in this study than previously reported. Sex differences were not found.

In an attempt to generate stable age-specific prevalence estimates for dementia, data from 11 European population-based studies were pooled (4). Crude prevalence ranged from about 6% to 9% across studies. Age-adjusted prevalence was about 6% for all causes of dementia, 4% for Alzheimer's disease, and 2% for vascular dementia. Prevalence was markedly related to age, almost doubling with every five additional years of age beyond 65. That is, approximately 1% of those aged 65 to 69 are affected with dementia, whereas almost 30% of those aged 90 and older; prevalence rates were higher among women than men. Moreover, Alzheimer's disease was by far the most common subtype of dementia, representing more than 50% of cases, and prevalence of Alzheimer's disease also increases dramatically with age from about 1% in those 65 to 69 to more than 20% in those 90 and older. Vascular dementia accounted for about 16% of cases, and its prevalence also increases with age, rising from less than 1% in those aged 65 to 69 to about 5% in those aged 90 and older. These estimates are generally consistent with other site-specific studies of dementia prevalence (3,4,7,34–36).

Notably, prevalence estimates are subject to variation due to differences in the methodology used across studies and can be difficult to interpret (33). However, the available prevalence studies yield at least two important conclusions: first, dementia affects a very large proportion of elderly persons and, like its incidence, the prevalence of dementia increases dramatically with age (1,2). Second, Alzheimer's disease is by far the most common subtype of dementia.

ECONOMIC IMPACT AND FUTURE TRENDS

Costs of Dementia Care

It is estimated that approximately 5 million Americans and 28 million persons worldwide currently suffer from dementia, and the public health and economic impact of dementia is staggering (1,2). According to the Global Burden of Disease estimates for the 2003 World Health Report, dementia contributed more than 11% of total years lived with disability among elderly persons (37). The contribution of dementia to disability exceeded that of stroke (almost 10%), musculoskeletal disorders (9%), cardiovascular disease (5%), and all forms of cancer combined (about 2%). Persons with dementia are heavy users of health care services, but the bulk of the burden of care of persons with dementia falls on family members and friends. Thus, dementia is associated with costs resulting from decreased productivity and health among family members and other care providers, in addition to costs of care for those with dementia (38). The Alzheimer's Association and the National Institute on Aging estimate that dementia spending currently exceeds $100 billion per year in the United States alone (39). Dementia is one of the costliest health conditions for which there is no cure and has been described as the pandemic of the twenty-first century.

The first worldwide estimate of combined direct and informal costs for dementia and Alzheimer's disease was released in 2006 (1,40). Direct costs refer to those for which fees are assessed and generally include professional health care services such as medications, hospital and doctor's visits, and nursing home stays. Informal costs are those related to care provided without associated financial fees; informal care is usually provided by family members or friends. The recent report estimated that $248 billion are spent annually worldwide for dementia care. To put this figure in perspective, only 18 of 216 countries in the world had Gross National Products above $248 billion in 2003.

The estimated $248 billion spent annually on dementia care assumes a worldwide prevalence of nearly 28 million persons with dementia and includes $156 billion for direct care costs and $92 billion for informal care costs. Notably, more than 90% of the costs are borne by the advanced economies, although only about 40% of prevalent cases live in advanced economies (1,2).

Future Trends

According to the Department of Health and Human Services Administration, there were about 36 million persons aged 65 years and older living in the United States in 2004 (41). At that time, elderly persons represented about 12% of the United States population, approximately one in eight Americans. However, persons older than 65 years represent the fastest growing segment of the population and it is estimated that there will be more than 71 million elderly persons by the year 2030, representing approximately 20% of the total U.S. population. Notably, the proportion of ethnic minorities among the elderly in the United States is also increasing, largely due to a dramatic increase in the number of Hispanic and African American persons older than 65 years. In accordance with the increase in the number of elderly persons, the prevalence of dementia in the United States is expected to triple by the year 2050, with particular increases in those aged 85 and older (36,42–44). Racial and ethnic minorities will bear a disproportionate share of the economic and social burden associated with dementia. According to the Alzheimer's Association, Medicare costs for people with Alzheimer's disease in the United States are expected to exceed $160 billion in 2010 and skyrocket to more than $1 trillion by 2050. The costs of Alzheimer's disease alone could overwhelm the United States health care system (39,41). Future projections of the worldwide occurrence of dementia also are startling. The number of persons aged 65 years and older worldwide is projected to increase even more dramatically than expected within the United States alone, more than doubling from about 420 million in 2000 to about 970 million in 2030 and more than 1 billion in 2050. The number persons with dementia worldwide is expected to increase dramatically, doubling approximately every 20 years to more than 40 million by 2020 and more than 80 million by 2040, assuming no changes in mortality and no effective intervention or preventative agent (1,2). Further, the rate of increase is predicted to be three to four times higher in developing than developed regions, and more than 70% of those affected in the year 2050 will be living in less developed regions. Because of the magnitude of the problem posed by dementia, identifying modifiable risk factors that prevent or delay disease onset is a major public health priority.

RISK FACTORS FOR DEMENTIA

Identifying risk factors for dementia is a challenging but critically important task. Much of the available information on dementia risk factors comes from studies of persons receiving medical attention or population-based studies of persons with prevalent disease; however, such studies are vulnerable to bias because only a limited and nonrandom fraction of persons with dementia come to the attention of the health care system. In addition, persons with dementia often cannot provide accurate medical and social history information needed to identify risk factors. Moreover, because prevalence is strongly related to survival, population-based studies of prevalent disease can lead to the identification of risk factors that are associated with survival with disease rather than actual risk of disease. Population-based studies of incident disease, in which risk factors are identified prior to disease onset and persons are followed over time to document incident disease, therefore are better suited to identifying true risk factors. Some data from such studies are available, although fewer of these studies exist as they are expensive, time consuming, and labor intensive. Despite these caveats, several factors, including age and apolipoprotein E allele status, have been shown to be associated with an increased risk of dementia; these are called promoting risk factors. Other factors, such as education, have been shown to be associated with a reduced risk of dementia; these are called protective factors.

The data on promoting and protective risk factors are reviewed in the following text and possible mechanisms by which they influence the development of dementia are discussed. It is important to note that, although some risk factors have been well studied, less data are available for others. In addition, the relationships between risk factors, common age-related neuropathologies such as Alzheimer's disease pathology, and cognitive impairment are complex. Risk factors can be associated with dementia via three pathways: they can initiate or cause pathological processes that lead to cognitive impairment and dementia, they can modify or alter the association of pathology with cognition, and/or they may be related to dementia but unrelated to common pathologic indices. In many cases, the neurobiologic basis of the association between the risk factor and dementia remains unknown. Nevertheless, an understanding of how risk factors relate to pathology to cause cognitive impairment and dementia is essential to our ultimate goal of alleviating or preventing dementia in the elderly. The discussion in the following text therefore includes findings from clinical–pathological studies, in which clinical data collected prior to death are related to pathological findings postmortem, with particular focus on the most common causes of dementia, Alzheimer's pathology (e.g., amyloid plaques and neurofibrillary tangles) and cerebral infarctions.

GENETIC FACTORS

Promoting
Genetics/apolipoprotein E ε4 allele status: The existence of alternative alleles (specific DNA sequence variants) at a single genetic locus is referred to as a genetic polymorphism. A polymorphism that invariably causes a disease is considered a mutation. Mutations in three genes are now known to cause Alzheimer's disease (amyloid precursor protein, presenilin 1, and presenilin 2) (45). Notably, however, these mutations account for only about 1% of Alzheimer's disease cases and are associated with early onset Alzheimer's disease. In contrast to mutations, other polymorphisms act as susceptibility factors (risk factors) for diseases with complex multifactorial etiologies but do not directly result in disease. Thus, such polymorphisms increase the likelihood that a person will develop a disease but are not deterministic. Several polymorphisms have been reported to be associated with an increased risk of Alzheimer's disease, but the apolipoprotein E gene is the only consistently replicated risk factor for the common form of Alzheimer's disease (onset after 65 years of age). Persons with one or more copies of the ε4 allele have about a two- to threefold greater risk of developing Alzheimer's disease compared with those without the ε4 allele (46–51); this association has been shown to vary by race in some studies, such that the association of ε4 with Alzheimer's disease is stronger among whites than African Americans (47,48,50). In addition, some, but not all, studies suggest that the allele also is associated with an increased risk of vascular dementia (51). The mechanism underlying the increased risk has not yet been fully elucidated but there appears to be an important link with Alzheimer's pathology. For example, the ε4 allele has been associated with the amount of Alzheimer's disease pathology in some clinical–pathological studies, and findings from a recent study provide evidence that the ε4 allele works through amyloid deposition and subsequent tangle formation to cause cognitive impairment (52–55). However, other data suggest that the allele may be associated more generally with neuronal repair and survival (e.g., neuron survival and synapses) rather than a specific association with age-related pathology (53). The ε4 allele also has been shown to increase the likelihood of cerebral infarction, which itself increases the likelihood of developing dementia (56,57). These findings suggest that the association between the ε4 allele and dementia is complex and that the allele interacts with other risk factors to cause cognitive impairment.

Protective
Genetics/apolipoprotein E ε2 allele status: In contrast to the ε4 allele, the presence of the ε2 allele is associated with a reduced risk of developing Alzheimer's

disease (45,48,58). Notably, there have been relatively few studies of this allele largely because the ε2 allele is not very common, but a meta-analysis reported that persons with an ε2 allele have about a 40% lower risk of Alzheimer's disease compared with those without the allele (48,59). Although various mechanisms have been proposed, clinical–pathological findings suggest that the apolipoprotein E (ApoE) genotype affects the risk of Alzheimer's disease primarily by affecting the accumulation of Alzheimer's pathology (54,55,60).

ENVIRONMENTAL OR EXPERIENTIAL FACTORS

Promoting

Age
The occurrence of dementia is highly related to age. Dementia is rare among persons younger than 65 years but quite frequent among those older than 65 years; about one in 10 individuals older than 65 years and nearly half of those older than 85 years are affected (1–4). Moreover, most studies suggest that dementia incidence continues to increase with age, even into very advanced age (22). Approximately one out of every 10 people older than 85 years develops Alzheimer's disease each year. Importantly, however, although age is commonly viewed as a risk factor for dementia, the extent to which age actually causes dementia is unclear. It is likely that age is a proxy for other as yet unidentified processes associated with disease occurrence.

Female sex
Several studies have shown that dementia is more common among women than men, particularly in those older than 80 years, although this sex difference is at least in part due to increased longevity among women (22,25). Thus, like age, the extent to which female sex is a true risk factor for dementia is unclear (25,61). Some researchers speculate that there could be a sex-specific vulnerability to dementia, possibly due to the decline in estrogen levels in women following menopause. In addition, findings from one clinical–pathological study suggest that Alzheimer's pathology may be more likely to be expressed as a clinical dementia syndrome in women than in men (62). Animal models also suggest that sex differences in amyloid precursor protein processing may predispose females to the development of Alzheimer's disease pathology (63). Although sex differences may exist, further research is needed to establish that the increased risk of dementia among women is not simply an artifact of increased longevity in women and related methodologic limitations (i.e., limited representation of men older than 80 years in comparative studies).

Race/ethnicity
There have been relatively few large population-based studies of dementia in multiracial and/or multiethnic communities and some, but not all, report that African Americans and Hispanics are more likely than non-Hispanic whites to develop dementia, including Alzheimer's disease and vascular dementia (7,9,16). In some studies, the observed racial differences persisted even after adjusting for the effects of education and other markers of socioeconomic status (16). Although

these findings have led some to conclude that racial differences are biologically determined, it is important to note that low education, poverty, and other markers of socioeconomic status are strongly associated with many common chronic diseases of elderly persons; this is true among members of all racial and ethnic groups. Thus, although these indicators may not affect health directly, they are indicators of access to resources and are almost certainly markers of other, currently unknown, factors that affect health. In the United States in particular, race is a powerful predictor of social class, and adjusting for education and income in statistical models does not necessarily account for all of the potential confounding effects of race. Moreover, discrepancies in cognitive test performance may be explained at least in part by methodologic issues associated with testing racial and ethnic minorities (64). Finally, other nongenetic medical or environmental risk factors may play a role in the association of race with dementia. Therefore, the data on the association of race/ethnicity and dementia should be interpreted with caution. Even if the findings of an increased risk among racial and ethnic minorities are accurate, it is still likely that the discrepancy can be explained, in large part, by modifiable social factors.

Cerebrovascular disease/stroke

Dementia due to cerebrovascular disease is most often considered either a pathogenetically distinct entity (i.e., vascular dementia) or a contributing cause of dementia (i.e., mixed dementia). However, cerebrovascular disease itself is associated with an increased risk of clinically diagnosed Alzheimer's disease and may influence the clinical expression of dementia (65–70). Although the mechanism by which cerebrovascular disease influences the risk of dementia is not entirely clear, stroke may lower the threshold of Alzheimer's disease (AD) pathology needed to result in clinical signs and symptoms of dementia or interact with Alzheimer's and other age-related pathologies to increase the likelihood of dementia. For example, one clinical–pathological study showed that, among persons with AD pathology, the risk of clinical dementia was greater among those with subcortical brain infarcts, suggesting that subcortical infarcts increased the likelihood that Alzheimer's pathology was expressed clinically (66). Another study showed that cerebral infarctions independently contributed to the likelihood of clinical dementia, but cerebral infarctions did not interact with AD pathology to increase the likelihood of dementia beyond their additive effect (57). Additional research is needed to further clarify exactly how cerebrovascular disease contributes to the risk of dementia, particularly AD.

Other vascular risk factors

The association of vascular risk factors with the risk of dementia has become a topic of great interest in recent years. Several factors, including high blood pressure, diabetes, heart disease, and hypercholesterolemia are associated with an increased risk of dementia (71–94). Blood pressure is the best studied, and high blood pressure in midlife has been consistently associated with an increased risk of AD and vascular dementia (71–74); results are less consistent for late-life blood pressure (76–78). Diabetes also has been fairly consistently associated with an increased risk of AD, as well as vascular dementia, and cholesterol studies suggest that high low-density lipoprotein (LDL) or low high-density lipoprotein (HDL) levels may be associated with an increased risk of dementia, although findings for cholesterol are inconsistent (79–94). The mechanisms underlying the associations of vascular risk factors with dementia are not fully understood. Vascular risk factors are associated with the development of cerebrovascular disease and likely increase dementia risk via cerebrovascular disease. In addition, vascular factors may lead to hypoperfusion, ischemia, and hypoxia in the brain, which may initiate the pathological process of AD (74,90). Clinical–pathological studies have examined the relation of specific vascular risk factors to pathologic changes in the brain, but findings are mixed. For example, some clinical–pathological studies on diabetes have reported relations between diabetes and AD pathology and cerebral infarctions, whereas others have not, and still another study reported an association of diabetes with cerebral infarctions but not AD pathology (92–94). It is likely that the associations of vascular factors with dementia are complex and multifactorial. Moreover, vascular factors appear to add to or interact with each other as well as other risk factors (e.g., cerebrovascular disease, ApoE) to cause cognitive impairment.

Obesity and the metabolic syndrome
In addition to the individual vascular factors described earlier, obesity and the metabolic syndrome (a clustering of several common disorders including obesity, hypertriglyceridemia, low HDL levels, hypertension, and hyperglycemia) appear to be associated with the risk of dementia, including AD and vascular dementia (95–101). Further, the association of the metabolic syndrome does not appear to be driven by the influence of one particular component. The mechanisms underlying the relationship between obesity, the metabolic syndrome, and dementia are unclear. Obesity has numerous adverse health effects, and both obesity and the metabolic syndrome are associated with other vascular risk factors and an increased risk of cerebrovascular disease (97–100). Thus, these conditions may increase the risk of dementia via cerebrovascular disease, or they may have other direct and indirect deleterious effects on the brain. For example, one study showed that the association of the metabolic syndrome with cognitive impairment was greatest in persons with high levels of circulating inflammatory markers, suggesting that some of the association may be modified by inflammation (101). Additional research is needed to further clarify the mechanism by which these conditions lead to an increased risk of dementia.

Change in body mass index and weight loss
In contrast to the findings on obesity, some studies, including a recent large prospective study, suggest that declining body mass index or weight loss are associated with an increased risk of dementia (102–104). Although it is possible that loss of body mass represents a true risk factor for dementia, a more likely explanation is that factors associated with the development of dementia also lead to loss of body mass, and decreased body mass therefore may be apparent prior to the onset of clinical dementia. Interestingly, recent work suggests that changes in body mass and weight may occur secondary to AD pathology or changes in brain structures known to be involved in AD (105). Loss of body mass index and weight therefore may reflect the consequence of pathologic processes such as Alzheimer's pathology that contribute to the subsequent development of dementia, rather than a true risk factor.

Depressive symptoms and loneliness
Depressive symptoms have been associated with an increased risk of dementia in several large prospective studies (106–109). The association between depressive symptoms and dementia is fairly strong; for example, one prospective study reported that the risk of developing AD increased by about 20% for each depressive symptom endorsed (109). One aspect of depressive symptoms is loneliness, which reflects one's sense of connectedness to others. A recent study found that loneliness was associated with risk of AD (110). The findings remained after controlling for depressive symptoms. The basis of these associations has not been established, however. One possibility is that depressive symptoms and loneliness are a consequence of incipient dementia or its underlying pathology rather than a true risk factor for dementia. However, longitudinal studies have not shown that either depressive symptoms or loneliness increase in old age, and clinical–pathological findings do not support a relation between depressive symptoms or loneliness and AD pathology or cerebral infarctions, the leading causes of dementia (108,110). Depressive symptoms and loneliness therefore may predict dementia via some other mechanism. Depressive symptoms may also modify the relation of other risk factors to dementia, including physical activity, social engagement, ApoE, diabetes, and other vascular factors. The association of depressive symptoms with dementia therefore is complex and deserves further investigation.

Neuroticism or proneness to psychological distress
In addition to depressive symptoms, personality traits such as neuroticism, proneness to psychological distress, and loneliness recently have been associated with an increased risk of dementia, particularly AD (111–113). In a recent study, persons with a high level of distress proneness, the tendency to be overwhelmed by stress, were more than twice as likely to develop AD as those not prone to distress (112). Further, the association of distress proneness with Alzheimer's pathology was examined in a subsample of participants who died and underwent brain autopsy, and distress proneness was unrelated to measures of Alzheimer's pathology. These results suggest that, like depressive symptoms and loneliness, neurobiologic mechanisms other than Alzheimer's pathology must underlie the association of this personality trait with dementia. For example, in animal models, chronic stress has been associated with a spectrum of neurobiological changes in brain regions critical for memory (114). These findings suggest that distress proneness may gradually compromise memory systems in the brain so that relatively less age-related neuropathology is needed to compromise function. Future research is needed to clarify the neurobiologic basis of the association of proneness to psychological distress with dementia.

Head trauma
Head trauma (usually defined as head trauma with loss of consciousness) has been associated with an increased risk of AD in many, but not all, studies (115–120). In particular, repeated and severe head trauma can cause a dementia syndrome distinct from AD, and some data suggest that even a single head injury from which an individual fully recovers also may be associated with a dementia syndrome. Several hypotheses have been offered to explain the association; for example, head trauma results in neuronal damage and reduced neuronal

reserve, which may lead to the accumulation and clinical expression of Alzheimer's pathology. Whether brain trauma in some way initiates a cascade of events leading to the accumulation of Alzheimer's pathology or reduces the capacity of the brain to tolerate AD or other age-related pathologies is unclear. An interaction between head injury and the presence of the ApoE ε4 allele has also been reported, suggesting that head injury interacts with other risk factors to cause cognitive impairment (117,120).

Parkinsonian and other motor signs

Large prospective studies of persons without Parkinson's disease have shown that Parkinsonian signs, including gait dysfunction, rigidity, tremor and bradykinesia, and other motor signs are associated with an increased risk of dementia, particularly AD (121–124). By contrast, one study showed that persons with gait abnormalities had a greater risk of vascular dementia but not AD (121). Little is known about the mechanisms underlying the association of motor dysfunction with dementia. However, motor dysfunction is common in aging and recent findings suggest that Alzheimer's pathology in areas of the brain that subserve motor function contribute to motor impairment both in persons with and without dementia (125). It is also possible for Alzheimer's pathology in regions that subserve cognitive functions to impair motor function, as motor performance ultimately involves control, planning, and execution of motor sequences. Thus, Parkinsonian signs and impaired motor function may predict the development of dementia because motor dysfunction is an early clinical sign of a pathologic process rather than a true risk factor.

Smoking

Cigarette smoking has been associated with an increased risk of dementia in some, but not all, studies (126–131). For example, findings from a recent large study of incident disease showed that current smoking was associated with an increased risk of AD, especially among persons without the ApoE ε4 allele (126). Although this finding is consistent with other recent prospective studies which that suggest that smoking is associated with an increased risk of dementia, findings are mixed and the association of smoking and dementia remains controversial (126–131). In addition, although current smoking appears to be most consistently associated with dementia, the extent to which current versus former smoking is related to cognition in old age is not entirely clear. The neurobiologic basis of the association of smoking and dementia is not well understood; studies have focused on the potential involvement of nicotine receptors in the neocortex.

Dietary fats and copper

Evidence from some prospective studies suggests that intakes of dietary fats and copper maybe associated with an increased risk of dementia (132–134). For example, in one large community-based study, persons with high intakes of either saturated or trans fats had about a two- to threefold increase in the risk of incident Alzheimer's disease (133). Subsequently, in the same population, high copper intake was found to be associated with a faster rate of cognitive decline but only among persons who also consumed a diet high in saturated and trans fats, suggesting that high dietary intake of copper combined with a diet high in saturated and trans fats maybe linked to cognitive impairment (134). The basis of these associations is not well understood. Dietary fats or copper may interfere with the clearance of Alzheimer's pathology from the brain or they may actually promote or accelerate the accumulation of Alzheimer's pathology, particularly amyloid. Copper also contributes to the production of hydrogen peroxide, a potent oxidant and neurotoxin. Thus, dietary fats and copper may influence the risk of dementia via their associations with Alzheimer's pathology and oxidative stress, although additional research is needed in this area.

Inflammatory markers

Inflammation may play an important role in the pathogenesis of AD, and findings from some prospective studies suggest that the level of systemic inflammation markers, particularly C-reactive protein and interleukin-6, are associated with an increased risk of dementia (135–137). One large study reported a threefold increase in the risk of AD among men with high levels of C-reactive protein (137). Others also have reported increases in the risk of AD among persons with C-reactive protein and interleukin-6 (alone and in combination), although one recent study found an association between inflammatory markers and the risk of vascular dementia but not AD (135). Several potential mechanisms underlie the association between inflammation and dementia; inflammation can occur as a consequence of neurodegeneration, or it may be part of a cascade of events that lead to the accumulation of Alzheimer's pathology, particularly amyloid deposition (138). Inflammation also is associated with vascular disease and may be related to dementia via cerebrovascular disease. Additional research is needed to further clarify the role of inflammation in the development of dementia and the basis of this association.

Protective

Education and cognitive activity

Years of formal education have been related to risk of dementia and AD in most, but not all, studies (139–143). years of formal education, occupation, and other markers of socioeconomic status are strongly associated with many common chronic diseases of elderly persons; it is possible, therefore, that this association is not specific for dementia. Moreover, several lines of evidence suggest that, in addition to education, cognitive activity and cognitive experiences across the life course affect cognitive function in old age (144–150); more specifically, greater participation in early life cognitive and leisure activities and cognitive activity in late adulthood are associated with a decreased risk of AD. Several potential mechanisms may underlie this association. First, it has been hypothesized that education, or variables related to education, may provide some type of reserve that protects against the clinical expression of disease despite the accumulation of pathology. In support of this hypothesis, clinical–pathological studies have shown that education reduces the association of AD pathology, particularly amyloid, with cognition (151). Another study reported that written language assessed in early adult life predicted both the level of cognitive function prior to death and AD pathology, raising the possibility that even early life experiences may affect the accumulation of disease pathology in late life (152). It is also possible that lifetime cognitive experiences influence the numbers of neurons and synapses that survive into adult life; in animal models, complex environmental experiences

in early life and adulthood have been associated with greater numbers of neurons and synapses, and findings from transgenic animal models link enriched
environments to altered amyloid deposition (153,154). More research is needed
to determine how education and cognitive activity, both of which are modifiable
risk factors for dementia, may modify or interact with other genetic and vascular
risk factors and common age-related pathologies to reduce the risk of dementia.

Social engagement and social networks

The relation between the extent of social ties or social engagement and dementia has been examined in several recent studies (155–158). Most, but not all,
showed that people with more extensive social networks had a decreased risk
of developing cognitive impairment and dementia. Little is known about the
potential neurobiological basis of this association, however. Although social networks could be directly related to the accumulation of AD pathology, it is more
likely that cognitive processing skills that allow people to develop and maintain
large social networks help provide a reserve against the development of cognitive
impairment, such that socially connected persons can tolerate greater amounts
of AD pathology prior to developing clinical dementia. In support of this idea, a
recent clinical–pathological study reported that large social networks reduced the
impact of AD pathology on the level of cognitive function in elderly persons (159).

Physical activity

Physical activity is a modifiable lifestyle factor that has been associated with a
reduced risk of AD in some, but not all, studies (160–164). The mechanisms linking physical activity to cognitive function are complex and poorly understood.
Physical activity has been related to overall cardiovascular health and also to
stroke, and physical activity may reduce the risk of dementia via its effects on
the vasculature of the brain. However, physical activity also has been related
to decreased production of Alzheimer's pathology in transgenic animal models
(165). More studies are needed to further establish the link between physical
activity and dementia and to determine the possible basis of this association.

Vitamins E, C, and antioxidants

Several population-based studies have examined the association between vitamins E and C and other antioxidants with the risk of dementia. The results of
these studies have been conflicting; for example, whereas some showed a protective effect for one or both of the vitamins E and C, others did not, and still
another reported that combined use of vitamin E and C supplements (but neither
one individually) was associated with a lower incidence of AD (166–171). More
recently, it has been suggested that dietary intake rather than supplement use is
associated with a reduced risk of dementia. For example, dietary intake of n-3
fatty acids and weekly consumption of fish have been associated with a reduced
risk of incident AD, but this association appears to hold only among individuals
without the apolipoprotein ε e4 allele (166,172). Oxidative injury has long been
thought to contribute to age-related diseases including AD, and vitamins are
thought to work via their antioxidant effects in the brain, in addition to potential
vascular benefits. Clinical–pathological data are lacking, however. Moreover, it is
noteworthy that the data on vitamins remain modest and difficult to interpret, in
part because vitamin users tend to be younger, more highly educated, have higher

incomes, and be more health conscious than nonusers. In addition, measurement of vitamin intake from food is very difficult to ascertain. Thus, more research is needed to establish the relationship between vitamins and antioxidants and dementia and the basis of this association.

Folate

Folate is an essential B vitamin that is widely recognized as important for the normal development of the nervous system. Although some observational studies have shown that folate intake is associated with a reduced risk of AD, findings are mixed (173–175). For example, a large study recently examined folate together with vitamins C, E, A, B6, and B 12, and only folate emerged as a protective factor against dementia; persons who ingested more folate than the recommended allowance (400 U/day) had about a 50% reduction in the risk of AD compared with those whose folate intake was below the recommended amount (174). By contrast, however, other large prospective studies have reported no benefit from folate. The potential mechanism of the possible association of folate with dementia is unclear; folate has been related to brain atrophy in humans, and animal studies suggest that folic acid deficiency may be related to amyloid toxicity, although folic acid deficiency is rare, especially among Americans. Folic acid supplementation generally is not recommended in elderly persons without known deficiency because of safety issues. Also, as noted earlier, studies on diet can be difficult to interpret due to confounding by healthy lifestyles and other factors.

Alcohol

Both total alcohol intake and wine consumption in particular have been associated with a reduced risk of dementia, although findings are not entirely consistent (176–179). Although some studies have reported a reduced risk of AD among persons who consume moderate amounts of alcohol, others have found that alcohol is associated with a reduced risk of vascular dementia but not AD, and still others have reported no benefit from alcohol. The protective effect of alcohol has been seen with varying levels of consumption but is most consistently associated with consumption of about one to three drinks/day; heavy consumption of alcohol has been associated with an increased risk of dementia as well as other negative health outcomes. Moderate alcohol use is associated with cardiovascular and cerebrovascular benefit, and it has been suggested that moderate levels of alcohol intake may help maintain brain vasculature and prevent small strokes. In support of this idea, one study reported that moderate alcohol was associated with fewer white matter abnormalities and infarcts on MRI among elderly individuals without prior cerebrovascular disease (177). Other data suggest that moderate alcohol intake might have direct effects on Alzheimer's pathology or favorably alter the release of acetylcholine, a neurotransmitter involved in learning and memory (178). In addition, wine has antioxidant properties and may offer some nutritional benefit.

Medications

Several medications, including estrogen, nonsteroidal anti-inflammatory agents, and statins have been examined for their potential to protect against dementia (180–187). Estrogen therapy is probably the best studied and has been associated with a reduced risk of dementia, particularly AD, in several observational studies (175,180–182). Moreover, some reported a dose–response relationship, whereby longer duration of estrogen therapy was associated with greater protection. Similar findings have been reported for nonsteroidal anti-inflammatory agents, with some studies reporting a reduced risk of dementia among users (particularly those using for more than two years), although conflicting findings do exist (184,185). Finally, some cross sectional or case-control studies have shown a protective effect for statins, but prospective cohort studies generally have not replicated those findings (175,186,187). It is noteworthy that clinical trials examining the potential for estrogen and nonsteroidal agents to prevent or delay the onset of dementia have not been successful (188,189). In clinical trials, hormone replacement and nonsteroidals have been associated with adverse health outcomes. Therefore, although some questions remain about the association of estrogen and nonsteroidals with dementia, clinical trials have been discontinued because of safety concerns. Clinical trials of statins are ongoing.

CONCLUSIONS
Dementia is extremely common among the elderly, currently affecting about 5 million Americans and 28 million persons worldwide. Dementia is associated with significant morbidity and mortality and ranks among the costliest incurable diseases. Recent estimates indicate that annual dementia spending exceeds $100 billion in the United States alone and approaches $250 billion worldwide. Future projections of the worldwide occurrence and costs of dementia are startling. Because of the projected increase in the aging population over the next several decades, the number of persons with dementia will rise dramatically, approximately doubling every 20 years to more than 40 million worldwide by 2020 and more than 80 million by 2040. Moreover, the rate of increase is predicted to be three to four times higher in developing than developed regions, and more than 70% of those affected in the year 2050 will be living in less developed regions. Without effective prevention or treatment, dementia is poised to overwhelm the United States health care system and devastate less developed economies. Dementia has been referred to as the pandemic of the twenty-first century.

AD and vascular dementia are the most common causes of dementia. AD accounts for more than two-thirds of all cases, whereas vascular dementia accounts for about one-fifth of all cases. Risk factors associated with an increased risk of AD and vascular dementia include age, the presence of the apolipoprotein e4 allele, cerebrovascular disease, vascular risk factors, depressive symptoms, and lifestyle factors, among others. Factors associated with a decreased risk of dementia include education, the presence of the apolipoprotein e2 allele, cognitive and social activity, diet, and lifestyle factors, among others. Although some risk factors appear to affect the risk of dementia via AD pathology, others affect the risk of dementia via cerebrovascular disease or other mechanisms. Moreover, risk factors may interact with or modify the presence of other risk factors, and the relationships between risk factors, common age-related pathologies, and dementia are complex. Additional research from prospective studies of incident disease is greatly needed to further identify the true risk factors for dementia and to establish the neurobiologic basic of the link between various risk factors and dementia. A clearer understanding of how risk factors relate to pathology to cause cognitive impairment and dementia is essential to our ultimate goal of reducing or preventing dementia in the elderly.

REFERENCES

1. Wimo A, Jonsson L, Winblad B. An estimate of the worldwide prevalence and direct costs of dementia in 2003. Dement Geriatr Cogn Disord 2006; 21(3):175–181.
2. Ferri CP, Prince M, Brayne C, et al. Global prevalence of dementia: A Delphi consensus study. Lancet 2005; 24(31):2112–2117.
3. Evans DA, Funkenstein HH, Albert MS, et al. Prevalence of Alzheimer's disease in a community population of older persons. Higher than previously reported. JAMA 1989; 262(18):2551–2556.
4. Lobo A, Laurier LJ, Fratiglioni L, et al. Prevalence of dementia and major subtypes in Europe: A collaborative study of population-based cohorts. Neurologic diseases in the elderly research group. Neurology 2000; 54(11, suppl 5):S4–S9.
5. Fratiglioni L, Laurier LJ, Andersen K, et al. Incidence of dementia and major subtypes in Europe: A collaborative study of population-based cohorts. Neurology 2000; 54(11, suppl 5):S1015.
6. Rothman K, Greenland S. Modern Epidemiology. 2nd ed. Philadelphia, PA: Lippincott-Raven, 1998.
7. Fitzpatrick AL, Kuller LH, Ives DG, et al. Incidence and prevalence of dementia in the Cardiovascular Health Study. J Am Geriatr Soc 2004; 52(2):195–204.
8. Di Carlo A, Baldereschi M, Amaducci L, et al. Incidence of dementia, Alzheimer's disease, and vascular dementia in Italy. The ILSA Study. J Am Geriatr Soc 2002; 50(1):41–48.
9. Evans DA, Bennett DA, Wilson RS, et al. Incidence of Alzheimer disease in a biracial urban community: Relation to apolipoprotein E allele status. Arch Neurol 2003; 60(2):185–189.
10. Ott A, Breteler MB, van Harskamp F, et al. Incidence and risk of dementia. The Rotterdam Study. Am J Epidemiol 1998; 147:574–580.
11. Ganguli M, Dodge HH, Chen P, et al. Ten-year incidence of dementia in a rural elderly US community population. The Movies Project. Neurology 2000; 54:1109–1116.
12. Rocca WA, Cha RH, Waring SC, et al. Incidence of dementia and Alzheimer's disease: A reanalysis of data from Rochester, Minnesota, 1975–1984. Am J Epidemiol 1998; 148:51–62.
13. The Canadian Study of Health and Aging Working Group. The incidence of dementia in Canada. Neurology 2000; 55:66–73.
14. Jorm AF, Jolley D. The incidence of dementia: A meta-analysis. Neurology 1998; 51:728–733.
15. Dubois MF, Hebert R. The incidence of vascular dementia in Canada: A comparison with Europe and East Asia. Neuroepidemiology 2001; 20:179–187.
16. Tang MX, Cross P, Andrews H, et al. Incidence of AD in African-Americans, Caribbean Hispanics, and Caucasians in northern Manhattan. Neurology 2001; 56(1):49–56.
17. Matthews F, Brayne C; MRC Investigators. The incidence of dementia in England and Wales: Findings from the five identical sites of the MRC CFA Study. PLoS Med 2005; 2:e193.
18. Ravaglia G, Forti P, Maioli F, et al. Incidence and etiology of dementia in a large elderly Italian population. Neurology 2005; 64(9):1525–1530.
19. Hebert LE, Scherr PA, Beckett LA, et al. Age-specific incidence of Alzheimer's disease in a community population. JAMA 1995; 273:1354–1359.
20. Fillenbaum GG, Heyman A, Huber MS, et al. The prevalence and 3-year incidence of dementia in older Black and White community residents. J Clin Epidemiol 1998; 51:587–595.
21. Andersen K, Nielsen H, Lolk A, et al. Incidence of very mild to severe dementia and Alzheimer's disease in Denmark: The Odense Study. Neurology 1999; 52:85–90.
22. Fratiglioni L, Viitanen M, von Strauss E, et al. Very old women at highest risk of dementia and Alzheimer's disease: Incidence data from the Kungsholmen Project, Stockholm. Neurology 1997; 48:132–138.
23. Andersen K, Launer LJ, Dewey ME, et al. Gender differences in the incidence of AD and vascular dementia. The EURODEM Studies EURODEM Incidence Research Group. Neurology 1999; 53:1992–1997.

24. Miech RA, Breitner JC, Zandi PP, et al. Incidence of AD may decline in the early 90s for men, later for women: The Cache County Study. Neurology 2002; 58:209-218.

25. Hebert LE, Scherr PA, McCann JJ, et al. Is the risk of developing Alzheimer's disease greater for women than for men? Am J Epidemiol 2001; 153(2):132–136.

26. Walsh JS, Welch HG, Larson EB. Survival of outpatients with Alzheimer-type dementia. Ann Intern Med 1990; 113(6):429–434.

27. Molsa PK, Marttila RJ, Rinne UK. Survival and cause of death in Alzheimer's disease and multi-infarct dementia. Acta Neurol Scand 1986; 74(2):103–107.

28. Wolfson C, Wolfson DB, Asgharian M, et al. Clinical Progression of Dementia Study Group. A reevaluation of the duration of survival after the onset of dementia. N Engl J Med 2001; 344(15):1111–1116.

29. Brookmeyer R, Corrada MM, Curriero FC, et al. Survival following a diagnosis of Alzheimer disease. Arch Neurol 2002; 59(11):1764–1767.

30. Larson EB, Shadlen MF, Wang L, et al. Survival after initial diagnosis of Alzheimer disease. Ann Intern Med 2004; 140(7):501–509.

31. Knopman DS, Rocca WA, Cha RH, et al. Survival study of vascular dementia in Rochester MN. Arch Neurol 2003; 60(1):85–90.

32. Fitzpatrick AL, Kuller LH, Lopez OL, et al. Survival following dementia onset: Alzheimer's disease and vascular dementia. J Neurol Sci 2005; 229–230:43–49.

33. Corrada M, Brookmeyer R, Kawas C. Sources of variability in prevalence rates of Alzheimer's disease. Int J Epidemiol 1995; 24:1000–1005.

34. Berr C, Wancata J, Ritchie K. Prevalence of dementia in the elderly in Europe. Eur Neuropsychopharmacol 2005; 15:463–471.

35. White L, Petrovitch H, Ross GW, et al. Prevalence of dementia in older Japanese-American men in Hawaii. The Honolulu-Asia Aging Study. JAMA 1996; 276:955–960.

36. Hebert LE, Scherr PA, Bienias JL, et al. Alzheimer disease in the US population: Prevalence estimates using the 2000 census. Arch Neurol 2003; 60(8):1119–1122.

37. World Health Organization. World Health Report 2003—Shaping the Future. Geneva, Switzerland: WHO, 2003.

38. Langa KM, Chernew ME, Kabeto MU, et al. National estimates of the quantity and cost of informal caregiving for elderly with dementia. J Gen Intern Med 2001; 16:770–778.

39. Alzheimer's Association statistics. www.alz.org.

40. Wimo A. Worldwide cost of Alzheimer's and dementia care estimated at $248 billion (U.S.). Paper presented at: 2006 International Conference on Alzheimer's disease; July 2006, Madrid, Spain.

41. Centers for Disease Control and Prevention. Trends in aging—United States and worldwide. MMWR Morb Mortal Wkly Rep 2003; 52:101–106.

42. Brookmeyer R, Gray S, Kawas C. Projections of Alzheimer's disease in the United States and the public health impact of delaying disease onset. Am J Public Health 1998; 88:1337–1342.

43. Hebert LE, Scherr PA, Bienias JL, et al. State-specific projections through 2025 of Alzheimer disease prevalence. Neurology 2004; 62(9):1645.

44. Hebert LE, Beckett LA, Scherr PA, et al. Annual incidence of Alzheimer disease in the United States projected to the years 2000 through 2050. Alzheimer Dis Assoc Disord 2001; 15:169–173.

45. Jellinger KA. Alzheimer 100—highlights in the history of Alzheimer research. J Neural Transco 2006; 113(11):1603–1623.

46. Tang M, Stern Y, Marder K, et al. The APOE-ε4 allele and the risk of Alzheimer disease among African Americans, whites, and Hispanics. JAMA 1998; 279:751–755.

47. Evans D, Beckett L, Field T, et al. Apolipoprotein E e4 and incidence of Alzheimer's disease in a community population of older persons. JAMA 1997; 277:822–824.

48. Farrer LA, Cupples LA, Haines JL, et al. Effects of age, sex, and ethnicity on the association between apolipoprotein E genotype and Alzheimer disease. A meta-analysis. APOE and Alzheimer Disease Meta Analysis Consortium. JAMA 1997; 278:1349–1356.

49. Strittmatter WJ, Roses AD. Apolipoprotein E and Alzheimer disease. Proc Natl Acad Sci U S A 1995; 92:4725–4727.

50. Murrell JR, Price B, Lane KA, et al. Association of apolipoprotein E genotype and Alzheimer disease in African Americans. Arch Neurol 2006; 63(3):431–434.
51. Baum L, Lam LC, Kwok T, et al. Apolipoprotein E epsilon4 allele is associated with vascular dementia. Dement Geriatr Cogn Disord 2006; 22(4):301–305.
52. McNamara MJ, Gomez-Isla T, Hyman BT. Apolipoprotein E genotype and deposits of Abeta40 and Abeta42 in Alzheimer disease. Arch Neurol 1998; 55:1001–1004.
53. Horsburgh K, Graham DI, Stewart J, et al. Influence of apolipoprotein E genotype on neuronal damage and apoE immunoreactivity in human hippocampus following global ischemia. J Neuropathol Exp Neurol 1999; 58:227–234.
54. Bennett DA, Wilson RS, Schneider JA, et al. Apolipoprotein E epsilon4 allele, AD pathology, and the clinical expression of Alzheimer's disease. Neurology 2003; 60(2):246–255.
55. Bennett DA, Schneider JA, Wilson RS, et al. Amyloid mediates the association of apolipoprotein E e4 allele to cognitive function in older people. J Neurol Neurosurg Psychiatry 2005; 76(9):1194–1199.
56. Schneider JA, Bienias JL, Wilson RS, et al. The apolipoprotein E epsilon4 allele increases the odds of chronic cerebral infarction [corrected] detected at autopsy in older persons. Stroke 2005 36(5):954–959.
57. Schneider JA, Wilson RS, Bienias JL, et al. Cerebral infarctions and the likelihood of dementia from Alzheimer disease pathology. Neurology 2004; 62(7):1148–1155.
58. Wilson RS, Bienias JL, Berry-Kravis E, et al. The apolipoprotein E epsilon 2 allele and decline in episodic memory. J Neurol Neurosurg Psychiatry 2002; 73(6):672–677.
59. Qiu C, Kivipelto M, Aguero-Torres H, et al. Risk and protective effects of the APOE gene towards Alzheimer's disease in the Kungsholmen project: Variation by age and sex. J Neurol Neurosurg Psychiatry 2004; 75(6):828–833.
60. Tiraboschi P, Hansen LA, Masliah E, et al. Impact of APOE genotype on neuropathologic and neurochemical markers of Alzheimer disease. Neurology 2004; 62(11):1977–1983.
61. Barnes LI, Wilson RS, Schneider JA, et al. Gender, cognitive decline, and risk of AD in older persons. Neurology 2003; 60:1777–1781.
62. Barnes LL, Wilson RS, Bienias JL, Schneider JA, Evans DA, Bennett DA. Sex differences in the clinical manifestations of Alzheimer disease pathology. Arch Gen Psychiatry 2005; 62(6):685–691.
63. Maynard CJ, Cappai R, Volitakis I, et al. Gender and genetic background effects on brain metal levels in APP transgenic and normal mice: Implications for Alzheimer beta-amyloid pathology. J Inorg Biochem 2006; 100(5–6):952–962.
64. Manly JJ, Byrd DA, Touradji P, et al. Acculturation, reading level, and neuropsychological test performance among African American elders. Appl Neuropsychol 2004; 11(1):37–46.
65. Snowdon D, Greiner L, Mortimer J, et al. Brain infarction and the clinical expression of Alzheimer disease. JAMA 1997; 277:813–817.
66. Esiri MM, Nagy M, Smith MZ, et al. Cerebrovascular disease and threshold for dementia in the early stages of Alzheimer's disease. Lancet 1999; 354:919–920.
67. Kalaria RN. The role of cerebral ischemia in Alzheimer's disease. Neurobiol Aging 2000; 21(2):321–330.
68. Honig LS, Tang MX, Albert S, et al. Stroke and the risk of Alzheimer disease. Arch Neurol 2003; 60(12):1707–1712.
69. Ivan CS, Seshadri S, Beiser A, et al. Dementia after stroke: The Framingham Study. Stroke 2004; 35(6):1264–1268.
70. Gamaldo A, Moghekar A, Kilada S, et al. Effect of a clinical stroke on the risk of dementia in a prospective cohort. Neurology 2006; 67(8):1363–1369.
71. Peila R, White LR, Petrovich H, et al. Joint effect of the APOE gene and midlife systolic blood pressure on late-life cognitive impairment: The Honolulu-Asia aging study. Stroke 2001; 32(12):2882–2889.
72. Launer LJ, Ross GW, Petrovitch H, et al. Midlife blood pressure and dementia: The Honolulu-Asia aging study. Neurobiol Aging 2000; 21:49–55.

73. Kivipelto M, Helkala EL, Laakso MP, et al. Apolipoprotein E epsilon4 allele, elevated midlife total cholesterol level, and high midlife systolic blood pressure are independent risk factors for late-life Alzheimer disease. Ann Intern Med 2002; 137:149–155.

74. Launer U. Demonstrating the case that AD is a vascular disease: Epidemiologic evidence. Ageing Res Rev 2002; 1:61–77.

75. Korf ES, White LR, Scheltens P, et al. Midlife blood pressure and the risk of hippocampal atrophy: The Honolulu Asia aging study. Hypertension 2004; 44:29–34.

76. Qiu C, Winblad B, Fratiglioni L. The age-dependent relation of blood pressure to cognitive function and dementia. Lancet Neurol 2005; 4:487–499.

77. Morris MC, Scherr PA, Hebert LE, et al. Association of incident Alzheimer disease and blood pressure measured from 13 years before to 2 years after diagnosis in a large community study. Arch Neurol 2001; 58(10):1640–1646.

78. Shah RC, Wilson RS, Bienias JL, et al. Relation of blood pressure to risk of incident Alzheimer's disease and change in global cognitive function in older persons. Neuroepidemiology 2006; 26(1):30–36.

79. Luchsinger JA, Tang MX, Stern Y, et al. Diabetes mellitus and risk of Alzheimer's disease and dementia with stroke in a multiethnic cohort. Am J Epidemiol 2001; 154(7):635–641.

80. Hayden KM, Zandi PP, Lyketsos CG, et al. Vascular risk factors for incident Alzheimer's disease and vascular dementia: The Cache County Study. Alzheimer Dis Assoc Disord 2006; 20(2):93–100.

81. Mielke MM, Zandi PP, Sjogren M, et al. High total cholesterol levels in late life associated with a reduced risk of dementia. Neurology 2005; 64(10):1689–1695.

82. Tan ZS, Seshadri S, Beiser A, et al. Plasma total cholesterol level as a risk factor for Alzheimer disease: The Framingham Study. Arch Intern Med 2003; 163(9):1053–1057.

83. Lindsay J, Laurin D, Verreault R, et al. Risk factors for Alzheimer's disease: A prospective analysis from the Canadian Study of Health and Aging. Am J Epidemiol 2002; 156(5):445–453.

84. Leibson CL, Rocca WA, Hanson VA, et al. Risk of dementia among persons with diabetes mellitus: A population-based cohort study. Am J Epidemiol 1997; 145:301–308.

85. Curb JD, Rodriguez BL, Abbott RD, et al. Longitudinal association of vascular and Alzheimer's demential, diabetes, and glucose tolerance. Neurology 1999; 52:971–975.

86. MacKnight C, Rockwood K, Awalt E, et al. Diabetes mellitus and the risk of dementia, Alzheimer's disease and vascular cognitive impairment in the Canadian Study of Health and Aging. Dement Geriatr Cogn Disord 2002; 14(2):77–83.

87. Peila R, Rodriguez BL, Launer LJ; Honolulu-Asia Aging Study. Type 2 diabetes, APOE gene, and the risk for dementia and related pathologies: The Honolulu-Asia Aging Study. Diabetes 2002; 51(4):1256–1262.

88. Xu WL, Qiu CX, Wahlin A, et al. Diabetes mellitus and risk of dementia in the Kungsholmen project: A 6 year follow up study. Neurology 2004; 63(7):1181–1186.

89. Arvanitakis Z, Wilson RS, Bienias JL, et al. Diabetes mellitus and risk of Alzheimer disease and decline in cognitive function. Arch Neurol 2004; 61(5):661–666.

90. Biessels GJ, Staekenborg S, Brunner E, et al. Risk of dementia in diabetes mellitus: A systematic review. Lancet Neurol 2006; 5(1):64–74.

91. Arvanitakis Z, Wilson RS, Bennett DA. Diabetes mellitus, dementia, and cognitive function in older persons. J Nutr Health Aging 2006; 10(4):287–291.

92. Beeri MS, Silverman JM, Davis KL, et al. Type 2 diabetes is negatively associated with Alzheimer's disease neuropathology. J Gerontol A Biol Sci Med Sci 2005; 60(4):471–475.

93. Heitner J, Dickson D. Diabetics do not have increased Alzheimer-type pathology compared with age-matched control subjects. A retrospective postmortem immunocytochemical and histofluorescent study. Neurology 1997; 49(5):1306–1311.

94. Arvanitakis Z, Schneider JA, Wilson RS, et al. Diabetes is related to cerebral infarction but not to AD pathology in older persons. Neurology 2006; 67(11):1960–1965.

95. Razay G, Vreugdenhil A, Wilcock G. Obesity, abdominal obesity and Alzheimer disease. Dement Geriatr Cogn Disord 2006; 22(2):173–176.
96. Razay G, Vreugdenhil A. Obesity in middle age and future risk of dementia: Midlife obesity increases risk of future dementia. BMJ 2005; 331(7514):455.
97. Kivipelto M, Ngandu T, Fratiglioni L, et al. Obesity and vascular risk factors at midlife and the risk of dementia and Alzheimer disease. Arch Neurol 2005; 62(10):1556–1560.
98. Gustafson D, Rothenberg E, Blennow K, et al. An 18-year follow-up of overweight and risk of Alzheimer disease. Arch Intern Med 2003; 163(13):1524–1528.
99. Vanhanen M, Koivisto K, Moilanen L, et al. Association of metabolic syndrome with Alzheimer disease: A population-based study. Neurology 2006; 67(5):843–847.
100. Kwon HM, Kim BJ, Lee SH, et al. Metabolic syndrome as an independent risk factor of silent brain infarction in healthy people. Stroke 2006; 37(2):466–470.
101. Yaffe K, Kanaya A, Lindquist K, et al. The metabolic syndrome, inflammation, and risk of cognitive decline. JAMA 2004; 292(18):2237–2242.
102. Stewart R, Masaki K, Xue OL, et al. A 32 year prospective study of change in body weight and incident dementia: The Honolulu Asia Aging study. Arch Neurol 2005; 62(1):55–60.
103. Barrett-Connor E, Edelstein S, Corey-Bloom J, et al. Weight loss precedes dementia in community-dwelling older adults. J Nutr Health Aging 1998; 2:113–114.
104. Buchman AS, Wilson RS, Bienias JL, et al. Change in body mass index and risk of incident Alzheimer disease. Neurology 2005; 65(6):892–897.
105. Buchman AS, Wilson RS, Schneider JA, et al. Body mass index in older persons is associated with Alzheimer's disease pathology. Neurology 2006; 67(11):1949–1954.
106. Dal Form G, Palermo MT, Donohue JE, et al. Depressive symptoms, sex, and risk for Alzheimer's disease. Ann Neurol 2005; 57(3):381–386.
107. Andersen K, Lolk A, Kragh-Sorensen P, et al. Depression and the risk of Alzheimer disease. Epidemiology 2005; 16(2):233–238.
108. Wilson RS, Schneider JA, Bienias JL, et al. Depressive symptoms, clinical AD, and cortical plaques and tangles in older persons. Neurology 2003; 61(8):1102–1107.
109. Wilson RS, Barnes LL, Mendel de Leon CF, et al. Depressive symptoms, cognitive decline, and risk of AD in older persons. Neurology 2002; 59(3):364–370.
110. Wilson RS, Krueger KR, Arnold SE, et al. Loneliness and risk of AD. Arch Gen Psychiatry 2007; 64(2):234–240.
111. Wilson RS, Evans DA, Bienias JL, et al. Proneness to psychological distress is associated with risk of Alzheimer's disease. Neurology 2003; 61(11):1479–1485.
112. Wilson RS, Arnold SE, Schneider JA, et al. Chronic psychological distress and risk of Alzheimer's disease in old age. Neuroepidemiology 2006; 27(3):143–153.
113. Wilson RS, Barnes LL, Bennett DA, et al. Proneness to psychological distress and risk of Alzheimer disease in a biracial community. Neurology 2005; 64(2):380–382.
114. Lucassen PJ, Heine VM, Muller MB, et al. Stress, depression and hippocampal apoptosis. CNS Neurol Disord Drug Targets 2006; 5(5):531–546.
115. Schofield PW, Tang M, Marder K, et al. Alzheimer's disease after remote head injury: An incidence study. J Neurol Neurosurg Psychiatry 1997; 62:119–124.
116. Mehta KM, Ott A, Kalmijn S, et al. Head trauma and risk of dementia and Alzheimer's disease: The Rotterdam Study. Neurology 1999; 53:1959–1962.
117. Sundstrom A, Nilsson LG, Cruts M, et al. Increased risk of dementia following mild head injury for carriers but not for non-carriers of the APOE epsilon4 allele. Int Psychogeriatr 2006; 19(1):1–7.
118. Fleminger S, Oliver DL, Lovestone S, et al. Head injury as a risk factor for Alzheimer's disease: The evidence 10 years on; a partial replication. J Neurol Neurosurg Psychiatry 2003; 74(7):857–862.
119. Plassman BL, Havlik RJ, Steffens DC, et al. Documented head injury in early adulthood and risk of Alzheimer's disease and other demential. Neurology 2000; 55(8):1158–1166.
120. Horsburgh K, McCarron MO, White F, et al. The role of apolipoprotein E in Alzheimer's disease, acute brain injury and cerebrovascular disease: Evidence of common mechanisms and utility of animal models. Neurobiol Aging 2000; 21(2):245–255.

121. Verghese J, Lipton RB, Hall CB, et al. Abnormality of gait as a predictor of non-Alzheimer's dementia. N Engl J Med 2002; 347(22):1761–1768.
122. Wilson RS, Schneider JA, Bienias JL, et al. Parkinsonianlike signs and risk of incident Alzheimer disease in older persons. Arch Neurol 2003; 60:539–544.
123. Wilson RS, Bennett DA, Gilley D, et al. Progression of Parkinsonism and loss of cognitive function in Alzheimer disease. Arch Neurol 2000; 57(6):855–860.
124. Marquis M, Moore MM, Howieson DB, et al. Independent predictors of cognitive decline in healthy elderly persons. Arch Neurol 2002; 59(4):601–606.
125. Schneider JA, Li JL, Li Y, et al. Substantia nigra tangles are related to gait impairment in older persons. Ann Neurol 2006; 59(1):166–173.
126. Aggarwal NT, Bienias JL, Bennett DA, et al. The relation of cigarette smoking to incident Alzheimer's disease in a biracial urban community population. Neuroepidemiology 2006; 26(3):140–146.
127. Hebert LE, Scherr PA, Beckett LA, et al. Relation of smoking and alcohol consumption to incident Alzheimer's disease. Am J Epidemiol 1992; 135(4):347–355.
128. Ott A, Slooter AJ, Hofman A, et al. Smoking and risk of dementia and Alzheimer's disease in a population-based cohort study: The Rotterdam Study. Lancet 1998; 351:1840–1843.
129. Merchant C, Tang MX, Albert S, et al. The influence of smoking on the risk of Alzheimer's disease. Neurology 1999; 52:1408–1412.
130. Tvas SL, Pederson LL, Koval JJ. Is smoking associated with the risk of developing Alzheimer's disease? Results from three Canadian data sets. Ann Epidemiol 2000; 10(7):409–416.
131. Tyas SL, White LR, Petrovitch H, et al. Mid-life smoking and late-life dementia: The Honolulu-Asia Aging Study. Neurobiol Aging 2003; 24(4):589–596.
132. Kalmijn S, Launer LJ, Ott A, et al. Dietary fat intake and the risk of incident dementia in the Rotterdam Study. Ann Neurol 1997; 42(5):776–782.
133. Morris MC, Evans DA, Bienias JL, et al. Dietary fats and the risk of incident Alzheimer disease. Arch Neurol 2003; 60(2):194–200.
134. Morris MC, Evans DA, Tangney CC, et al. Dietary copper and high saturated and trans fat intakes associated with cognitive decline. Arch Neurol 2006; 63(8):1085–1088.
135. Ravaglia G, Forti P, Maioli F, et al. Blood inflammatory markers and risk of dementia: The Conselice Study of Brain Aging. Neurobiol Aging 2007; 28(12):1810–1820.
136. van Oijen M, de Maat MP, Kardys I, et al. Polymorphisms and haplotypes in the C-reactive protein gene and risk of dementia. Neurobiol Aging 2007; 28(9):1361–1366.
137. Schmidt R, Schmidt H, Curb JD, et al. Early inflammation and dementia: A 25-year follow-up of the Honolulu-Asia Aging Study. Ann Neurol 2002; 52(2):168–174.
138. Zhang Y, Hayes A, Pritchard A, et al. Interleukin-6 promoter polymorphism: Risk and pathology of Alzheimer's disease. Neurosci Lett 2004; 362(2):99–102.
139. Evans D, Hebert L, Beckett L, et al. Education and other measures of socioeconomic status and risk of incident Alzheimer disease in a population of older persons. Arch Neurol 1997; 54:1399–1405.
140. Stern Y, Gurland B, Tatemichi T, et al. Influence of education and occupation on the incidence of Alzheimer's disease. JAMA 1994; 271:1004–1010.
141. Cobb JL, Wolf PA, Au R, et al. The effect of education on the incidence of dementia and Alzheimer's disease in the Framingham Study. Neurology 1995; 45:1707–1712.
142. Caamano-Isorna F, Corral M, Montes-Martinez A, et al. Education and dementia: A meta-analytic study. Neuroepidemiology 2006; 26(4):226–232.
143. Karp A, Kareholt I, Oui C. Relation of education and occupation-based socioeconomic status to incident Alzheimer's disease. Am J Epidemiol 2004; 159(2):175–183.
144. Wilson RS, Mendes De Leon CF, Barnes LL, et al. Participation in cognitively stimulating activities and risk of incident Alzheimer disease. JAMA 2002; 287(6):742–748.
145. Wilson RS, Bennett DA, Bienias JL, et al. Cognitive activity and cognitive decline in a biracial community population. Neurology 2003; 61(6): 812–816.
146. Wilson RS, Scherr PA, Hoganson G, et al. Early life socioeconomic status and late life risk of Alzheimer's disease. Neuroepidemiology 2005; 25(1):8–14.

147. Hall KS, Gao S, Unverzagt FW, et al. Low education and childhood rural residence: Risk for Alzheimer's disease in African Americans. Neurology 2000; 54:95–99.
148. Snowdon D, Kemper S, Mortimer J, et al. Linguistic ability in early life and cognitive function and Alzheimer's disease in late life. JAMA 1996; 275:528–532.
149. Wilson RS, Scherr PA, Bienias JL, et al. Socioeconomic characteristics of the community in childhood and cognition in old age. Exp Aging Res 2005; 31(4):393–407.
150. Wilson RS, Bennett DA, Bienias JL, et al. Cognitive activity and incident AD in a population-based sample of older persons. Neurology 2002; 59(12):1910–1914.
151. Bennett DA, Schneider JA, Wilson RS, et al. Education modifies the association of amyloid but not tangles with cognitive function. Neurology 2005; 65(6):953–955.
152. Snowdon DA, Greiner LH, Markesbery WR. Linguistic ability in early life and the neuropathology of Alzheimer's disease and cerebrovascular disease. Findings from the Nun Study. Ann N Y Acad Sci 2000; 903:34–38.
153. Jankowsky JL, Melnikova T, Fadale DJ, et al. Environmental enrichment mitigates cognitive deficits in a mouse model of Alzheimer's disease. J Neurosci 2005; 25(21):5217–5224.
154. Lazarov O, Robinson J, Tang YP, et al. Environmental enrichment reduces Abeta levels and amyloid deposition in transgenic mice. Cell 2005; 120(5):701–713.
155. Bassuk SS, Glass TA, Berkman LF. Social disengagement and incident cognitive decline in community-dwelling elderly persons. Ann Intern Med 1999; 131:165–173.
156. Fratiglioni L, Wang HX, Ericsson K, et al. Influence of social network on occurrence of dementia: A community-based longitudinal study. Lancet 2000; 355:1315–1319.
157. Barnes LL, Mendes de Leon CF, Wilson RS, et al. Social resources and cognitive decline in a population of older African Americans and whites. Neurology 2004; 63:2322–2326.
158. TE Seeman, TM Lusignolo, M Albert, et al. Social relationships, social support, and patterns of cognitive aging in healthy, high-functioning older adults: MacArthur studies of successful aging. Health Psychol 2001; 20:243–255.
159. Bennett DA, Schneider JA, Tang Y, et al. The effect of social networks on the relation between Alzheimer's disease pathology and level of cognitive function in old people: A longitudinal cohort study. Lancet Neurol 2006; 5(5):406–412.
160. Rovio S, Kareholt 1, Helkala EL, et al. Leisure-time physical activity at midlife and the risk of dementia and Alzheimer's disease. Lancet Neurol 2005; 4(11):705–711.
161. Sturman MT, Morris MC, Mendes de Leon CF, et al. Physical activity, cognitive activity, and cognitive decline in a biracial community population. Arch Neurol 2005; 62(11):1750–1754.
162. Podewils LJ, Guallar E, Kuller LH, et al. Physical activity, APOE genotype, and dementia risk: Findings from the Cardiovascular Health Cognition Study. Am J Epidemiol 2005; 161(7):639–651.
163. Lautenschlager NT, Almeida OP. Physical activity and cognition in old age. Curr Opin Psychiatry 2006; 19(2):190–193.
164. Abbott RD, White LR, Ross GW, et al. Walking and dementia in physically capable elderly men. JAMA 2004; 292(12):1447–1453.
165. Briones TL. Environment, physical activity, and neurogenesis: Implications for prevention and treatment of Alzheimer's disease. Curr Alzheimer Res 2006; 3(1):49–54.
166. Morris MC, Evans DA, Bienias JL, et al. Consumption of fish and n-3 fatty acids and risk of incident Alzheimer disease. Arch Neurol 2003; 60(7):940–946.
167. Morris MC, Evans DA, Bienias JL, et al. Dietary intake of antioxidant nutrients and the risk of incident Alzheimer disease in a biracial community study. JAMA 2002; 287(24):3230–3237.
168. Masaki K, Losonezy KG, Ismirlian G, et al. Association of vitamin E and C supplement use with cognitive function in elderly men. Neurology 2000; 54:1256–1272.
169. Laurin D, Foley DJ, Masaki KH, et al. Vitamin E and C supplements and risk of dementia. JAMA 2002; 288(18):2266–2268.
170. Cherubim A, Martin A, Andres-Lacueva C, et al. Vitamin E levels, cognitive impairment and dementia in older persons: The InCHIANTI study. Neurobiol Aging 2005; 26(7):987–994.

171. Morris MC, Evans DA, Tangney CC, et al. Relation of the tocopherol forms to incident Alzheimer disease and to cognitive change. Am J Clin Nutr 2005; 81(2):508–514.
172. Huang TL, Zandi PP, Tucker KL, et al. Benefits of fatty fish on dementia risk are stronger for those without APOE epsilon4. Neurology 2005; 65(9):1409–1414.
173. Morris MC, Evans DA, Schneider JA, et al. Dietary folate and vitamins B-12 and B-6 not associated with incident Alzheimer's disease. J Alzheimers Dis 2006; 9(4):435–443.
174. Corrada M, Kawas C, Hallfrisch J, et al. Reduced risk of Alzheimer's disease with high folate intake: The Baltimore Longitudinal Study of Aging. Alzheimer Dement 2005; 1:11–18.
175. Kawas CH. Medications and diet: Protective factors for AD? Alzheimer Dis Assoc Disord 2006; 20(3, suppl 2):S89–S96.
176. Letenneur L. Risk of dementia and alcohol and wine consumption: A review of recent results. Biol Res 2004; 37(2):189–193.
177. Mukamal KJ, Chung H, Jenny NS, et al. Alcohol use and risk of ischemic stroke among older adults: The cardiovascular health study. Stroke 2005; 36(9):1830–1834.
178. Truelsen T, Thudium D, Gronbaek M. Amount and type of alcohol and risk of dementia: The Copenhagen City Heart Study. Neurology 2002; 59(9):1313–1319.
179. Luchsinger JA, Tang MX, Siddiqui M, et al. Alcohol intake and risk of dementia. J Am Geriatr 2004; 52(4):540–546.
180. Baldereschi M, Di Carlo A, Lepore V, et al. Estrogen-replacement therapy and Alzheimer's disease in the Italian Longitudinal Study on Aging. Neurology 1998; 50:996–1002.
181. Kawas C, Resnick S, Morrison A, et al. A prospective study of estrogen replacement therapy and the risk of developing Alzheimer's disease: The Baltimore Longitudinal Study of Aging. Neurology 1997; 48:1517–1521.
182. Zandi PP, Carlson MC, Plassman BL, et al. Hormone replacement therapy and incidence of Alzheimer disease in older women: The Cache County Study. JAMA 2002; 288(17):2123–2129.
183. Zandi PP, Anthony JC, Khachaturian AS, et al. Reduced risk of Alzheimer disease in users of antioxidant vitamin supplements: The Cache County Study. Arch Neurol 2004; 61(1):82–88.
184. Stewert WF, Kawas C, Corrada M, et al. Risk of Alzheimer's disease and duration of NSAID use. Neurology 1997; 48:626–632.
185. Veld BA, Launer LJ, Hoes AW, et al. NSAIDs and incident Alzheimer's disease. The Rotterdam Study. Neurobiol Aging 1998; 19:607–611.
186. Zandi PP, Sparks DL, Khachaturian AS, et al. Do statins reduce risk of incident dementia and Alzheimer disease? The Cache County Study. Arch Gen Psychiatry 2005; 62(2):217–224.
187. Li G, Higdon R, Kukull WA, et al. Statin therapy and risk of dementia in the elderly: A community-based prospective cohort study. Neurology 2004; 63(9):1624–1628.
188. Cole GM, Morihara T, Lim GP, et al. NSAID and antioxidant prevention of Alzheimer's disease: Lessons from in vitro and animal models. Ann N Y Acad Sci 2004; 1035:68–84.
189. Roberts RO, Cha RH, Knopman DS, Petersen RC, Rocca WA. Postmenopausal estrogen therapy and Alzheimer disease: Overall negative findings. Alzheimer Dis Assoc Disord 2006; 20(3):141–146.

Diagnosis of mild cognitive impairment and dementia

Maria Kataki

MILD COGNITIVE IMPAIRMENT

Mild cognitive impairment (MCI) refers to a transitional state between the cognition of normal aging and mild dementia in which people experience memory loss, yet they do not meet currently accepted criteria for dementia or clinically probable Alzheimer's disease.

From a diagnostic perspective, the concept of MCI has been recognized as being heterogeneous (1–4). Most research has been conducted on the amnestic MCI, which, as its name implies, represents a primary memory disorder with relative preservation of other cognitive domains (1,5). The diagnosis of MCI has been made if the patient meets the following criteria: (*i*) memory complaint, (*ii*) normal activities of daily living, (*iii*) normal general cognitive function, (*iv*) abnormal memory for age, and (*v*) not demented (1).

Amnestic MCI can be subdivided into a single domain subtype with memory deficit or a multiple domain subtype that includes memory impairment along with some impairment in other cognitive domains such as language, executive function, and visuospatial skills. Another subtype of MCI is nonamnestic, which similarly can be subdivided into single and multiple domains subtypes. Most studies indicate that the amnestic subtype progresses to Alzheimer's disease (AD) while the nonamnestic subtype likely progresses to non-AD dementias. Given the association between depression and impairments in executive function, the nonamnestic subtypes of MCI may be the most pertinent in late-life mood disorders. Individuals developing frontotemporal dementia would also likely present as nonamnestic MCI. A similar construct cognitive impairment, no dementia (CIND) has also been used in recent epidemiological studies to describe this transitional state between normal and dementia conditions.

The prevalence and classification of MCI in the Cardiovascular Health Study Cognition Study, a multicenter population study that included 3608 participants, was 19% (465 of 2470 participants); prevalence increased with age from 19% in participants younger than 75 years to 29% in those older than 85 years. The prevalence of MCI at the Pittsburg Center was 22%; prevalence of the amnestic-type was 6% and of the MCI multiple cognitive deficits-type was 16% (5).

MCI Pathology

Clearly, most of the patients afflicted with MCI had a "transitional state of evolving AD"rather than advanced (Braak stage V–VI) disease based on a neuropathological study of 34 cases that determined the pathologic substrates of dementia in cases with prior diagnosis of MCI. Of interest, however, 2 of the MCI patients had progressed to the point of Braak stage V AD, while almost half of the

MCI brains studied showed features of argyrophilic grain disease. In addition, there were many concomitant multiple pathologic abnormalities, including argyrophilic grain disease, hippocampal sclerosis, and vascular lesions (6,7). Most patients with MCI did not meet the neuropathologic criteria for AD, but their pathologic findings suggested a transitional state of evolving AD, as reported in another study of 66 individuals. In that study, 15 who had memory impairment beyond that allowed for aging, but who were not demented, were studied along with 28 clinically healthy individuals and 23 patients with probable AD for comparison. All the patients with MCI had pathologic findings involving medial temporal lobe structures, likely accounting for their memory impairment. The neuropathologic features of MCI matched the clinical features and seemed to be intermediate between the neurofibrillary changes of aging and the pathologic features of very early AD (8).

There is a frequent occurrence of hippocampal atrophy on MRI imaging in amnestic MCI compared with cognitively intact controls. It has also been shown that the degree of hippocampal atrophy on MRI can predict the rate of conversion from MCI to AD, and hippocampal atrophy seen in MCI can be correlated with autopsy evidence of atrophy and neuronal loss (9).

MCI Diagnosis

AD and MCI cannot be diagnosed by neuropsychological tests alone, and clinical judgment is always required. First, performance on neuropsychological tests is affected by many factors, including education, age, cultural background, and illnesses other than AD. Second, neuropsychological measures cannot fully distinguish among different types of dementia, because there is substantial overlap in neuropsychological profiles. The usefulness of any battery for identifying cases of MCI will depend on its composition, size, and supporting data. A brief battery, including measures of new learning, delayed recall, attention, and executive function, could provide valuable information for screening and diagnosis if interpreted properly (10). In order to avoid the impracticality in the primary care setting of many currently available cognitive instruments and to reduce barriers to screening, we developed a brief cognitive screening instrument called the Self-Administered Gerocognitive Examination (SAGE) as a screening instrument for MCI and early dementia (11).

ALZHEIMER'S DISEASE

AD is now universally recognized as the major dementing disorder of aging. AD epitomizes the age-dependent disorders of late life with the prevalence doubling every 5 years of age, at least between ages 65 and 85.

Pathology of AD

AD was first identified and named in 1906 by Dr. Alois Alzheimer, a German neuropathologist. He had treated a middle-aged woman who exhibited symptoms of memory loss and disorientation. Five years later, the patient died after suffering hallucinations and symptoms of dementia. The manifestations and course of the disease were so unusual that Dr. Alzheimer was unable to classify her in any of the existing diagnostic categories. Postmortem examination of the brain revealed microscopic and macroscopic lesions and distortions, including neuritic plaques and neurofibrillary tangles (12–15). The existence of this new entity was quickly confirmed by other investigators, and by 1910 there was a consensus to name this novel form of presenile dementia "Alzheimer's disease"; the senium then considered to begin at age 60! (12).

Ultrastructural studies resolved the half-century debate and confirmed that "senile dementia"is the same entity as Alzheimer's presenile dementia and provided the basis of subsequent molecular characterization of the abnormal fibrous proteins characteristic of AD. These dramatic ultrastructural changes were identical in subjects whose onset of their dementia was in the presenium and in subjects whose onset of dementia occurred in the senium. Molecular chemistry has also confirmed that the chemical constitution of the amyloid fibril and paired helical filament is identical in brains of Alzheimer patients with onset in the presenium. Thus, the identity of AD in both presenile and senile patients became established (12).

Health care professionals now know that while there is a strong and as yet incompletely understood relationship between aging and AD, they are not the same conditions (16).

Clearly AD is associated with abnormal accumulation of a breakdown product of the amyloid precursor protein known as beta-amyloid, especially in the insoluble form. Amyloid appears to be toxic to cells in vitro, and abnormal accumulation may actually cause cell loss. No one knows why beta-amyloid accumulates, but it may be secondary to abnormal processing within neurons. Tau protein is part of the cytoskeleton of neuronal cells. In damaged cells (e.g., after heat shock), its expression is increased. Tau protein is found in the neurofibrillary tangles of patients with AD. Tau appears to be hyperphosphorylated in cells destined to develop neurofibrillary tangles. It may be an early marker of cells with abnormal cytoskeletal function and abnormal metabolism.

AD Demographics

In 2004 there were more than 4.5 million people in the United States and 22 million people worldwide with AD, the most common form of dementia. Three percent of people aged 65 years or older are diagnosed with AD; the incidence doubles every 5 years thereafter. Forty-seven percent of the population aged 85 years or older has the disease. The number of adults older than 65 years of age is steadily increasing; by the year 2030, adults older than 65 years of age are expected to constitute approximately 20% of the U.S. population (17). Because of global population aging, Edward Truschke, former president of the Alzheimer's Association, stated, "We have an imminent worldwide epidemic if a cure is not found." Thirty-five to seventy-five percent of residents in long-term care facilities have been diagnosed with AD or another senile dementia for which there is no cure. The annual cost of caring for and treating patients with AD is approximately $100 billion (18). The total estimated worldwide cost of dementia is $604 billion in 2010 (18).

Diagnosing AD

The misdiagnosis of depression as dementia was first described by Kiloh (19) in 1961 as "pseudodementia." During the 1970s, differentiation of the dementia syndrome from major depression was studied by a number of psychiatrists (20), and in 1980, the American Psychiatric Association, in the third edition of its *Diagnostic and Statistical Manual* (DSM-III) (21) set clear-cut operational criteria for the two disorders. These criteria limited the diagnosis of dementia to individuals who were alert and awake and who had experienced a decline in functional abilities secondary to cognitive impairment, with evidence of such cognitive impairment in at least two areas of cognition. Clinicians using this definition of dementia were able to diagnose a dementia syndrome with greater than 95% accuracy and differentiate not only dementia from depression but also dementia from amnestic syndromes and delirium. The success of the DSM-III criteria for the diagnosis of dementia led to the formation of a task force by the National Institute of Neurological and Communicative Disorders and Strokes (NINCDS) and the Alzheimer's Disease and Related Disorders Association (ADRDA) to establish criteria for the diagnosis of AD (22). Definite diagnosis of AD depends on neuropathological confirmation. However, their criteria for probable AD have turned out to have an accuracy of 85% to 95% based on subsequent clinical-pathological analyses.

Obviously it is not possible to biopsy the brains of suspected AD patients to make the definite diagnosis. Other methods of diagnosing the disease are necessary. A probable diagnosis of AD can be made based on the medical history, physical examination, a full mental status examination, diagnostic studies, and assessment for the presence of delirium and depression. The observation of signs and symptoms and the ruling out of other disease processes support the diagnosis even in the absence of pathology reports. The earlier the diagnosis is made, the greater the benefit managing the clinical course of the illness.

There are other medical conditions that present similar clinical manifestations as AD. Some of these conditions may be reversible with appropriate treatment. A person suspected of having AD or any dementia should be given a complete work-up by practitioners who are experienced in the diagnosis and treatment of dementias. Someone who has personal knowledge of the patient should be available to answer questions that assist in establishing a diagnosis. Knowing the type of dementia is helpful to establish a prognosis.

The goals of the diagnostic process are to make a specific diagnosis; avoid implementing the wrong treatment as a result of misdiagnosis; identify any psychiatric or systemic illness; determine the type of dementia; determine the extent of impairment or the stage of the disease; avoid labeling a person with a diagnosis of dementia or AD when it does not exist; define the practical and psychosocial needs of the patient, the family, and primary caregivers; and plan for the future.

A complete and thorough history is imperative to making an accurate diagnosis. The family history may identify genetic or familial illness. Information about abrupt or gradual onset, progressive or fluctuating course, and gradual worsening or step-wise progression can be of diagnostic value. Early symptoms of AD include forgetfulness for recent events or newly acquired information, often causing the patient to repeat himself/herself. Other early features are disorientation, especially to time and difficulty with complex cognitive functions such as mathematical calculations or organization of activities that require several steps. Advanced AD includes a history of progression and pervasive memory loss sufficient to impair everyday activities, disorientation to place and/or aspects of person (e.g., age), inability to keep track of time, and problems with personal care (23).

As AD progresses, various mood and behavioral disorders may become prominent in many patients and may require intervention and treatment with medications. Some of these behavioral manifestations may lead to reconsideration of the diagnosis of AD. Lewy body dementia may be more likely in the presence of visual hallucinations and extrapyramidal symptoms. Pick's disease may be entertained with the presence of significant personality changes. The most common pathological behaviors in patients with AD are apathy (70%), agitation (60%), motor abnormalities (40%), nighttime behavioral disturbances (30%), delusions (25%), disinhibited behaviors (20%), hallucinations (10%), and euphoria (2%) (24).

Histories should be obtained to rule out other potential causes of cognitive loss and dementia. Knowing about impaired vision and hearing is important. People with hearing impairments often deny their problem and will answer questions inappropriately, thus appearing confused. Visually impaired people may have problems navigating their environment and may also appear disoriented. Proper nutrition improves brain health. Altered nutrition is not uncommon among elder adults and typically is related to living circumstances, diminished appetite, functional deficits, and economic factors. Dehydration is common among the elderly as thirst is not sharply experienced and fear of incontinence also hinders the consumption of adequate fluids.

Anemia, hypoglycemia, hyperglycemia, hypoproteinemia, and vitamin deficiencies often present with clinical manifestations similar to AD. The aging process causes diminished liver and kidney function. This loss may interfere with the absorption and metabolism of medications. Adverse effects of drugs such as cimetidine, digoxin, and diazepam often present through behavioral changes. A thorough assessment of the medication regimen should be included in the history. The patient and the family should be interviewed regarding all prescription medications, over-the-counter medications, eye drops and topical medications, medications prescribed by someone else, herbal and vitamin preparations, alcohol, addictive and chemical substances.

After the complete history is obtained, a thorough physical and neurological examination is performed. It may also suggest physical or neurological conditions that could affect mentation (25).

A Clinical Practice Guideline, Recognition and Initial Assessment of Alzheimer's Disease and Related Dementias (26) suggested in 1996 that laboratory tests should be carried out only after it has been confirmed that the patient has impairment in multiple domains that is not lifelong and that these impairments represent a decline from previous level of functioning. The routine evaluations should include: complete blood count, urine analysis with culture and sensitivity if indicated, erythrocyte sedimentation rate, blood chemistries including electrolytes and blood sugar level, vitamin B_{12} and folate, liver function studies, kidney function studies, thyroid function studies, syphilis serology, enzyme-linked immunosorbent assay for detecting AIDS, chest x-ray, and electrocardiogram. By 1999, the Report of the Council on Scientific Affairs of the American Medical Association (27) cited the need to rule out metabolic and structural causes for cognitive disorders and suggested performing the above tests without the prior restrictions. By 2001, the American Academy of Neurology established practice recommendations for the diagnosis and management of dementia. According to these guidelines, it is considered standard of care to obtain thyroid and vitamin B_{12} laboratories and, in case of risk factors, to conduct a screening for sexually transmitted diseases (23).

Imaging of AD

The advent of newer imaging techniques has provided the means of obtaining a presumptive diagnosis, especially when combined with other testing modalities.

Magnetic resonance imaging (MRI) is now able to measure, with considerable accuracy, the size of intracerebral structures, such as the hippocampus, that atrophies over time in those with AD (28). Patients with AD have a decreased volume of their hippocampus when compared to nonaffected individuals. In addition, patients with some degree of atrophy are more liable to develop AD. MRI easily identifies cerebral atrophy and it is a useful tool to pick up other abnormalities that are associated with decreased cognition or dementia. Computerized tomography (CT) can also help in the diagnosis by identifying structural changes such as infarcts or mass lesions that could produce cognitive changes. The American Academy of Neurology states that structural neuroimaging with either a noncontrast CT or MRI in the initial evaluation of patients with dementia is appropriate (29). Single photon emission tomography (SPECT) and positron emission tomography (PET) are imaging techniques that provide information about cerebral function and regional cerebral blood flow. The ability to image the regional metabolism of the brain and locate areas of diminished function has been of particular importance in advancing the ability to diagnose AD. These techniques also help to differentiate AD from other causes of dementia with typical findings in AD showing hypometabolism on PET and hypoperfusion on SPECT in parietal and temporal cortices (30–32). One of the benefits of these imaging tests is the ability to help identify people in the early stages of AD or those with MCI who may benefit from treatments that are now being offered or may soon be developed.

Among the most promising techniques to assist in diagnosis of AD was a study conducted at the University of Pittsburg, where a compound was developed that adheres to amyloid plaques in the brain and can be detected by PET imaging. The compound, known as Pittsburg Compound B (PIB), may allow for the differential diagnosis of patients with dementia and help with an earlier detection of those who are at risk for advancing AD (33). A study from Los Angeles reported the development of another compound called 18-F-FDDNP that adheres both to amyloid plaques and tangles of abnormal tau protein in the brains of AD patients. These and other similar compounds being developed are sure to aid in early diagnosis of AD.

Cognitive Evaluation of AD

Mental status examinations provide additional information for developing a more complete clinical picture. They offer a baseline for monitoring the progression of the disease and can be used to reassess cognition in people who have delirium or depression on initial evaluation. There are several brief mental status examinations that are typically used. The Mini-Mental State Examination (MMSE) (34) includes items to assess verbal memory, orientation, language, constructional praxis, and attention. The test is scored from 0, indicating severe impairment, to 30 if the patient makes no errors. Patients with AD generally score 26 or less, although performance is clearly affected by age and education as well as disease state (34). Another widely used screening test is the Short Blessed Test (35), which ranges from 0, for a subject who makes no errors, to 28; AD patients usually score

6 or more. Other brief screening tests such as the Mental Status Questionnaire and the Short Probable Mental Status Questionnaire (36) have items that overlap to a large extent with the MMSE and the Short Blessed Test. The SAGE, mentioned earlier, is scored from 0 (worst) to 22 (best) with 14 or lower usually indicating dementia.

Longer instruments for use in clinical settings usually cover the same cognitive domains but in greater detail. One very useful battery which takes approximately 45 to 50 minutes to administer was developed by the Consortium to Establish a Registry for Alzheimer's Disease (CERAD), a group composed of investigators from AD research programs in the United States funded by the U.S. National Institute on Aging (37). The CERAD battery contains more extensive tests of verbal memory, including immediate and delayed recall, language tests of naming and verbal fluency, and drawings to test constructional praxis. Another widely used test that can be administered in about 30 to 40 minutes is the Alzheimer's Disease Assessment Scale (ADAS) (38). Some of the items included in the ADAS, which also assess memory, language, praxis, orientation, and attention, are used in the CERAD battery. The ADAS is slightly shorter, however, and also includes a set of clinician-rated items to assess the severity of noncognitive disturbances such as agitation, psychosis, and depressed mood. Because the ADAS was designed as an outcome measure for drug treatment trials, it provides specific rules for calculating overall severity scores for both cognitive and noncognitive symptoms. Both the CERAD battery and the ADAS are more comprehensive than the brief screening tests, particularly in their assessment of memory functions. Other sophisticated instruments designed to evaluate the cognitive symptoms of dementia include the Mattis Dementia Rating Scale (DRS) (39) and the short Kurtz test (SKT) (40,41).

Genetics of AD

In early onset familial AD, some families show a mutation in the gene that encodes amyloid precursor protein on chromosome 21. Other families show mutations on chromosome 14 (in the gene for presenilin-1) or chromosome 1 (in the gene for presenilin-2). It is likely that other genes will be linked to the early onset familial form of AD. These mutations are rare and account for less than 5% of AD cases. Late onset familial AD is linked to chromosome 19. It has been demonstrated that the particular inherited form of apolipoprotein E (APOE) (coded by a gene in chromosome 19) determines the age-dependent risk and age of onset for AD in these patients. APOE is a cholesterol-carrying blood protein that comes in three forms: APOE $\varepsilon2$, $\varepsilon3$, $\varepsilon4$. We inherit one APOE allele from each parent. Patients who inherit one or more $\varepsilon4$ alleles are at greater risk of getting AD, but only about 50% of AD patients have $\varepsilon4$. Other families have been linked to variant forms of alpha-2 macroglobulin on chromosome 12. These gene associations likely represent inherited risk factors rather than genetic forms of AD. It is not clear if there is a genetic component to all cases of AD. Patients with a family history of AD in even one primary relative appear to be at increased risk of getting AD themselves and the risk is higher if both parents have AD. Cases that seem to be sporadic are common, although the APOE genotype is a clear risk factor for both sporadic and late onset familial cases. Multiple genetic factors probably account for a predisposition for AD.

Risk Factors of AD

Well-described risk factors for AD include increased age, the presence of APOE ε4, serious head injury in APOE ε4-positive people, aging, postmenopausal estrogen deficiency, positive family history (independent of APOE genotype), elevated serum homocysteine levels, and low education level. Aluminum exposure is frequently cited as a risk factor, but no sound evidence supports the association.

Protective Factors of AD

While definite proof is lacking, estrogen replacement early in the menopause, anti-inflammatory drugs (including nonsteroidal agents), antioxidants, and the use of statin drugs have been proposed to reduce the risk of AD and are under study. In most studies, neurofibrillary tangles correlate best with the severity of dementia. Synaptic density has been shown to have an inverse correlation with severity of dementia, at least in some brain regions. Because education seems to increase synaptic density, some have suggested that education may have a protective effect against the manifestation of AD cognitive changes (42).

Differential Diagnosis of AD

Early on, normal aging needs to be distinguished from AD. In addition, dementia with Lewy bodies, Parkinson's disease (PD), progressive supranuclear palsy, and vascular dementias are sometimes difficult to distinguish from AD. They are caused by different pathology than the plaques and tangles of AD but they may affect similar brain regions. Clinical correlations are extremely important in such cases.

DIFFERENTIAL DIAGNOSIS OF DEMENTIA

Most common causes of dementia are as follows:

- Alzheimer's disease
- Vascular dementia
- Alcoholism
- Parkinson's disease
- Drug/medication intoxication

    Less common causes of dementia are as follows:

- Vitamin deficiencies—thiamine: Wernicke's encephalopathy, B_{12} pernicious anemia, nicotinic acid
- Endocrine and other organ failure: Hypothyroidism, adrenal insufficiency and Cushing's syndrome, hypo- and hyperparathyroidism, renal failure, liver failure, pulmonary failure
- Chronic infections: HIV, neurosyphilis, papovavirus (progressive multifocal leucoencephalopathy), prion (Creutzfeldt–Jacob and Gerstmann–Straussler–Scheinker diseases), tuberculosis, fungal and protozoal, Whipple's disease
- Head trauma and diffuse brain damage: Dementia pugilistica, chronic subdural hematoma, postanoxia, postencephalitis, normal-pressure hydrocephalus
- Neoplastic: Primary brain tumor, metastatic brain tumor, paraneoplastic limbic encephalitis
- Toxic disorders: Drug, medication, and narcotic poisoning, heavy metal intoxication, dialysis dementia (aluminum), organic toxins

- Psychiatric: Depression (pseudodementia), schizophrenia, conversion reaction
- Degenerative disorders: Huntington's disease, Pick's disease, dementia with Lewy bodies, progressive supranuclear palsy (Steel–Richardson syndrome), multisystem degeneration (Shy–Drager syndrome), hereditary ataxias (some forms), motor neuron disease (amyotrophic lateral sclerosis, ALS; some forms)
- Miscellaneous: Sarcoidosis, vasculitis, cerebral autosomal dominant arteriopathy with subcortical infarcts and leucoencephalopathy (CADASIL), acute intermittent porphyria, recurrent nonconvulsive seizures
- Additional conditions in children or adolescents: Hallervorden–Spatz disease, subacute sclerosing panencephalitis, metabolic disorders (e.g., Wilson's and Leigh's diseases, leukodystrophies, lipid storage diseases, mitochondrial mutations) (43).

FRONTOTEMPORAL DEMENTIAS

Frontotemporal dementia (FTD) usually affects people in the age range of 35 to 75 years old. Postmortem investigation has reported a relative frequency of FTD of 3% to 10% of all dementias (44). About 20% to 40% of FTD patients have a positive family history (45).

Two recent studies have addressed the prevalence of FTD. Ratnavalli et al. (46) reported a prevalence of 15 per 100,000 in a population between 45 and 64 years of age, while Russo et al. (47), who studied the prevalence of FTD in the Netherlands, reported an overall prevalence of FTD of 1.1 in 100,000 with a maximum prevalence of 9.4 per 100,000 for ages 60 to 69 years. Overall FTD is estimated to account for 20% of degenerative dementia cases with presenile onset (48). Two recent studies have reported that the incidence rates for FTD (new cases per 100,000 person-years) were 2.2 for ages 40 to 49 years, 3.3 for ages 50 to 59 years, and 8.9 for ages 60 to 69 years. In comparison, the corresponding rates for AD were 0.0, 3.3, and 88.9, respectively (49,50). While the age of onset tends to be less than in patients with AD, it does not seem to vary for familial versus sporadic cases. The median age of onset of FTD is about 58 years with 22% of the patients having an age of onset after age 65.7 (51).

In a recent study by Hodges et al. in 2003 (52), median survival period from symptom onset was found to be 6 +/− 1.1 years for FTD and 3 +/−0.4 years for FTD-motor neuron disease (FTD-MND). The median survival period for the entire group was 3 years from the time of diagnosis, and 75% were dead within 6 years. This short survival period was attributable partly to delayed diagnosis; on average, 3 years elapse between symptom onset and diagnosis. Some of the factors associated with a decreased survival period in FTD include the presence of amyotrophic lateral sclerosis (ALS), specific degeneration of frontal-subcortical circuits, and tau-negative cases. They also found that patients with semantic dementia (SD) had significantly longer survival period compared to other subsets of FTD (52,53).

Diagnosing FTD

Patients with FTD should have a neuropsychiatric assessment, neuropsychological testing, and neuroimaging study to clarify the diagnosis. On neuropsychological testing, orientation and recall of recent personal events is good, but performance on anterograde memory tests can be variable. Patients tend to do poorly on recall-based tasks but they improve with clueing. An amnestic memory condition is not usually observed. A reduction in spontaneous conversation is common. Subjects also perform well on visuospatial tests when the organizational aspects are minimized. The Folstein Mini-Mental State Examination (MMSE) (54) is unreliable for the detection and monitoring of patients with FTD, who frequently perform normally even when requiring nursing home care (55).

There have been several different classifications proposed to make the clinical diagnosis of FTD. The Lund and Manchester Group (56) initially established diagnostic criteria for FTD in 1994. Patients were required to present with at least two of the following signs or symptoms: loss of personal awareness, strange eating habits, perseveration or changes in mood. In addition, they had to have one of the following features: frontal executive dysfunction, reduced speech, or normal visuospatial ability. Neary et al. in 1998 (57) developed another set of diagnostic criteria, and specifically divided FTD into three prototypic syndromes. They have been delineated above as frontal-variant FTD (FvFTD), semantic dementia (SD), and progressive nonfluent aphasia (PNFA). McKhann et al. in 2001 (45) sought to further define clinical criteria for FTD that can be easily used by clinicians in order to make a prompt diagnosis of FTD. They proposed the following criteria for FTD:

1. The development of behavioral or cognitive deficits manifested by either
   a. early and progressive change in personality, characterized by difficulty in modulating behavior, often resulting in inappropriate responses or activities or
   b. early and progressive change in language, characterized by problems with expression of language or severe naming difficulty and problems with word meaning.
2. The deficits outlined in 1a or 1b cause significant impairment in social or occupational functioning and represent a significant decline from a previous level of functioning.
3. The course is characterized by a gradual onset and continuing decline in function.
4. The deficits outlined in 1a or 1b are not due to other nervous system conditions (e.g., cerebrovascular accident), systemic conditions, or substance abuse-induced conditions.
5. The deficits do not occur exclusively during a delirium.
6. The disturbance is not better accounted for by another psychiatric diagnosis.

Imaging of FTD

Neuroimaging can also be helpful in distinguishing FTD from other types of cognitive disorders. Typically, structural imaging shows anterior temporal and frontal atrophy, while functional imaging shows decreased perfusion of frontal and temporal lobes (58). MRI scans indicate that both PNFA and FvFTD show frontotemporal atrophy. The focus of the atrophy is in the left perisylvian region in PNFA patients, in the left anterior temporal lobe in SD patients, and usually in both frontal lobes in FvFTD patients. In contrast, the mesial temporal lobes are atrophic in AD patients (59). Imaging abnormalities in FvFTD usually appear later in the disease course. Technetium-hexamethylpropylene-amineoxine single-photon-emission-computed-tomography (Tc-HMPAO-SPECT) scanning can detect hypoperfusion in the ventromedial frontal region even before atrophy is evident. In the later stages of the disease, atrophy of the frontal and anterior temporal lobes becomes more apparent (55). According to a recent report studying SPECT differences in FTD patients with different symptoms, patients with right frontal involvement meet the consensus criteria more frequently than patients with greater involvement in other areas (60).

Neurochemistry of FTD

Neurochemical changes in the behavioral presentation of FTD contrast with those of AD. There is evidence of less cholinergic deficit and more serotonergic disturbance in FTD than in AD. In fact, acetylcholinesterase and choline acetyltransferase activities are well preserved in FTD. Serotonin dysfunction is linked with impulsivity, irritability, affective change, and changes in eating behavior. These are all common features of FTD. Additionally, the serotonergic system has wide distribution in the frontal lobes, which are commonly affected in FTD. Using functional imaging, serotonin binding has shown to be reduced in the frontal cortex in FTD. Monoaminergic and dopaminergic alterations have also been reported in the literature (61).

Clinical Features of FTD

FTD results in behavioral, cognitive, and neurological impairments. Three major clinical presentations are described below. Generally, in terms of behavioral alterations, patients often tend to lack appropriate social cognition and emotions. Patients with FTD commonly present either with disinhibition and overactivity or apathy and blunted affect (62). Some behavioral abnormalities seen in patients with FTD have been compared to those presented by patients with antisocial personality disorder. Functional imaging studies have shown abnormalities in individuals with acquired sociopathy that involve the same areas affected in FTD. These include the anterior temporal lobe, ventromedial frontal lobe, and orbitofrontal cortex (63). It has also been suggested that these patients suffer from "moral agnosia," which could be related to an inability to differentiate right from wrong or from the loss of the capacity to reason (64). Patients with FTD show marked deficiencies in executive functioning and working memory (62). Other frequently encountered cognitive abnormalities include deficits in attention, poor abstraction, difficulty shifting mental set, and perseveration (48). Interestingly, related to preserved parietal-occipital lobe functioning in many, spatial skills seem to remain unaffected in these patients (62).

Neurological signs are usually absent early in the disease, although patients may display primitive reflexes. With disease progression, some patients develop parkinsonian signs of akinesia and rigidity, which can be prominent. They may also have repetitive motor behaviors and muscular rigidity (62). A minority of patients develops neurological signs consistent with MND (48).

The symptoms of FTD reflect the distribution of the pathological changes rather than the precise histological subtype. The degree of frontal versus temporal pathology can account for additional variability in the presenting symptoms of FTD (60). Complicating matters further, patients may initially present with symptoms consistent with one particular FTD syndrome but then progress to a different FTD subtype (44). The three major clinical presentations of FTD include: (*i*) a frontal or behavioral variant (FvFTD); (*ii*) a temporal, aphasic variant, also called semantic dementia (SD); and (*iii*) a progressive aphasia (PA), typically nonfluent in type.

Frontal Variant FTD

FvFTD is characterized by the insidious onset of personality changes, behavioral abnormalities, and poor insight. The division of frontal lobe function into three separate areas (orbitobasal, medial, and dorsolateral) offers a way to understand the clinical presentation of FvFTD. Orbitobasal involvement leads to some of the most common symptoms encountered in this disorder. These include disinhibition, poor impulse control, antisocial behavior, and stereotypical behavior. Examples of stereotypical, or ritualized behaviors, include insisting on eating the same food at exactly the same time daily, cleaning the house in precisely the same order, or simple repetitive behaviors such as foot-tapping. Ritualized acts may also include the use of a "catch-phrase"and a change in food preference (55). A patient's decline in social conduct can include breaches of interpersonal etiquette and tactlessness. Verbally inappropriate sexual comments and gestures are common (65).

Apathy is correlated with the severity of medial frontal-anterior cingulate involvement (55). Dietary changes are frequent and typically take the form of overeating, that is, hyperorality, with a preference for sweet foods (55). Patients also exhibit emotional blunting. Speech output is attenuated and mutism eventually develops. Echolalia and perseveration may be present.

The most common cognitive deficit in FvFTD is an impairment of executive function or working memory (65), which is indicative of frontal and prefrontal cortex involvement. Other frequently encountered cognitive abnormalities include attentional deficits, poor abstraction, difficulty shifting mental set, and perseverative tendencies (48). Deficits in planning, organization, and other aspects of executive function become universal as the disease progresses, and this reflects the involvement of the dorsolateral prefrontal cortex (55).

Within the clinical subtypes of FvFTD, there is marked heterogeneity of clinical presentations, often as a result of differential involvement of brain regions. Some patients are disinhibited, fatuous, purposelessly overactive, easily distracted, socially inappropriate, and lacking in concern. At the other extreme, others are bland, apathetic, inert, lacking volition, mentally rigid, and perseverative (48). Social behavior has been shown to be more disrupted in patients with predominantly right-hemisphere pathology (48). Moreover, McMurtray (60) demonstrated that patients with frontal predominate FTD showed hypoactivity and apathy, whereas patients with temporal predominate FTD showed hypomania-like behavior. Decreased insight was associated with right frontal hypoperfusion, while decreased hygiene and grooming with left frontal hypoperfusion. Patients with left hemisphere FTD had early speech and language difficulty but greater normal behavior, whereas patients with right hemisphere FTD had normal speech and language but more frequent inappropriate behavior (60).

Semantic Dementia

Temporal FTD, also known as semantic dementia (SD), is associated with bilateral atrophy of the middle and inferior temporal neocortex (62). The most common initial presentation in these patients is an abnormality of language, which includes loss of memory for words or loss of a word's meaning (65). Patients with SD are often unaware of their difficulties with comprehension. Speech is fluent, but patients tend to use substitute phrases such as "thing" or "that." Patients lose the ability to name and understand words and to recognize the significance of faces, objects, and other sensory stimuli. They also show deficits on nonverbal tasks using visual, auditory, and other modalities, suggesting that the key impairment in SD is a breakdown in conceptual knowledge rather than a specific problem with language. Working memory and autobiographical memory, at least for the recent past, tend to be preserved. However, patients with SD perform poorly on standard anterograde verbal memory tests, such as word-list learning (66).

Behavioral symptoms may occur early or late in the clinical course. Patients with SD may present as less apathetic and more compulsive than those with FvFTD (65). They may show interpersonal coldness and impairments in emotional processing. Patients with more marked right temporal lobe involvement tend to present with significant changes in personality, such as emotional disturbances, bizarre alterations in dress, and limited, fixed ideas (60). Snowden et al. (48) compared behavioral patterns and functional imaging in patients with FvFTD to those with SD. Whereas lack of emotional responsiveness was pervasive in FvFTD, it was often more selective in SD and particularly affected the capacity to show fear. Apathetic FvFTD patients also had a higher pain threshold, whereas patients with SD had an exaggerated response to pain. Overall, emotional, repetitive, and compulsive behaviors discriminated FvFTD from SD with an accuracy of 97%.

Progressive Nonfluent Aphasia
PNFA is a disorder predominantly of expressive language, in which severe problems in word retrieval occur in the context of preserved word comprehension. This disorder is associated with asymmetric atrophy of the left hemisphere (62). Patients have changes in fluency, pronunciation, and word finding difficulty. They do not present with behavioral problems until later in the disease (65). In a study that assessed discourse in patients with both semantic dementia and PNFA, patients with PNFA had the sparsest output producing narratives and had the fewest words per minute (67).

Pathology of FTD
The typical changes seen in FTD are atrophy of the prefrontal and anterior temporal regions of the neocortex. Routine histology shows microvacuolation of the outer cortical laminae due to large neuronal cell loss, or transcortical gliosis (62). Pathologically, FTD is heterogeneous; some cases may show tau- or ubiquitin-associated TAR DNA-binding protein 43 (TDP-43)-positive inclusions (68), or they may lack distinctive histological features (69). Sensitive methods for detecting tau, ubiquitin, and TDP-43 abnormalities are essential in the neuropathological evaluation of FTD (46,68).

Tau-protein is involved in the regulation of microtubule assembly and disassembly. These tau abnormalities may lead to aggregation or disruption of microtubules, which in turn affects the intraneuronal transport system (70). Tau has been the subject of intense study because it is the major constituent of the neurofibrillary tangles that are a key pathologic finding in AD (71). Ubiquitin inclusions are a common feature in many neurodegenerative diseases. Proteins tagged with ubiquitin are usually destined for digestion by proteasomes (72).

In 2001, an international group of scientists reassessed neuropathological criteria for the diagnosis of FTD. They recommended classifying neurodegenerative disorders associated with FTD into five distinct neuropathological categories, based on presence or absence of tau-positive and ubiquitin-positive inclusions, predominance of microtubule-binding repeats in insoluble tau, and presence of MND-type inclusions. However, they emphasized that only probabilistic statements could be made when examining the causal relationship between neuropathological findings and clinical manifestations of neurodegenerative disorders, as it is unclear exactly how neurodegenerative diseases cause specific clinical syndromes (45).

Kertesz (44) followed 60 patients who met criteria for behavioral variants of FTD to autopsy. They reported that the most common histological variety was MND-type inclusion, followed by corticobasal degeneration, Pick's disease, dementia lacking distinctive histopathology, and progressive supranuclear palsy. They also reported that tau-negative patients had an earlier age of onset. Forman et al. (73) showed that specific clinical features in patients with FTD predict the underlying pathology in 90 patients with a pathological diagnosis of FTD. They reported that taupathies were more frequently associated with an extrapyramidal disorder, whereas patients with ubiquitin-positive inclusions were more likely to present with social and language dysfunction as well as with motor neuron disorder. A growing consensus holds that the clinical presentation of FTD offers clues to underlying histopathology. FTD-MND is associated with TDP-43 protein only, while PNFA is more likely to be related to tau, and SD is most often linked to TDP-43-positive cases. Hippocampal sclerosis is a common pathologic finding in FTD and may be more common in TDP-43-positive cases. The reliability of clinicopathologic correlation varies, however, depending on the clinical presentation.

Genetics of FTD

Most cases of FTD are associated with either tau-positive (MAPT gene chromosome 17) or TDP-43-positive inclusions within neurons and oftentimes glia (associated genes IFT74 mutation on chromosome 9, PGRN mutations on chromosome 17, VCP mutations on chromosome 9, CHMP2B on chromosome 3) (68).

In 1998, mutations in the microtubule-associated protein tau gene (MAPT) on chromosome 17 were found in some familial FTD cases and they were classified as FTDP17 (74–77). For hereditary FTD, more than 50 different tau mutations have now been identified in several families. While the frequency of tau mutations in sporadic FTD is low, in patients with a family history of FTD the frequency of tau mutations ranges from 9.4% to 10.5%.

In the summer of 2006, mutations were found in progranulin (GRN) gene also on chromosome 17 in FTD families that did not have tau mutations (78–80). FTDP17 cases with MAPT mutations all have aggregated tau in neurons or glia while cases with GRN mutations have ubiquitin and aggregated TDP-43. There are also additional cases of FTD without MAPT or GRN mutations that have tau or ubiquitin inclusions.

Degenerative Parkinsonian Syndromes

Degenerative disorders usually have an insidious onset and gradual progression. A positive family history of a similar clinical disorder implicates an autosomal dominant or familial variant of a degenerative disorder. Characterizing the type, timing, and topography of parkinsonian motor signs and associated cognitive, neuropsychiatric, or other clinical manifestations is important for differential diagnosis.

Motor profiles
In Parkinson's disease with dementia (PDD), progressive supranuclear palsy (PSP), and multisystem atrophies (MSA), parkinsonian motor signs typically dominate the initial presentation, with neuropsychiatric and cognitive symptoms often being less prominent in early manifestations. Other conditions, including dementia with Lewy bodies (DLB) and corticobasal degeneration (CBD), have more variable initial presentations with respect to motor, cognitive, and neuropsychiatric features. Motor characteristics of parkinsonian dementia syndromes may be categorized into three general types: typical parkinsonian signs, atypical parkinsonian signs, or parkinsonian plus other motor signs.

Cognitive profiles
Cognitive deficits associated with parkinsonian dementia syndromes generally fall under heading of "subcortical"dementia, as first applied to PSP by Albert in 1974 (81). The syndrome of subcortical dementia primarily reflects aberrant information processing, in contrast to more content-specific deficits in language (aphasia) and perceptual processing (agnosia) associated with the prototypical cortical dementia, Alzheimer's disease (AD).

Cortical and subcortical dementia syndromes are further distinguished by the nature of short-term memory deficits. While impaired delayed spontaneous recall of word-list is characteristic of both cortical and subcortical dementias, providing clues or testing recognition by multiple choice will typically aid recall in a subcortical dementia (retrieval deficit), but not AD (learning deficit). Tests of divided attention (e.g., saying months in reverse order), verbal fluency (e.g., the number of grocery items named in 60 seconds, normal 18 ± 6), and clock-drawing may be useful for detecting attentional, executive, and visuospatial deficits.

Neuropsychiatric profiles
Apathy, reflecting impaired motivation or diminished interest in hobbies or social activities, is a common feature of parkinsonian dementia syndromes. Depression and anxiety are other common manifestations in PDD, affecting about 30% to 40% of such individuals. While florid visual hallucinations, typically of animals and children, are often a prominent clinical manifestation of DLB, psychosis is relatively uncommon in other parkinsonian dementias.

Molecular profiles
Degenerative parkinsonian dementia conditions may be parsed into two broad molecular families: alpha-synucleinopathies (PDD, DLB, MSA) and taupathies (PSP, CBD, some forms of FTD), reflecting an expanded molecular-genetic focus of clinicopathological correlation (82). A systemic approach to classifying multiple pathological features and their clinical correlates is essential to understanding the spectral nature of neurodegenerative conditions. Beyond PDD, and to some extent DLB, which are responsive to neurotransmitter-based therapies, increased knowledge regarding the molecular bases of neurodegenerative parkinsonian

disorders is needed to identify in vivo diagnostic markers and effective disease-specific interventions.

DEMENTIA WITH LEWY BODIES

The dementia with Lewy bodies (DLB) Consortium has revised criteria for the clinical (83) and pathological diagnosis of DLB incorporating new information about the core clinical features and suggesting improved methods to assess them. REM sleep behavior disorder, severe neuroleptic sensitivity, and reduced striatal dopamine transporter activity on functional neuroimaging are given greater diagnostic weighting as features suggestive of a DLB diagnosis. Lewy body disease includes both the syndrome in which Parkinsonism precedes dementia by over a year, the syndrome in which the movement disorder and cognitive disorder occur within a year of one another, or the situation where the cognitive disorder is dominant. DLB is more complex than just a combination of a dementing illness and PD. The disorder of thinking in DLB includes memory impairment. In many DLB patients, it is subtly different from AD in that attention and concentration are somewhat more affected and memory somewhat less intensely affected in DLB compared to AD. These problems can range from mild to severe. The mobility disorder in DLB can be very much like typical PD, but more often than not, walking and balance problems predominate in DLB. Tremor is less common. Slowness of movement and thinking is characteristic of DLB. Patients suffering from DLB have a tendency to fall and lose their balance with some frequency. In some, though, the walking and balance problems may be minimal at the beginning of the disorder. Thus, the absence of prominent motor abnormalities does not rule out DLB (84). Diagnosis is established based on the Third Consensus Criteria for Lewy Body Dementia (85).

Third Consensus Criteria for Lewy Body Dementia

1. Central feature essential for a diagnosis of possible or probable DLB:
   - Dementia defined as progressive cognitive decline of sufficient magnitude to interfere with normal social or occupational function.
   - Prominent or persistent memory impairment may not necessarily occur in the early stages but is usually evident with progression.
   - Deficits on tests of attention, executive function, and visuospatial ability may be especially prominent.
2. Core features (two core features are sufficient for diagnosis of probable DLB, one for possible DLB):
   - Fluctuating cognition with pronounced variations in attention and alertness
   - Recurrent visual hallucinations that are typically well formed and detailed
   - Spontaneous features of Parkinsonism
3. Suggestive features (if one or more of these is present in the presence of one or more core features. A diagnosis of probable DLB should not be made on the basis of the following suggestive features alone):
   - REM sleep behavior disorder
   - Severe neuroleptic sensitivity
   - Low dopamine transporter uptake in basal ganglia demonstrated by SPECT or PET imaging

4. Supportive features (commonly present but not proven to have diagnostic specificity):
   - Repeated falls and syncope
   - Transient, unexplained loss of consciousness
   - Severe autonomic dysfunction, for example, orthostatic hypotension, urinary incontinence
   - Hallucinations in other modalities
   - Systematized delusions
   - Depression
   - Relative preservation of medial temporal lobe structures on CT/MRI scans
   - Generalized low uptake on SPECT/PET perfusion scan with reduced occipital activity
   - Abnormal (low uptake) meta-iodo benzyl guanidine (MIBG) myocardial scintigraphy
   - Prominent slow wave activity on EEG with temporal lobe transient sharp waves
5. A diagnosis of DLB is less likely:
   - In the presence of cerebrovascular disease evident as focal neurologic signs or on brain imaging
   - In the presence of any other physical illness or brain disorder sufficient to account in part or in total for the clinical picture
   - If Parkinsonism only appears for the first time at a stage of severe dementia
6. Temporal sequence of symptoms:
   DLB should be diagnosed when dementia occurs before or concurrently with Parkinsonism (if it is present). The term Parkinson's disease dementia (PDD) should be used to describe dementia that occurs in the context of well-established PD. In a practice setting, the term that is most appropriate to the clinical situation should be used and generic terms such as Lewy body disease (used for PDD or DLB) are often helpful. In research studies in which distinction needs to be made between DLB and PDD, if the existing 1-year rule between the onset of dementia and Parkinsonism is true, then DLB continues to be recommended. Adoption of other time periods will simply confound data pooling or comparison between studies. In other research settings that may include clinico-pathologic studies and clinical trials, both clinical phenotypes may be considered collectively under categories such as LB disease or alpha-synucleinopathy. (*Source*: From Ref. 85).

DLB is a clinical diagnosis. Neuropsychological testing may be helpful in the context of a good clinical history and examination. There are other laboratory tests that are of limited value but they are both optional and modest in the additional information they provide.

Pathology of DLB and PDD

Most neuropathologists now characterize Lewy body pathology by the topography and frequency of Lewy bodies (consisting of the protein alpha-synuclein) and Lewy neuritis using ubiquitin and particularly alpha-synuclein immunocytochemistry. The syndrome of DLB is often associated with limbic or neocortical-predominant Lewy bodies (83,85,86). The same pathology is also present in patients with PDD. Clearly further work in this area is necessary to better understand the pathologic substrate for the dementia syndrome associated with Lewy bodies.

DLB was originally defined as a clinicopathologic entity with a specific constellation of clinical features, and a descriptive approach was proposed for assessing neuropathology. The only neuropathologic requirement for DLB was the presence of Lewy bodies somewhere in the brain of a patient with a clinical history of dementia. Other pathologic features, for example, senile plaques and neuron loss, could occur, but they were not inclusive or exclusive to the diagnosis. In many, but not all, cases the neuropathologic findings conform to those previously described as limbic (Lewy bodies in limbic regions only) or diffuse (Lewy bodies in multiple cortical areas) Lewy body disease. New recommendations are proposed to take into account the extent of both Lewy-related and AD-type pathologies in assessing the degree of certainty that the neuropathologic findings explain the DLB clinical syndrome. The scheme proposed should provide increased diagnostic specificity, since cases in which Lewy bodies are detected in the setting of extensive AD-type pathology that is likely to obscure the clinical features of the DLB syndrome are now classified as having a low likelihood of DLB. Lewy bodies and Lewy neuritis are pathologic aggregations of alpha-synuclein. They are also associated with intermediate filaments, chaperone proteins, and elements of the ubiquitin-proteasome system, which are not specific for Lewy bodies and are also found in conjunction with other neuronal inclusions.

While hematoxylin and eosin histologic staining may be adequate for detection of Lewy bodies in the brainstem, as seen with classic PD, it is not sufficient for detection of cortical Lewy bodies and it is incapable of detecting Lewy neuritis. To avoid confusion, ubiquitin immunohistochemistry, which unequivocally stains Lewy bodies and Lewy neuritis, can only be recommended in cases with minimal concurrent AD-type pathology, since ubiquitin is also present in neurofibrillary tangles that are characteristic of AD pathology. Rather than ubiquitin immunohistochemistry, it is now more appropriate to use immunohistochemical staining for alpha-synuclein since this has been shown to be the most sensitive and specific method currently available for detecting Lewy bodies and Lewy-related pathology.

PROGRESSIVE SUPRANUCLEAR PALSY

PSP (Steele–Richardson–Olszewski syndrome) is distinguished clinically from PD by the absence of a rest tremor, greater axial (neck and trunk) than limb rigidity, more severe speech and swallowing difficulties as a result of the supranuclear palsy, a greater degree of gait and balance impairment, and limitation in voluntary downward gaze (supranuclear gaze palsy). Prevalence estimates of PSP based on community studies are as high as 6.4 per 100,000 and clinicopathological studies often find it misdiagnosed as PD.

Standardized clinical criteria for diagnosing PSP, derived from symptoms in pathologically proven cases, have been proposed. High sensitivity and specificity for these criteria have been demonstrated in an independent clinical sample with autopsy-confirmed diagnosis (87).

National Institute of Neurological Disorders and Stroke clinical criteria for PSP are as follows (88):

– Probable PSP: (a) Gradually progressive disorder; (b) onset at age 40 years or older; (c) vertical (upward or downward) gaze ophthalmoparesis; and (d) marked instability and falls in the first year of symptom onset.
– Possible PSP: (a) and (b) as above and either vertical supranuclear ophthalmo- paresis or slowing of vertical saccades and marked instability with falls within 1 year of symptom onset.

Early postural instability and falls, vertical supranuclear palsy with downgaze paresis, and akinetic-rigid symmetrical Parkinsonism are the most common clinical features. Myoclonus, resting tremor, and pyramidal tract signs are rare. Cognitive symptoms reflecting frontal lobe dysfunction and a subcor- tical dementia typically appear later. Most, but not all, will develop clinically significant dementia. Apathy, dysphoria, and anxiety are common neuropsy- chiatric concomitants of PSP. Pathological laughing and crying (pseudobulbar affect) frequently are present and need to be distinguished from a primary mood disturbance.

Symptomatic pharmacological therapy of PSP has had very limited suc- cess. While occasional, modest, and transient benefits in motor function have been observed with L-dopa and other dopaminergic agonists, adverse effects (i.e., orthostatic hypotension, psychosis) often outweigh the benefits. Similar observa- tions with donepezil have been reported in a placebo-controlled, double-blind study involving 21 patients with PSP, which showed modest improvement in memory test scores that was offset by deterioration in functional mobility (89). Depression, anxiety, and pseudobulbar affect may respond to antidepressants, which are generally well tolerated.

The histopathological hallmark of PSP is globose neurofibrillary tangles, composed of aggregated 4R tau protein, that accumulate in prefrontal cortex and a number of subcortical regions, principally the globus pallidus, substantia nigra, and subthalamic nucleus (90). Tau-reactive tangles also occur in glial cells and reactive gliosis and neuronal loss are variable features. Gross atrophy of the midbrain tegmentum may be evident on MRI imaging, although cortical atrophy is an exclusionary feature, being more characteristic of CBD, among these disorders.

CORTICOBASAL DEGENERATION

The disorder, now commonly referred to as CBD, was initially described by Reibeiz and colleagues in 1968 as "corticodentonigral degeneration with neu- ronal achromasia". CBD is a relatively rare but distinctive parkinsonian demen- tia syndrome characterized by unilateral or asymmetric signs of parkinsonian rigidity, myoclonus, and apraxia, often associated with circumscribed higher cor- tical deficits. Limb dyspraxia occurs in a majority of subjects, and many also will exhibit alien-hand phenomena. During the course of the disease, virtually all patients with CBD will develop unilateral parkinsonian features or a gait dis- order. In a large multicenter case series of 147 patients, dementia occurred in 25% of subjects, although most (93%) exhibited some evidence of higher cortical dysfunction (e.g., cortical sensory loss, agnosia, executive dysfunction) over the disease course (91).

Pharmacological treatment of parkinsonian motor signs in CBD has shown a modest response rate to L-dopa, with about 25% of treated subjects showing some benefit (92). Clonazepam may be useful for treating myoclonus and dystonia in some patients. Limited clinical experience with cholinesterase inhibitor therapy in CBD generally has been unrewarding (93).

The pathological hallmarks of CBD are gliosis and large, achromatic neurons (neuronal achromasia) that are distributed asymmetrically in discrete (frontal or parietal) cortical areas and in subcortical regions affected in PSP. Focal unilateral or asymmetric cortical atrophy may be evident on structural or functional imaging (94). Gross pathological similarities between CBD, PSP, and FTD have been seen, and a specific tau polymorphism has been shown to link PSP and CBD (95).

MULTISYSTEM ATROPHY

Multisystem atrophy (MSA) refers to a degenerative parkinsonian disorder with variable associated features, including autonomic, cerebellar, and pyramidal tract dysfunction. The prevalence of MSA has been estimated to be 4.4 per 100,000, making it slightly less common than PSP (96).

Three clinical variants of MSA were initially recognized as: (*i*) striatonigral degeneration (SND), (*ii*) Shy–Drager syndrome (SDS), and (*iii*) olivopontocere-bellar atrophy (OPCA) (97). All share a common pathological substrate of alpha-synuclein-containing glial cytoplasmic inclusions, which are distributed variably in the cortex, subcortical regions, cerebellum, spinal cord, and dorsal root ganglia. More recently, consensus diagnostic criteria for MSA have suggested two main types based on the predominant clinical feature: (*i*) MSA-Parkinson features and (*ii*) MSA-cerebellar features. Most cases of MSA have some degree of Parkin-sonism and autonomic dysfunction, and about half will have either cerebellar or pyramidal tract dysfunction. Accordingly, previously described cases of SND and SDS are now classified as MSA-Parkinson, and sporadic OPCA conforms to MSA-cerebellar. In MSA-Parkinson, neuronal loss is typically severe in the putamen and substantia nigra compared to PD and is generally distinguished on clinical grounds by the absence of a resting tremor, more severe autonomic dys-function, and evidence of pyramidal tract involvement (e.g., spasticity + Babinski sign) (98). A blunted response of growth hormone release to arginine challenge shows promise in distinguishing MSA-Parkinson from idiopathic PD.

Cognitive functioning in MSA-Parkinson is relatively preserved, although executive deficits characteristically are observed on formal neuropsychological testing. While patients with MSA-Parkinson initially may respond to L-dopa to a limited degree, the duration of benefit is typically short-lived, and treatment in many cases is not well-tolerated. REM sleep behavior disorder is also asso-ciated with MSA just as in PD and DLB, leading to the observation that REM sleep behavior disorder may be a common manifestation of synucleinopathies. Early, severe dysautonomia, including orthostatic hypotension, impotence, uri-nary incontinence, constipation, and hyperhidrosis is also common in MSA. Orthostatic hypotension may be particularly disabling and can be exacerbated by L-dopa and other dopaminergic drugs. Fludrocortisone (Florinef) and midodrine (ProAmitine) often provide a measure of symptomatic relief.

MSA-cerebellar (formally sporadic OPCA) is distinguished primarily by dysarthria and ataxia with marked cerebellopontine atrophy on MRI brain imag-ing. Parkinsonian motor signs and autonomic dysfunction are present to a variable degree. Impaired saccadic eye movements and vertical gaze palsy also may occur. MSA-cerebellar as with MSA-Parkinson has only been described as a sporadic disorder; no familial cases have been reported. This stands in contrast to hereditary forms of OPCA, which are pathologically distinct and form a class of spinocerebellar ataxias-based trinucleotide repeat sequences. Beyond the presence of multiple affected family members in the latter, distinguishing clinical signs of hereditary forms of OPCA include concomitant optic atrophy, retinal degeneration, neuropathic signs, or spastic paraparesis.

VASCULAR DEMENTIA

Vascular dementia is often considered the second or third most common cause of dementia accounting from 10% to 20% of dementia cases, depending on the criteria used for diagnosis. Most cases of vascular dementia can be attributed to multiple cerebral infarcts (strokes), a single strategically located infarction, global hypoxia or anoxia, and hemorrhages. In those with multiple infarctions, the infarctions may be large cortical and/or subcortical infarctions. They may be related to large vessel disease or multiple small infarctions related to small vessel disease.

Demographic risk factors for vascular dementia include advanced age and being of certain ethnic groups (Asians and African-Americans). Men may have an increased risk though studies have not been consistent. Similar to AD, it appears that higher education is a protective factor (99). It would seem reasonable that vascular dementia risk factors would include risk factors for cerebral vascular disease and heart disease. Clinical studies show good evidence that hypertension, smoking, hypercholesterolemia, diabetes are all significant risk factors for vascular dementia (99). The risk of dementia is nine times higher among persons with a history of stroke, especially those with a left hemispheric stoke or a large dominant hemispheric stroke. Also, the odds of becoming demented from infarctions is related to the size and number of infarctions (100,101). Minorities and those with low educational level may also have a higher risk.

Similar to the role of genetics in stroke, the genetic factors associated with vascular dementia are currently not clear. Of note, however, some genetic diseases like CADASIL predispose to stroke and therefore vascular dementia. CADASIL is an autosomal dominant disease due to a notch 3 mutation on chromosome 19. CADASIL results in a deposition of an abnormal substance within blood vessels and causes recurrent subcortical ischemic strokes and hypoperfusion. About half of the patients have a progressive dementia, depression, or psychiatric features. Other symptoms include gait disturbance, incontinence, pseudobulbar palsy, seizures, and hemiplegic migraine. Imaging shows multiple deep infarctions and periventricular white matter lesions. Most patients are symptomatic before the age of 45 and if migraines are present, typically, they begin before the age of 30. Of note, dementia can develop in the absence of discrete vascular events (100).

Vascular dementia caused by multiple subcortical infarctions produces a lot of white matter disease referred to as leukoencephalopathy and older terms including Binswanger's disease and subcortical arteriosclerotic dementia. CADASIL, amyloid angiopathy, and vasculitis conditions can also cause small vessel infarcts. The original term "multi-infarct dementia"has been largely replaced by "vascular dementia"to reflect these varied possibilities. In addition, there is a spectrum of underlying pathologic etiologies (e.g., atherothrombotic disease, lacunar disease, embolic disease, hypoperfusion which results in global hypoxia or global ischemia due to watershed infarcts, hemorrhagic vascular dementia due to trauma, subdural, subarachnoid hemorrhage, intracerebral hemorrhage, or venous occlusions) but the common result is a decrease or cessation of blood flow or oxygen of sufficient duration and/or severity to cause cellular or tissue injury (102,103).

Vascular disease in isolation or perhaps more commonly in association with AD pathology (mixed dementia) is a significant contributor to cognitive impairment of older individuals (101). While multiple lacunar infarction and even strategically located single subcortical infarctions (e.g., thalamic) may certainly cause dementia, the role of "silent infarction," "ischemic white matter changes," and "periventricular white matter changes"(leukoencephalopathy or leukoaraiosis) in the causation of dementia remains controversial and under investigation (104). Many older persons have apparently benign forms such that there is no cognitive impairment; whereas others have more pronounced changes consistent with what used to be termed Binswanger's disease (104). A recent study, however, has shown that white matter hyperintensities and lacunes are independently associated with cognition in older persons living independently. These authors propose that white matter changes should be considered when evaluating cognitive function (105). "Silent"cerebral infarctions located in strategic areas of the brain have also been associated with cognitive impairment. "Silent"infractions tend to be smaller and less often multiple then clinically evident infarctions (101). While the role of these infarcts in dementia has been controversial, a recent study showed that their presence on MRI is associated with accelerated cognitive decline and incident dementia in a population (106). In addition, the total size of infarction and total number of infarctions increase the likelihood of dementia due to stroke (101). The role of these infarctions in mixed dementia and vascular cognitive impairment without dementia continues to be investigated.

Diagnosis and Clinical Features of Vascular Dementia
The most important clinical sign for a diagnosis of vascular dementia is a history or neurologic examination consistent with a focal neurological event confirmed by neuroimaging, which occurred proximate to the onset of cognitive impairment. Of note, the signs of vascular dementia will depend on the location of the ischemia and the presence or absence of concomitant AD.

Subcortical ischemic vascular dementia often involves multiple subcortical injuries and typically involves basal ganglia. Characteristic symptoms often include psychomotor retardation, forgetfulness, and changes in speech and mood (107). Other clinical signs may include urinary incontinence and gait disturbance (normal pressure hydrocephalus should be excluded), rigidity, hypokinesia, and hemimotor dysfunction. Large vessel vascular disease is associated with aphasia, hemianopia, hemimotor or sensory dysfunction, reflex asymmetry, and hemiplegic gait.

Persons with vascular dementia often show a different pattern of cognitive impairment than those with AD. The term "vascular cognitive impairment" has been proposed instead of vascular dementia to emphasize that cognitive impairment in vascular disease may not be characterized by the typical pattern or severity of classic Alzheimer's-type dementia (108). Rather than the well-known episodic memory loss as seen in AD, those with vascular dementia tend to have prominent frontal/executive dysfunction and usually have less language impairment than is seen in AD (104). Since the MMSE does not test executive function well, it may therefore not be the best screening test for the diagnosis of vascular dementia (107).

Vascular dementia is often associated with a step-wise progression with sudden episodes of abrupt decline and then stabilization until the next stroke-like episode. However, many with vascular cognitive impairment may have a more gradual and progressive course that mimics other degenerative diseases like AD. In addition, because mixed vascular dementia is often combined with AD, signs and symptoms may overlap and the clinical diagnosis may prove to be difficult (109). Confusional states can be seen after stroke in about 25% of individuals and may represent preexisting cognitive decline or complications from the stroke (infectious, metabolic, and epileptogenic).

Diagnosis of vascular dementia is typically based on cognitive loss, a history of stroke or clinical signs of stroke documented by imaging, and a temporal link between the event and the dementia (103,107). The patient may or may not improve after the event and though a stepwise progression may be noted. This is not a necessary diagnostic criterion for diagnosis. The Hachinski Ischemic Scale (Table 1) has been used extensively for the diagnosis of vascular dementia, and while it has a fairly high sensitivity and specificity, it is relatively insensitive to mixed disease and does not take into account neuroimaging. If this scale is used, the most important components of the scale include stepwise deterioration, fluctuating course, history of hypertension, history of stroke, and the presence of focal neurologic impairment. The higher the score, the more likely the dementia has a vascular component (101).

Evaluation for Vascular Dementia

MRI and or CT scanning are important in the diagnostic work-up for possible vascular dementia. When stroke is a suspected etiology for dementia, MRI may be preferable to CT since MRI shows more details over CT, especially in subcortical regions. If the scan shows only cortical atrophy, the diagnosis of vascular dementia is unlikely. On the other hand, multiple infarctions generally support the diagnosis. The clinical relevance of the frequent MRI findings of periventricular white matter abnormalities and subcortical white matter hyperintensities in individual patients is unclear and remains under research investigation.

Table 1 Hachinski Ischemic Scale[a]

Abrupt onset of neurological symptoms	2
Stepwise deterioration	1
Fluctuating course of symptoms	2
Nocturnal confusion	1
Relative preservation of personality	1
Depression	1
Prominent somatic complaints	1
Emotional incontinence (pseudobulbar palsy)	1
History of hypertension	1
History of stroke	2
Evidence of associated atherosclerosis	1
History of focal neurological symptoms	2
Evidence of focal neurological signs	2

[a]7 or more points suggest vascular dementia and 4 or fewer points suggest degenerative dementia.
Source: From Ref. 110.

In addition to the MRI, persons with vascular cognitive impairment or dementia should be worked up as a person with any other form of cerebrovascular disease, that is, sources of emboli should be excluded, including the use of carotid ultrasound for occlusive disease or source of emboli and echocardiogram for cardiac source of emboli. The person should also be evaluated for arrhythmias.

If a person with vascular dementia is without risk factors for vascular disease or is young, other etiologies should be sought, for example, fibromuscular dysplasia, protein C or S deficiency, antiphospholipid syndromes, primary disorders of blood vessels, CADASIL, and vasculitis. In the older age group in addition to the traditional etiologies for stroke, clinicians should be vigilant for symptoms or temporal arteritis (e.g., headache, fatigue, visual loss) and consider ordering a sedimentation rate and a temporal artery biopsy if clinically indicated.

Treatment of Vascular Dementia

Treatment of vascular dementia alone or in combination with AD (e.g., mixed dementia) focuses on the prevention of further vascular events as well as trying to improve current symptomatology. If the diagnosis suggests small vessel disease, hypertension and diabetes should be controlled. Controlling other risk factors for vascular disease such as cessation of smoking, improving weight control, and managing cholesterol levels is also likely to be beneficial. Antiplatelet therapy, if there are no contraindications, is indicated for prevention of recurrent stroke. Anticoagulation may be indicated if there is evidence of a source of emboli.

In addition to preventative measures, treatments for AD (e.g., cholinesterase inhibitors) have been tested on vascular dementia subjects. Thus far, clinical trials have shown that cholinesterase inhibitors are beneficial in persons with vascular dementia as well as in those with mixed dementias (AD plus vascular dementia).

Management and treatment of behavior and other psychosocial issues (see also chap. 4) may be treated accordingly to models created for AD (105).

OTHER CAUSES OF DEMENTIA

Prion disorders such as Creutzfeldt–Jacob disease (CJD) are rare conditions (about 1 per million population) that produce dementia. CJD is a rapidly progressive disorder associated with dementia, focal cortical signs, rigidity, and myoclonus, causing death usually in less than 1 year from the first symptoms. The rapidity of progression seen with CJD is uncommon in AD so that distinction between the two disorders is not difficult. However, CBD and DLB, more rapid degenerative dementias with prominent abnormalities in movement, are more likely to be mistaken for CJD. The differential diagnosis for CJD also usually includes other rapidly progressive dementing conditions such as viral or bacterial encephalitides, Hashimoto's encephalitis, CNS vasculitis, lymphoma, or paraneoplastic syndromes. The markedly abnormal periodic EEG discharges and cortical and basal ganglia abnormalities on diffusion-weighted MRI are unique diagnostic features of CJD. Transmission from infected cattle to the human population in the United Kingdom has caused a small epidemic of variant CJD in young adults.

Normal pressure hydrocephalus (NPH) is a relatively uncommon syndrome. Historically, many of the individuals who have been treated for NPH have suffered from other dementias, particularly AD, multi-infarct dementia, or DLB. For NPH the clinical triad includes an abnormal gait (ataxic or apraxic), dementia (usually mild to moderate), and urinary incontinence. Neuroimaging studies reveal enlarged lateral ventricles (hydrocephalus) with little or no cortical atrophy. This syndrome is a communicating hydrocephalus with a patent aqueduct of Sylvius in contrast to congenital aqueduct stenosis, where the aqueduct is small. In many cases, periventricular edema is present. Lumbar puncture opening pressure is in the high normal range, and the cerebrospinal fluid (CSF) protein, sugar concentrations, and cell count is normal. NPH is presumed to be caused by obstruction to normal flow of CSF over the cerebral convexity and delayed absorption into the venous system. The indolent nature of the process results in enlarged lateral ventricles but relatively little increase in CSF pressure. There is presumed stretching and distortion of white matter tracts in the corona radiata, but the exact physiologic cause of the clinical syndrome is unclear. Some patients have a history of conditions producing scarring of the basilar meninges (blocking upward flow of CSF) such as previous meningitis, subarachnoid hemorrhage, or head trauma. Others with longstanding but asymptomatic congenital hydrocephalus may have adult-onset deterioration in gait or memory that is confused with NPH. In contrast to AD, the NPH patient has an early and prominent gait disturbance and no evidence of cortical atrophy on CT or MRI. A number of attempts have been made to use various special studies to improve the diagnosis of NPH and predict the success of ventricular shunting. These include radionuclide cisternography (showing a delay in CSF absorption over the convexity) and various attempts to monitor and alter CSF flow dynamics, including a constant-pressure infusion test. None has proven to be specific or consistently useful. There is sometimes a transient improvement in gait or cognition following lumbar puncture (or serial punctures) with removal of 30 to 50 mL of CSF, but this finding also has not proven to be consistently predictive of post-shunt improvement. AD often masquerades as NPH, because the gait may be abnormal in AD and cortical atrophy sometimes is difficult to determine by CT or MRI early in the disease. Hippocampal atrophy on MRI is a clue favoring AD. Approximately 30% to 50% of patients identified by careful diagnosis as having NPH will show improvement with a ventricular shunting procedure. Gait may improve more than memory. Transient, short-lasting improvement is common. Patients should be carefully selected for this operation, because subdural hematoma and infection are known complications.

Dementia can accompany chronic alcoholism. This may be a result of associated malnutrition, especially of B vitamins and particularly thiamine. However, other poorly defined aspects of chronic alcohol ingestion may also produce cerebral damage. A rare idiopathic syndrome of dementia and seizures with degeneration of the corpus callosum has been reported primarily in male Italian drinkers of red wine (Marchiafava–Bignami disease). Thiamine (vitamin B_1) deficiency causes Wernicke's encephalopathy. The clinical presentation is a malnourished individual (frequently but not necessarily alcoholic) with confusion, ataxia, and diplopia from ophthalmoplegia. Thiamine deficiency damages the thalamus, mamillary bodies, midline cerebellum, periaqueductal grey matter of the midbrain, and peripheral nerves. Damage to the dorsomedial thalamic region correlates most closely with the memory loss. Prompt administration of parenteral thiamine (100 mg intravenously for 3 days followed by daily oral dosage) may reverse the disease if given in the first days of symptom onset. However, prolonged untreated thiamine deficiency can result in an irreversible dementia/amnestic syndrome (Korsakoff's psychosis) or even death. In Korsakoff's syndrome, the patient is unable to recall new information despite normal immediate memory, attention span, and level of consciousness. Memory for new events is seriously impaired, whereas memory of knowledge prior to the illness is relatively intact. Patients are easily confused, disoriented, and incapable of recalling new information for more than a brief interval. Superficially, they may be conversant, entertaining, and able to perform simple tasks and follow immediate commands. Confabulation is common, although not always present, and may result in obviously erroneous statements and elaborations. There is no specific treatment because the previous thiamine deficiency has produced irreversible damage to the medial thalamic nuclei and mamillary bodies. Mamillary body atrophy may be visible on high-resolution MRI.

Vitamin B_{12} deficiency, as can occur in pernicious anemia, causes a macrocytic anemia and may also damage the nervous system. Neurologically, it most commonly produces a spinal cord syndrome (myelopathy) affecting the posterior columns (loss of position and vibratory sense) and corticospinal tracts (hyperactive tendon reflexes with Babinski responses). It also damages peripheral nerves, resulting in sensory loss with depressed tendon reflexes. Damage to cerebral myelinated fibers may also cause a dementia syndrome. The mechanism of neurologic damage is unclear but may be related to a deficiency of S-Adenosylmethionine (required for methylation of myelin phospholipids) due to reduced methionine synthase activity or accumulation of methylmalonate, homocysteine, and propionate, providing abnormal substrates for fatty acids synthesis and myelin. The neurologic signs of vitamin B_{12} deficiency are usually associated with macrocytic anemia but on occasion may occur in its absence. Treatment with parenteral vitamin B_{12} (1000 µg intramuscularly daily for a week, weekly for a month, and monthly for life for pernicious anemia) stops progression of the disease if instituted promptly, but reversal of advanced nervous system damage will not occur (43).

DEMENTIA OF DEPRESSION

Not all clinical researchers are in agreement about the term depression when applied to older patients with a mood disturbance. There is likely to be an agreement when one takes a syndromal approach to depression, calling on the *Diagnostic and Statistical Manual of Mental Disorders,* Fourth Edition (111) to identify symptom clusters such as those seen with major depression.

Clinical presentations of depression in old age have considerable variability, suggesting the need for a broad approach to assessment of co-occurring depression and cognitive impairment. There is a range of depressive symptoms and associated behavioral manifestations that occur in the context of cognitive impairment. In the early stages of impairment, the most commonly seen symptoms include irritability, impatience, apathy, hopelessness, changes in temperament, and thoughts about death. Other areas that should be assessed might include changes in personality, appetite changes, sleep apnea and sleep disturbances, as well as childhood traumatic events, depression history, and background characteristics that could predict cognitive impairment.

Dementia of depression is characterized by variable onset, often abrupt, and is reversible with treatment. Duration varies between weeks to several months to years. Sensorium remains clear. Attention span can be normal but they are easily distracted. Selective memory impairment can be identified. Problem solving and thinking are usually unimpaired but patients often express hopelessness and helplessness. The dementia of depression often coincides with major life changes (112).

In contrast to the theory that depression represents a prodrome to dementia, there is a growing evidence that depression may represent an independent risk factor predisposing to dementing disorders even when depressive symptoms occur more than 10 years before the onset of dementia. Depression is also a risk factor for vascular dementia (113–115).

REFERENCES

1. Petersen RC, Smith GE, Waring SC, et al. Mild cognitive impairment: Clinical characterization and outcome. Arch Neurol 1999; 56:303–308.
2. Petersen RC. Mild cognitive impairment or questionable dementia. Arch Neurol 2000; 57:643–644.
3. Petersen RC, Doody R, Kurz A, et al. Current concepts in mild cognitive impairment. Arch Neurol 2001; 58:1985–1992.
4. Petersen RC. Conceptual overview. In: Petersen RC, ed. Mild Cognitive Impairment: Aging to Alzheimer's Disease. New York, NY: Oxford University Press Inc, 2003: 1–14.
5. Lopez OL, Jagust WJ, DeKosky ST, et al. Prevalence and classification of mild cognitive impairment in the Cardiovascular Health Study Cognition Study: Part 1. Arch Neurol 2003; 60:1385–1389.
6. Vinters HV. Neuropathology of amnestic mild cognitive impairment. Arch Neurol 2006; 63:645–646.
7. Jicha GA, Parisi JE, Dickson DW, et al. Neuropathologic outcome of mild cognitive impairment following progression to clinical dementia. Arch Neurol 2006; 63:647–681.
8. Petersen RC, Parisi JE, Joseph E, et al. Neuropathologic features of amnestic mild cognitive impairment. Arch Neurol 2006; 63:665–672.
9. Jack CR Jr, Petersen RC, Xu YC, et al. Prediction of AD with MRI-based hippocampal volume in mild cognitive impairment. Neurology 1999; 52:1397–1403.
10. Petersen RC, Stevens JC, Ganguli M, et al. Practice parameter: Early detection of dementia: Mild cognitive impairment (an evidence based review). Report of the Quality Standards Subcommittee of the American Academy of Neurology. Neurology 2001; 56:1133–1142.
11. Scharre DW, Change S-I, Murden RA, et al. Self-Administered Gerocognitive Examination (SAGE): A brief cognitive assessment instrument for Mild Cognitive Impairment (MCI) and early dementia. Alzheimer Dis Assoc Disord 2010; 24:64–71.
12. Katzman R, Brown T, Fuld P, et al. Valiation of a short orientation-memory-concentration test of cognitive impairment. Am J Psychiatry 1983; 140:734–739.
13. Bick KL. The early story of Alzheimer's disease. In: Terry RD, Katzman R, Bick KL, eds. Alzheimer's Disease. New York: Raven Press, 1994:1.
14. Newton RD. The identity of Alzheimer's disease and senile dementia and their relationship in senility. J Ment Sci 1948; 94:225.
15. Neumann MA, Cohn R. Incidence of Alzheimer's disease in a large mental hospital: Relation to senile psychosis and psychosis with cerebral arteriosclerosis. Arch Neurol Psychiatry 1953: 69:615.
16. Morris JC. Alzheimer's disease: Unique, Differentiable, and Treatable. Presented at the 52nd Annual Meeting of the American Academy of Neurology, San Diego, California, April 29–May 6, 2000.
17. U.S. Census Bureau. www.census.gov/population/statbrief/gebnet.htm. Accessed 10/8/10.
18. Thies W. The Human and Societal Costs of Alzheimer's Disease. http://www.ama-assn.org/ama/pub/article/12202–8331.html. Accessed 03/2004.
19. Kiloh LG. Pseudodementia. Acta Psychiatr Scand 1961; 37:336.
20. Folstein MF, McHugh PR, Dementia syndrome of depression. In: Katzman R, Terry RD, Bick KL, eds. Alzheimer's Disease. New York: Raven Press, 1978:87.

21. American Psychiatric Association Task Force on Nomenclature and Statistics, ed. Diagnostic and Statistical Manual of Mental Disorders (DSM-III). 3rd ed. Washington, DC: American Psychiatric Association, 1980.
22. McKhann G, Drachman D, Folstein M, et al. Clinical diagnosis of Alzheimer's disease: Report of the NINCDS-ADRDA Work Groups under the auspices of Department of Health and Human Services Task Force on Alzheimer's Disease. Neurology 1984; 34:939–944.
23. Doody RS. Dementia. In: Loren Rolak ed. Neurology Secrets. 5th ed. Philadelphia, PA: Elsevier Mosby, 2010:235.
24. Daniel ES. Alzheimer's disease. In: Rakel RE, Bope ET, eds. Conn's Current Therapy. Philadelphia, PA: W.B Saunders Co., 2004:891–898.
25. Daly MP. Diagnosis and management of Alzheimer's disease. J Am Board Fam Pract 1999; 12(5):375–384
26. Agency for Health Care Policy and Research. Recognition and Initial Assessment of Alzheimer's Disease and Related Dementias. No 97-R123. Rockville, MD: U.S. Department of Health and Human Services, 1996.
27. Guttman R, Altmann RD, Nielsen NH. Alzheimer's disease. Arch Neurol 1999; 8:347–353.
28. Grudman M, Petersen RC, Ferris SH, et al. Mild cognitive impairment can be distinguished from Alzheimer's disease and normal aging for clinical trials. Arch Neurol 2004; 61:59–66.
29. American Academy of Neurology. http://www.neurology.org/cgi/content/full/56/9/1143.
30. Alzheimer's Disease Education and Referral Center (ADEAR). Progress Report on Alzheimer's Disease. Research Advances at NIH. National Institute on Aging. U.S. Department of Health and Human Services, 2003. http://www.nia.nih.gov/alzheimers. ADEAR Center, Silver Spring, MD 20907-8250.
31. Bonte FJ, Harris TS, Roney CA, et al. Differential diagnosis between Alzheimer's and frontotemporal disease by the posterior cingulate sign. J Nucl Med 2004; 45(5):771–774.
32. Scarmeas N, Zarahn E, Anderson KE, et al. Cognitive reserve-mediated modulation of positron emission tomographic activations during memory tasks in Alzheimer disease. Arch Neurol 2004; 61:73–78.
33. Abstract in 9th International Conference on Alzheimer's Disease and Related Disorders, Philadelphia, Pennsylvania in July 2004. Lancet Neurology 2004; 3(9):510 (ICAD) PMID 15344278.
34. Folstein M, Anthony JC, Parhad I, et al. The meaning of cognitive impairment in the elderly. J Am Geriatr Soc 1985; 33:228–335.
35. Blessed G, Tomlinson BE, Roth M. The association between quantitative measures of dementia and of senile change in the cerebral gray matter of elderly subjects. Br J Psychiatry 1968; 114:797–811
36. Pfeiffer E. A Short Portable Mental Status Questionnaire for the assessment of organic brain deficit in elderly patients. J Am Geriatr Soc 1975; 23:433–441.
37. Morris JC, Heyman A, Mohs RC, et al. and the CERAD investigators. The Consortium to Establish a Registry for Alzheimer's Disease (CERAD). Part I. Clinical and neuropsychological assessment of Alzheimer's disease. Neurology 1989; 39:1159–1165.
38. Rosen WG, Mohs RC, Davis KL. A new rating scale for Alzheimer's disease. Am J Psychiatry 1984; 141:1356–1364.
39. Coblentz JM, Mattis S, Zingesser LH, et al. Presenile dementia: Clinical aspects and evaluation of cerebrospinal fluid dynamics. Arch Neurol 1973; 29:299–308
40. Erzigkeit H. The SKT-a short cognitive performance test as an instrument for the assessment of clinical efficacy of cognitive enhancers. In: Bergener W, Riesberg B, eds. Diagnosis and Treatment of Senile Dementia, Springer-Verlag: Heidelberg, 1989: 164.
41. Mohs RC. The use of tests and instruments in the evaluation of patients with dementia. In: Khachaturian ZS, Radebaugh TS, eds. Alzheimer's Disease Cause(s), Diagnosis, Treatment and Care. Boca Raton, FL: CRC Press, 1996:97.

42. Terry R, Masliah E, Salmon DP, et al. Physical basis of cognitive alterations in Alzheimer's disease: Synapse loss is the major correlate of cognitive impairment. Ann Neurol 1991; 30:572–580.
43. Bird TD, Miller BL. Dementia. In: Harrison's online, 17th edition, chapter 365, part sixteen, section 2: Diseases of the Central Nervous System.
44. Kertesz A. Frontotemporal dementia: One disease, or many? Probably one, possibly two. Alzheimer Dis Assoc Disord 2005; 19:S19–S24.
45. McKhann GM, Albert MS, Grossman M, et al. Clinical and pathological diagnosis of frontotemporal dementia: Report of the Work Group on Frontotemporal Dementia and Pick's Disease. Arch Neurol 2001; 58:1803–1809.
46. Ratnavalli E, Brayne C, Dawson K, et al. The prevalence of frontotemporal dementia. Neurology 2002; 58:1615–1621.
47. Rosso SM, Donker Kaat L, Baks T, et al. Frontotemporal dementia in the Netherlands, patient characteristics and prevalence, estimates from a population-based study. Brain 2003; 126:2016–2022.
48. Snowden JS, Bathgate D, Varma B, et al. Distinct behavioral profiles in frontotemporal dementia and semantic dementia. J Neurol Neurosurg Psychiatry 2001; 70:323–332.
49. Knopman DS, Petersen RC, Edland SD, et al. The incidence of frontotemporal lobar degeneration in Rochester, Minnesota, 1990 through 1994. Neurology 2004; 62:506–508.
50. Warren JD, Schott JM, Fox N. Brain biopsy in dementia. Brain 2005; 128:2016–2025.
51. Piguet O, Brooks WS, Halliday GM, et al. Similar early clinical presentations in familial and non-familial frontotemporal dementia. J Neurol Neurosurg Psychiatry 2004; 75:1743–1745.
52. Hodges JR, Davies R, Xuereb J, et al. Survival in frontotemporal dementia. Neurology 2003; 61:349–354.
53. Roberson ED, Hesse JH, Rose KD, et al. Frontotemporal dementia progresses to death faster than Alzheimer disease. Neurology 2005; 65:719–725.
54. Folstein MF, Folstein SE, McHugh PR. Mini-Mental State: A practical method for grading the cognitive state of patients for the clinician. J Psychiatr Res 1975; 12:189.
55. Hodges JR. Frontotemporal dementia (Pick's disease): Clinical features and assessment. Neurology 2001; 56:S6–S10.
56. Consensus Statement. Clinical and neuropathological criteria for frontotemporal dementia. The Lund and Manchester Groups. J Neurol Neurosurg Psychiatry 1994; 57:416–418.
57. Neary D, Snowde JS, Gustafson L, et al. Frontotemporal lobar degeneration: A consensus on clinical diagnostic criteria. Neurology 1998; 51:1546–1554.
58. Talbot PR, Snowden JS, Lloyd JJ, et al. The contribution of single photon emission tomography to the clinical differentiation of degenerative cortical brain disorders. J Neurol 1995; 242:579–586.
59. Pasquier F, Fukui T, Sarazin M, et al. Laboratory investigations and treatment in frontotemporal dementia. Ann Neurol 2003; 54:S32–S35.
60. McMurtray AM, Chen AK, Shapira JS, et al. Variations in regional SPECT hypoperfusion and clinical features in frontotemporal dementia. Neurology 2006; 66:517–522.
61. Lebert F, Stekke W, Hasenbroekx C, et al. Frontotemporal dementia: A randomised, controlled trial with trazodone. Dement Geriatr Cogn Disord 2002; 17:355–359.
62. Neary D, Snowden J, Mann D. Frontotemporal dementia. Lancet Neurol 2005; 4:771–780.
63. Mendez MF, Shapira JS. Loss of insight and functional neuroimaging in frontotemporal dementia. J Neuropsychiatry Clin Neurosci 2005; 17:413–416.
64. Mendez M. What frontotemporal dementia reveals about the neurobiological basis of morality. Med Hypotheses 2006; 67:411–418.
65. Boxer AL, Miller BL. Clinical features of frontotemporal dementia. Alzheimer Dis Assoc Disord 2005; 19:S3–S6.
66. Knibb JA, Hodges. Semantic dementia and primary progressive aphasia. A problem of categorization? Alzheimer Dis Assoc Disord 2005; 19:S7–S14.
67. Ash S, Moore P, Antani S, et al. Trying to tell a tale: Discourse impairments in progressive aphasia and frontotemporal dementia. Neurology 2006; 66:1405–1413.

68. Yener GG, Rosen HJ, Papatriantafyllou J. Frontotemporal degeneration. Continuum Lifelong Learning Neurol 2010; 16(2):191–211.
69. Mariani C, Defendi S, Mailland E, et al. Frontotemporal dementia. Neurol Sci 2006; 27:S35–S36.
70. Sjogren M, Andersen C. Frontotemporal dementia—A brief review. Mech Ageing Dev 2006; 127:180–187.
71. Kosik KS, Joachim CL, Selkoe DJ. Microtubule-associated protein tau (tau) is a major antigenic component of paired helical filaments in Alzheimer's disease. Proc Natl Acad Sci USA 1986; 83:4044–4048.
72. Wilhemsen KC. Genetics of non-Alzheimer dementias. AAN Syllabus 2008.
73. Forman MS, Farmer J, Johnson JK, et al. Frontotemporal dementia: Clinicopathological correlations. Ann Neurol 2006; 59:952–962.
74. Poorkaj P, Bird T, Wijsman E, et al. Tau is a candidate gene for chromosome 17 frontotemporal dementia. Ann Neurol 1998; 43:815–825.
75. Hutton M, Dendon CL, Rizzu P, et al. Association of missense and 5′-splicec-site mutations in tau with the inherited dementia FTDP-17. Nature 1998; 393:702–705.
76. Goedert M, Crowther A, Spillantini MD. Tau mutations cause frontotemporal dementias. Neuron 1998; 21:955–958.
77. Clark LN, Poorkaj P, Wszolek ZK, et al. Pathogenic implications of mutations in the tau gene in pallido-ponto-nigral degeneration and related chromosome 17-liked neurodegenerative disorders. Proc Natl Acad Sci U S A 1998; 95:13103–13107.
78. Cruts M, Gijselinck I, van der Zee J, et al. Null mutations in progranulin cause ubiquitin-positive frontotemporal dementia linked to chromosome 17q21. Nature 2006; 442:920–924.
79. Baker M, Mackenzie IR, Pickering-Brown SM, et al. Mutations in Progranulin cause tau-negative frontotemporal dementia linked to chromosome 17. Nature 2006; 442:916–919.
80. Gass J, Cannon A, Mackenzie IR, et al. Mutations in progranulin are a major cause of ubiquitin-positive frontotemporal lobar degeneration. Hum Mol Genet 2006; 15:2988–3001.
81. Albert ML, Feldman RG, Willis AL. The subcortical dementia of progressive supranuclear palsy. J Neurol Neurosurg Psychiatry 1974; 37:121–130.
82. Kaufer DI, Dekosky ST. Diagnostic classification: Relationship to the neurobiology of dementia. In: Charney DS, Nestor E, Bunney BS, eds. Neurobiology of Mental Illness. New York: Oxford University Press, 1999:641–649.
83. McKeith IG, Galasko D, Kosaka K, et al. Consensus guidelines for the clinical and pathologic diagnosis of dementia with Lewy bodies (DLB): Report of the consortium on DLB international workshop. Neurology 1996; 47:1113–1124.
84. Knopman D. Diagnostic issues for frontotemporal lobar degenerations, vascular dementia, Lewy body dementia and normal pressure hydrocephalus. AAN Syllabus 2007.
85. McKeith G, Dickson DW, Lowe J, et al. for the Consortium on DLB. Diagnosis and management of dementia with Lewy bodies: Third report of the DLB consortium. Neurology 2005; 65:1863–1872.
86. McKeith I, O'Brien J. Dementia with Lewy bodies. Aust N Z J Psychiatry 1999; 33:800–808.
87. Lopez OL, Litvan I, Catt KE, et al. Accuracy of four clinical diagnostic criteria for the diagnosis of neurodegenerative dementias. Neurology 1999; 53:1292–1299.
88. Hauw JJ, Daniel SE, Dickson D, et al. Preliminary NINDS neuropathological criteria for Steele-Richardson-Olzewski syndrome (progressive supranuclear palsy). Neurology 1994; 44:2015–2019.
89. Litvan I, Phipps M, Pharr VL, et al. Randomized placebo-controlled trial of donepezil in patients with progressive supranuclear palsy. Neurology 2001; 57:467–473.
90. Sergeant N, Wattez A, Delacourte A. A neurofibrillary degeneration in progressive supranuclear palsy and corticobasal degeneration: Tau pathologies with exclusively "exon 10" isoforms. J Neurochem 1999; 72:1243–1249.
91. Kompoliti K, Goetz CG, Boeve BF, et al. Clinical presentation and pharmacological therapy in corticobasal degeneration. Arch Neurol 1998; 55:957–961.

92. Kompoliti K, Goetz CG, Litvan I, et al. Pharmacological therapy in progressive supranuclear palsy. Arch Neurol 1998; 55:1099–1052.
93. Kaufer DI. Parkinsonian Dementias. Lecture and chapter in the syllabus of the 60th Annual Meeting of the American Academy of Neurology, April 12–19, 2008, Chicago, IL. www.abstracts2view.com/aan2008chicago.
94. Boxer AL, Geschwind MD, Belfor N, et al. Patterns of brain atrophy that differentiate corticobasal degeneration syndrome from progressive supranuclear palsy. Arch Neurol 2006; 63:81–86.
95. Houlden H, Baker M, Morris HR, et al. Corticobasal degeneration and progressive supranuclear palsy share a common tau haplotype. Neurology 2001; 56:1701–1706.
96. Schrag A, Ben-Shlomo Y, Quinn NP. Prevalence of progressive supranuclear palsy and multisystem atrophy: A cross-sectional study. Lancet 1999; 354:1771–1775.
97. Wenning GK, Ben-Schlomo Y, Magalhaes M, et al. Clinical features and natural history of multiple system atrophy in 100 cases. Brain 1994; 117:835–845.
98. Gilman S, Low PA, Quinn N, et al. Consensus statement of the diagnosis of multiple system atrophy. J Neurol Sci 1999; 163:94–98.
99. Gorelick PB. Status of risk factors for dementia associated with stroke. Stroke 1997; 28:459–463.
100. Adams HP, Hachinski V, Norris J. Ischemic Cerebrovascular disease. In: Gilman S, series ed. Contemporary Neurology Series. New York: Oxford University Press, 2001:29.
101. Schneider JA, Wilson RS, Cochran EJ, et al. Relation of cerebral infarctions to dementia and cognitive function in older persons. Neurology 2003; 60:1082–1089.
102. Schneider JA. Two common non Alzheimer's dementias. Vascular dementia and dementia with Lewy bodies. Lecture and chapter in the syllabus of the 60th Annual Meeting of the American Academy of Neurology, April 12–19, 2008, Chicago, IL. www.abstracts2view.com/aan2008chicago.
103. Chui H, Mack W, Jackson, et al. Clinical criteria for the diagnosis of vascular dementia: A multicenter study of comparability and interrater reliability. Arch Neurol 2000; 57:191–196
104. Nyenhius DL, Gorelick PB. Vascular dementia: A contemporary review of epidemiology, diagnosis, prevention and treatment. J Am Geriatr Soc 1998; 46:1437–1448.
105. van der Flier WM, van Straatan EC, Barkhof F, et al. Small vessel disease and general cognitive function in nondisabled elderly. The LADIS Study. Stroke 2005; 36:2116–2120.
106. Vermeer SE, Prins ND, den Heijer T, et al. Silent brain infarcts and the risk of dementia and cognitive decline. N Engl J Med 2003; 348:1215–1222.
107. Roman GC, Erkinjuntti T, Wallin A, et al. Subcortical ischemic vascular dementia. Lancet Neurol 2002; 1:426–436.
108. Looi JCL, Sachdev PS. Differentiation of vascular dementia from AD on neuropsychological tests. Neurology 1999; 53:670–678.
109. Adams and Victor's Principles of Neurology, 8th ed. New York: McGraw-Hill, 2005.
110. Hachinski VC. Stroke and vascular cognitive impairment. Stroke 2006; 37:2220–2241.
111. American Psychiatric Association Task Force on Nomenclature and Statistics, ed. Diagnostic and Statistical Manual of Mental Disorders (DSM-IV). 4th ed. American Psychiatric Association, 2000.
112. Foreman MD, Fletcher K, Mion LC, et al. Assessing cognitive function. Geriatr Nurs 1996; 17:228–232.
113. Butters MA, Becker JT, Nebes RD, et al. Changes in cognitive functioning following treatment of late-life depression. Am J Psychiatry 2000; 157:1949–1954.
114. Speck CE, Kukull WA, Brenner DE, et al. History of depression as a risk factor for Alzheimer's disease. Epidemiology 1995; 6:366–369.
115. Jorm AF, van Duijn CM, Chandra V, et al. EURODEM Risk Factors Research Group. Psychiatric history and related exposures as risk factors for Alzheimer's disease: A collaborative re-analysis of case-control studies. Int J Epidemiol 1991; 20 (suppl 2):S58–S61.

Pharmacotherapy of cognition

David S. Geldmacher

INTRODUCTION

Pharmacotherapy has been available to address the progressive cognitive decline of Alzheimer's disease since the mid-1990s. Despite meeting regulatory criteria for approval, the utility of these therapies has been controversial, and they remain undervalued by many prescribers (1). In approaching therapy for cognition in Alzheimer's disease (AD), it is important to recognize that improvement in current symptoms is not the only model for successful treatment. A therapy that reduces or delays progression, even if it does not lead to clinically evident improvement, can be a meaningful benefit to patients (1,2). The idea of "benefit" without symptomatic "improvement" will continue to be important as new drug treatments enter the field. Many of the potential treatments under development are hypothesized to reduce neuronal death and slow disease progression rather than provide short-term symptomatic improvements.

Conceptually, symptomatic therapy maximizes neuronal function without affecting the rate of neuronal loss. There are several ways of viewing a symptomatic benefit in a progressive disease like AD: (*i*) patients might be expected to think and function better on treatment than they would without drug, even if they decline to be worse than when treatment began; (*ii*) patients have a reduced risk for reaching a certain amount of decline in a defined period of time; or (*iii*) patients have a increase in the time required to decline a set amount. Discontinuation of an effective symptomatic should result in rapid losses in ability, with the patient returning to the functional level where they would have been had they never been treated. This theoretically predicted effect has been observed with the cholinesterase inhibitor drugs in AD, but not with agents hypothesized to exert a more disease-modifying role (3).

ASSESSING THERAPEUTIC OUTCOME

A major challenge in AD therapeutics is assessing the outcome of treatment. In hypertension and diabetes mellitus, clinicians determine the effectiveness of therapy by using objective numbers that reflect the underlying pathophysiologic processes. Because there are no biological intermediaries for AD that can be routinely measured in clinical settings, assessments of treatment response in AD are typically dependent on subjective information. Even "objective" measures of cognition, like the Mini-Mental State Examination (MMSE) (4), are only surrogates for the underlying pathophysiology. These instruments are not ideal for capturing either important aspects of the cognitive deficits in AD (like executive function) or quasi-cognitive improvements that may result from medication (like improved initiation of activities). Furthermore, they are dependent on the patient's understanding of the test's demands, motivation to cooperate with testing, and ability to organize voluntary responses. The AD patient's reduced insight and memory also limit a clinician's ability to assess the impact of treatment by reviewing the course of events with the patient. Vital outcome information must therefore be obtained from surrogates, most often family members in a caregiving role.

Cognitive response to treatment is assessed differently in clinical trials and practice settings. In clinical trials, cognition is usually measured on standardized neuropsychological instruments, especially the Alzheimer's Disease Assessment Scale cognitive subtest (ADAS-cog) (5). In practice, many clinicians do not use standardized instruments at all; but among those that do, the MMSE is most commonly employed. The MMSE is heavily weighted toward memory and orientation. These cognitive domains are relatively insensitive to current treatments for AD. Ideally, outcome measures should reflect the specific cognitive or psychometric effects of the neurotransmitters affected by the drug being used. Although memory loss is the defining symptom of AD, it may not be the most treatment-responsive. For example, attentional abilities, rather than memory, appear to respond most robustly to cholinergic drugs (6,7). Attention-demanding tests, like Trail-making tests, serial subtraction, or reciting the months in reverse order, might therefore be a more efficient way to measure of response to the commonly prescribed cholinesterase inhibitor drugs in AD. Despite their shortcomings, regulatory bodies and many prescribers continue to focus on response on broad, but nonspecific batteries like the MMSE or specific memory tests as the defining element of treatment success.

Although impossible to quantify, the caregiver's subjective report on cognitive abilities should also be considered. The demands on cognition in the patient's usual environment are often far more intricate than any tests the clinician can present and measure in the office. Caregiver-reported cognitive improvements (or worsening) that fall below the threshold of detection on bedside testing should be weighed carefully, because of their considerable ecological validity. Interestingly, caregivers identify more robust treatment responses in open-label trials than prescribers report, even in the same patient (8). Furthermore, physicians acknowledge that available instruments do not capture important aspects of treatment response in AD (9).

AVAILABLE DRUGS

Cholinesterase Inhibitors

Rationale
AD is characterized by extensive cell loss in the deep cerebral nuclei with long projections to the cerebral cortex, including the raphe nucli (serotonin) and locus cereleus (norepinephrine), as well as the basal nuclei of the forebrain, including the nucleus basalis of Meynert. Basal forebrain nuclei house the cell bodies of neurons that produce the neurotransmitter acetylcholine (ACh). Axons from these cells synapse throughout the cerebral cortex, especially the frontal lobe, and also project to hippocampal structures. Reduced synaptic concentration of ACh is hypothesized to result from the loss of presynaptic neurons. The target regions are vital to attention, learning, and memory, which are cornerstone deficits in the clinical expression of AD. These observations have been summarized as the "cholinergic hypothesis" of AD. Facilitating cortical ACh activity to improve

cognition was therefore an early goal in AD drug development. Neither attempts to supplement production of ACh with precursor molecules nor activate ACh receptors with pharmacological agonists proved useful in well-conducted clinical trials. In contrast, inhibition of ACh catabolism with acetylcholinesterase inhibitor agents has been supported as an effective cholinomimetic treatment for AD in multiple prospective trials.

Acetylcholinesterase (AChE) is an intrasynaptic enzyme that rapidly hydrolyzes ACh into acetate and choline. AChE inhibition acts prolong the availability of the transmitter to the post-synaptic receptor. There are several subforms of AChE. There is also a closely related cholinesterase, butyrylcholinesterase, which is less specific to ACh. The relevance of the AChE subtypes and butyrylcholinesterase in AD treatment remains unknown.

Studies

Four acetylcholinesterase inhibitor (AChEI) agents have been released for marketing in the United States for treatment of AD: donepezil (Aricept, Eisai/Pfizer, approved 1996), rivastigmine (Exelon, Novartis, approved 2000), and galantamine (Reminyl, Razadyne, Janssen, approved 2001). The first agent of this class to be approved, tacrine (Cognex, Parke-Davis, approved 1993), is no longer in general use because of dosing, tolerability, and safety concerns. Different mechanisms of action have been purported for the available agents, but these appear to have a greater impact on ease of use and tolerability than measures of efficacy on dementia symptoms.

At of the end of 2006, donepezil was approved in the United States as treatment for AD symptoms at all levels of severity or stages. The other AChEIs are approved for treatment of the symptoms of mild or moderate AD in the United States. The scientific validity of limiting treatment availability by stage of disease is questionable and few, if any, drugs for other illnesses are regulated for use in patients with specified levels of disease severity. Determining the stage of AD is not straightforward. In clinical trials leading to approval, patients were required to have scores of 10 to 26 on the MMSE as well as a clinician's global rating of mild or moderate dementia severity. Unfortunately, the MMSE is not reliable as a sole source for judging overall dementia severity. Global measures like the Clinical Dementia Rating (10) and other interview-based instruments are better tools for classifying dementia stages than cognitive test scores alone, because they also incorporate assessments of function and behavior in the overall staging. Time-consuming, these staging instruments are generally not practical in clinical settings. More informal staging processes, on the basis of clinician's experience, are typically employed to determine suitability for AD therapy in practice. Therefore, patients with scores outside the 10 to 26 range receive these therapies, and prospective studies suggest that they may benefit from treatment in a manner similar to those with mild and moderate AD, as restrictively defined in the clinical trials leading to FDA approval.

Efficacy in mild–moderate AD. ChEIs provide statistically significant treatment benefits for patients with mild-to-moderate AD. Double-blind, placebo-controlled studies ranging from three to 24 months duration suggest improved cognition compared with baseline values over the short-term and statistically significant differences between treated and placebo groups over long-term follow-up. The

Table 1 Efficacy of AChEI Drugs in Mild–Moderate Alzheimer's Disease

Drug	Duration (month)	Dose (mg/day)	Drug-placebo difference (ADAS-cog)	References
Donepezil	3	5	2.7	(52)
		10	3.0	
	6	5	2.8	(53)
		10	3.1	
	6	5	2.5	(54)
		10	2.9	
Galantamine	6	16	3.9	(55)
		24	3.8	
	5	16	3.3	(56)
		24	3.6	
	6	24	2.9	(57)
Rivastigmine	6	6–12	4.9	(58)
	6	6–12	2.6	(59)

Results from intent-to-treat analyses of published, double-blind, placebo-controlled trials of FDA-approved doses and using ADAS-cog as the cognitive outcome measure are depicted.

pattern of efficacy is nearly indistinguishable across the different agents (11). A comparison of cognitive outcomes from these studies is depicted in Table 1. The average magnitude of the drug-placebo difference is about 3 points on the 70 point ADAS-cog. Study samples had baseline ADAS-cog scores of ~25/70 (higher scores represent more impairment on the ADAS-cog). The mean treatment effect (i.e., the arithmetic difference between treated and placebo groups) is generally of a consistent size from three months on. This means that if true improvement from baseline is going to be observed on cognitive measures, it is most likely in the first three months of treatment. Open-label observations suggest, but cannot confirm, that the therapeutic effects are sustained through three to five years of treatment (12–14).

It is important to note that averages are very misleading for predicting any individual's response to treatment in AD. To date, no predictors of individual response have been identified. Also, symptomatic expression and severity of the disease vary widely between affected individuals. A further complication in attempting to generalize group treatment responses to individual patients is that the treatment sensitivity of outcome measures varies with disease severity. This is reflected in the use of the Severe Impairment Battery (SIB)(15) rather than the ADAS-cog in studies of more severely affected individuals.

Although the studies leading to approval of AChEIs principally included patients with mild-to-moderate AD (and mean MMSE of about 20), similar cognitive benefit has been demonstrated at other levels of disease severity. Donepezil provided benefit on ADAS-cog, but not a specific verbal memory test when tested in patients with early AD (MMSE 21–26) (16). A more global pattern of benefit was seen with donepezil in moderate-to-severe AD (MMSE 5–17) (17). A small study of rivastigmine in patients with "advanced moderate" AD (MMSE ≤14) revealed similar outcomes (18). More recently, donepezil also showed a benefit relative to placebo in cognitive performance among patients with severe AD (MMSE 1–10) (19).

MMSE as an outcome.   Several studies have employed the MMSE as one of their primary cognitive outcomes. This is particularly pertinent for studies with longer treatment duration. A one-year double-blind placebo-controlled trial showed that donepezil-treated patients were maintained with an average of no decline, while those on placebo showed a mean decline of ~2.5 points (20). Mohs and colleagues reported a much more complicated design, in which patients were withdrawn from analysis at the time they showed specified levels of decline in daily function. This resulted in a shorter mean interval of observation and a treatment effect of about 1 MMSE point. The controversial AD 2000 study (21) also demonstrated benefit of donepezil versus placebo on MMSE. The magnitude of effect was approximately 0.8 points at two years. The interpretation of this effect size is complicated by a study design with less specific enrollment criteria, double-randomization, high dropout rates, and a 12-week planned treatment interruption after 48 weeks of therapy.

A blinded-rater comparison of donepezil and galantamine (conventional release) in patients with mild-to-moderate AD revealed no overall difference between agents on the MMSE, with mean times to decline below baseline in the 9 to 12 month range (22). Similarly, a two-year comparison trial of donepezil and rivastigmine in moderate-to-severe patients identified a mean MMSE decline of about 2.5 points from baseline and no difference between agents on the MMSE or the SIB (23). The magnitude of decline observed during two years of AChEI therapy is similar to the decline of the placebo group in an unrelated one-year trial (20). Taken together, these results suggest a mean treatment effect of 1 to 2 points on the MMSE that probably persists for two or more years. Unfortunately, this effect size is within the test–retest variability of the MMSE and reinforces that MMSE is not ideal for measuring treatment response to AChEI drugs in AD.

Dosing.   The standard dosing approach to AChEIs is shown in Table 2. The AChEIs demonstrate a dose–response relationship in reference to cognition. Though most studies of donepezil were not designed to discern a difference in efficacy between 5 mg/day and 10 mg/day dosing, a meta-analysis revealed that effects obtained with 10 mg/day donepezil were significantly superior to those with the 5 mg/day dose (24). Galantamine is effective at doses of 16 to 32 mg daily, with no clear additional benefit of 32 mg over 24 mg. There is also

Table 2   Dosing of AChEIs

Drug	Initial dose (oral)	Minimum effective dose	Target dose range	Alternate forms
Donepezil	5 mg daily	5 mg	5–23 mg daily	Oral dissolving tablet
Galantamine	4 mg twice daily	8 mg twice daily	8–12 mg twice daily	Oral solution (4 mg/mL)
Galantamine (extended release)	8 mg daily	16 mg daily	24–32 mg daily	
Rivastigmine	1.5 mg twice daily	3 mg twice daily	3–6 mg twice daily	Oral solution (2 mg/mL)
Rivastigmine (transdermal)	4.6 mg/24 hours (transdermal patch)	9.4 mg/24 hours	9.4 mg/24 hours	

Table 3 Proportion of AchEI-Treated Patients Achieving Specific Outcomes of 4-and 7-Point Improvements on ADAS-cog (Six-Month Studies)

Drug	Dose	Proportion (%) showing ADAS-cog improvement equal to:			References
		7	4	0	
Donepezil	Placebo	8	28	59	(53)
	5 mg	15	40	83	
	10 mg	26	58	82	
Galantamine	Placebo	6	17	44	(55)
	24 mg	19	34	64	
	32 mg	20	33	58	
Galantamine	Placebo	6	15	40	(57)
	24 mg	15	31	65	
	32 mg	20	35	64	
Rivastigmine	Placebo	2	7	27	(58)
	6–12 mg	12	25	56	
Rivastigmine	Placebo	6	19	45	(59)
	6–12 mg	18	29	55	

Proportions are cumulative (i.e., patients showing 7-point improvements are also included in 4-point and 0-point columns).

dose-dependent response with rivastigmine. Patients receiving 6 to 12 mg of rivastigmine daily show improvements relative to placebo, which are not evident at lower doses of 1 to 4 mg daily. Retrospective analysis suggests an additional direct dose–response relationship for doses within the 6 to 12 mg/day range.

Frequency of response
Another way to define response to treatment with AChEIs is the proportion of individuals showing a specified level of improvement during double-blind placebo-controlled trials. These data are reported in the prescribing information for each AChEI in the United States and are depicted in Table 3. Regardless of the specific study or agent being tested, these results suggest that a patient receiving maximum approved doses of the AChEI is about three times more likely to show a 7-point improvement on the ADAS-cog than an untreated individual. If absence of decline, rather than improvement from the starting point, is used as the measure of efficacy treated, patients appear to be 25% to 50% more likely to be stable than untreated ones. This can be difficult to discern in clinical settings, however, because nearly half of the placebo group failed to decline in most of the trials. Nonetheless, the data suggest that more patients improve and more patients maintain stable test scores on treatment with AChEIs.

In a large cohort (5462 AD patients) beginning open-label AChEI treatment in community settings, approximately 18% showed a 2-point or greater improvement from their baseline MMSE; about 16% of the enrolled patients sustained ≥ 2 point MMSE improvements at nine months of follow-up. A ≥ 2 point improvement at three months of treatment was strongly predictive of continued positive response at nine months (25).

Frequency of response can also be inferred by calculating the risk of rapid decline. In separate, but complementary, open-label studies, use of ChEIs more than doubled the likelihood of *slow* decline (26) and persistent exposure to ChEIs reduced the likelihood of *rapid* decline by more than half (27).

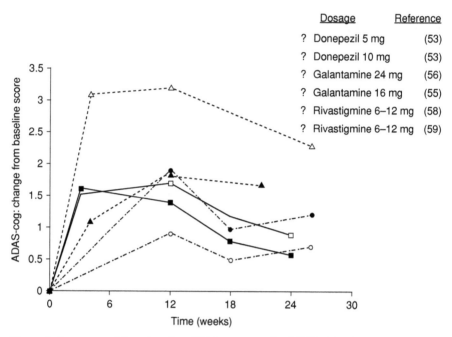

Figure 1 Improvement from baseline ADAS-cog score for AChEI trials of five to six months duration. Similarities in time course of response and magnitude of effects suggest no meaningful differences in initial cognitive efficacy between agents.

Timing of response

Peak cognitive responses to AChEI therapy are seen after 4 to 12 weeks of therapy. See Figure 1. The reason for the delay is unclear. Most studies did not assess cognitive outcomes until at least four weeks, so measurement artifact may contribute to the observation. Also, based on titration schedules or long half-lives, AChEIs may not reach steady state at therapeutic brain concentrations for two or more weeks. Family observations and clinical trials both suggest response latency of weeks. This raises the possibility that compensatory brain processes may influence the time course to response. This is the case for other neurotransmitter-mediated treatment approaches like antidepressants. There is a similar lag to loss of efficacy upon discontinuation of AChEIs. For example, discontinuing donepezil 10 mg for three weeks after 12 weeks of treatment was not associated with the persistent loss of efficacy observed following discontinuation of the agent for six weeks after six months of therapy (28). The differences between the long-term adverse effects of three weeks versus six weeks of discontinuation can not be explained by donepezil's half-life, since blood levels should approach zero in only two weeks.

Magnitude of response

Patients, and especially their families, should be counseled regarding realistic expectations for cognitive outcomes to AChEI therapy. The data from clinical trials and observational studies indicate that dramatic reversal of memory impairment is unlikely. Cholinesterase inhibition thus should not be expected to progressively improve cognition relative treatment initiation, but rather delay or forestall an inevitable decline by a period of time, with convergent evidence suggesting an average of one-year delay. A subset of patients exceeding this level of benefit can be identified by a prominent response during the first few months of treatment, a level of response that is also associated with fewer medical co-morbidities (25). Delaying cognitive decline remains a valuable goal. It is associated with preservation of daily function (29), i.e., "holding one's own," and may result in a significant delay in institutionalization, which is a commonly voiced goal among families facing dementia (30).

Duration of benefit
The duration of benefit with AChEIs is unknown, but a randomized, placebo-controlled study in the United Kingdom, sponsored by the National Health Service, showed that patients who received long-term donepezil treatment had cognitive and functional outcomes superior to placebo for at least two years (21). Numerous open-label or other forms of observational studies suggest that patients chronically treated with AChEIs show less than predicted levels of decline, with follow-up periods up to five years (31). One of these showed a correlation between time on AChEI treatment and time to nursing home placement over a reliable observational period of about three years (32).

Tolerability
Most patients taking AChEIs will experience few adverse effects; a large population-based study suggests an overall rate of adverse AChEI-related events of about 14% over nine months (25). All common AChEI side effects can be anticipated as the result of cholinergic augmentation, with the most frequent ones affecting the gastrointestinal tract. These may include loose stool or diarrhea, nausea, vomiting, or anorexia. In clinical trials, these complications are expressed in 5% to 15% of patients, most commonly during initial dosing or after a dose increase. AChEIs carry class warnings for gastrointestinal side effects, bladder outflow obstruction, seizures (although seizures may also be caused by AD), syncope, and asthma/obstructive pulmonary disease. The United States prescribing information for rivastigmine includes an additional warning regarding the potential for significant nausea, vomiting, and weight loss. Dose reduction is warranted if these symptoms are intolerable to the patient. Occasionally, muscle cramping, increased oronasal secretions, or urinary incontinence can occur.

Some patients will experience sleep disturbance, often with strikingly vivid dreams. Although the phenomenon appears to be most common with donepezil, comparative studies do not substantiate a differential impact on sleep between available agents. If sleep and dream problems emerge, they may be ameliorated by using morning dosing for the once daily agents, or moving evening dosing earlier in the day. Alternatively, switching to another member of the class may be justified.

Bradycardia is another expected complication of AChE inhibition, through its tonic effects on parasympathetic vagal nerve transmission. The bradycardia is not generally associated with reduced cardiac output, and orthostatic and hypotensive symptoms are uncommon in AD patients unless they are taking concomitant drugs with negative cardiac inoptropic effects. Syncope is therefore unusual, being seen in ~2% of clinical trials patients. When syncope occurs in AChEI-treated patients, cardiac causes are most commonly identified (33).

Observational studies conducted in routine clinical practice supplement the tolerability data collected in the more restricted environment and homogeneous patient populations of controlled clinical trials. Naturalistic observational studies may provide a more realistic estimate of safety and tolerability than what is seen in carefully selected clinical trials samples. Rates of donepezil discontinuation due to adverse events were 5% to 6% in two large, three-month observational studies (34,35). Over a 12-month period, the rate of donepezil discontinuation due to adverse events was higher (~12%). The higher rate is most likely related to greater window of time for adverse events to occur (36). For rivastigmine, the six-month discontinuation rate was also about 5% accounting for about 40% of all discontinuations (37). A nine-month study of all AChEIs showed an overall rate of adverse event-related discontinuation of about 5% with significantly higher rates of adverse reactions for galantamine and rivastigmine in comparison to donepezil (25). Similarly, a large head-to-head study of donepezil and rivastig-mine found a higher rate of gastrointestinal side effects, especially nausea and vomiting, associated with rivastigmine; the majority of these problems emerged, as expected, during the dose-titration phase of treatment and were less prob-lematic after stable maintenance of dosing of rivastigmine was achieved (23). Rivastigmine transdermal's rate of GI side effects is similar to placebo. Adverse event rates were similar for donepezil and galantamine (conventional release) in another one-year head-to-head study (22).

Discontinuation

No carefully controlled studies of AChEI treatment cessation have been reported. However, AChEIs are not known to have a major effect on neuronal survival. This is supported by the observation that discontinuation of the drug led to short-term decline in cognitive test scores and global function, such that test performance was at placebo levels within six weeks of the cessation of donepezil treatment (28). Patients should be expected to decline during prolonged treatment as neurons continue to die. Long-term follow-up of clinical trials patients strongly suggests, however, that a patient on treatment is likely to have improved cognition when compared with his or her projected condition at the same point in time if left untreated (31). Therefore, decline in cognition or function from baseline levels is not, by itself, an indication for discontinuing therapy.

The primary indications for cholinesterase inhibitor discontinuation are perceived lack of efficacy and intolerable side effects. Social factors including cost of drug therapy and patient resistance to treatment may also influence the duration of treatment.

If the clinician or family decide that the treatment should be discontinued, careful monitoring of the short-term outcomes of discontinuation is warranted. If acceleration in the pace of decline is seen in the first few weeks after discon-tinuation, resumption of treatment should be considered. Because of consistent clinical observations that once a function is lost to AD it is rarely restored, early resumption of treatment is important when rapid functional decline is observed upon withdrawal.

Despite the historic limitation of AChEIs to mild and moderate stages of dementia, evidence from well-controlled trials indicates there are individuals who will continue to show benefits even in the severe stages of the illness (17,19).

Since cognitive assessments are limited by dementia severity, one clinically useful end point to consider as a trigger for discontinuation is when the patient is no longer contributing meaningfully to basic activities such as dressing, feeding, grooming, toileting, or bathing. In these patients, the same pattern of carefully observing cognition and function after discontinuation of therapy is warranted. Even at this severe level of dysfunction, some individuals will show further rapid progression of cognitive impairment (e.g., not recognizing caregivers or familiar surroundings) upon treatment withdrawal. They may also experience declines in function or worsening of behavior without clear changes in cognition. Any of these changes represents an indication to resume therapy.

NMDA Receptor Modulation

Antagonists of the N-methyl-d-aspartate (NMDA) class of glutamate receptors are the other class of medications FDA-approved for use in AD. Memantine (*Namenda*, Forest Laboratories) is the only drug in the class currently available. It was approved in the United States during 2004 for use in moderate–severe dementia attributable to AD.

Rationale and mechanism of action

Memantine is an uncompetitive, low-affinity, open-channel antagonist of the NMDA receptor. The receptor is a glutamate-triggered calcium channel. A glutamatergic hypothesis of neuronal dysfunction in AD is the proposed mechanism for memantine's efficacy in AD (38). The hypothesis is largely inferential, with relatively little direct evidence in humans with AD. Elements of the model include an increase in resting synaptic glutamate concentrations or a change in resting membrane potential due to neuronal bioenergetic failure. The net effect of either of these is hypothesized to be excessive calcium flow through the receptor channel. Memantine does not appear to affect the glutamate binding site. Rather, it displaces the magnesium cation that normally occupies the channel. Memantine's effect is attributed to its different voltage response characteristics compared to magnesium ions. By being less likely to displacement at reduced membrane potentials, it reduces net calcium influx. This may normalize membrane potential and allow neurons to be more sensitive to physiologic inputs, and may also facilitate intracellular processes underlying memory, such as long-term potentiation. An additional proposed component of the model is based on the concept of calcium-mediated neuronal death, sometimes described under the concept of excitotoxicity. Conditions associated with acute, excessive, calcium influx into neurons including trauma and ischemia result in cellular dysfunction and death through calcium-mediated apoptotic pathways. However, the direct evidence for calcium-mediated neurotoxicity in AD is limited, and the current FDA-labeling for memantine specifically states that memantine is not known to act through "neuroprotective" mechanisms.

Studies

Cognitive outcomes in two primary studies conducted on patients classified to have moderate and severe levels of dementia due to AD led to approval of memantine in the United States (39,40). In contrast to most studies of AChEIs, which used the Clinical Dementia Rating (10) as the instrument to establish stages, memantine studies used the Global Deterioration Scale (41). The use of different staging schemes means that severity cannot be directly compared between studies. Specifically, individuals classified as "moderate" on one staging scale might be graded as "severe" on a different scale. This has implications for efficacy since the glutamatergic hypothesis implies that AD-related excessive glutamate activity correlates with dementia severity.

In a seven-month randomized, placebo-controlled study of patients with moderate-to-severe AD, treatment with memantine produced significantly better outcomes than placebo on cognition as measured by the SIB (39). Both the memantine and placebo groups exhibited a decline in cognition compared to baseline. When added to existing chronic donepezil therapy, memantine treatment results in stabilized cognitive test scores and less worsening than observed in patients treated with donepezil plus placebo over six months (40). For these studies, mean MMSE on entry was 11 to 14. Patients begun on memantine after six months of placebo showed improvements in cognition. After six months, their mean SIB cognitive test scores were indistinguishable from patients who had taken uninterrupted memantine therapy for 12 months (42).

More recently, a six-month trial of memantine in patients with milder stages of AD (mean MMSE on entry $\sim$17) was reported (43). In the primary intent-to-treat analysis, a statistical difference between treatment groups was identified with an effect size of 1.9 points on the ADAS cog. Effect sizes in the observed cases were smaller ($\sim$1 point) and did not reach statistical significant at the six-month follow-up.

Dosing
The approved dosage for memantine is 10 mg twice daily. Most clinical trials were conducted with a titration schedule that began with 5 mg daily and increased by 5 mg/day each week to reach a target dose of 10 mg twice daily. One study conducted in nursing home patients used a lower target of 10 mg daily and found global results similar to those seen with a 20 mg total daily dose but did not specifically assess cognitive outcomes (44). Dose reductions are recommended for patients with serious renal and hepatic compromise.

Frequency of response
Response frequencies have been reported for patients adding memantine or placebo to chronic donepezil treatment in patients with moderate and severe AD (45). Patients adding memantine were more likely to improve or maintain cognition (63% versus 53%; $p < 0.05$). The same study reported significantly greater likelihood of showing any improvement (57% versus 46%) and $\geq$8 point improvements on the SIB (16% versus 8%).

Timing of response
Improvement in mean cognitive test scores (relative to placebo) is evident within four weeks in all studies of memantine in AD reporting cognitive outcomes to date (39,40,43). In the clinical trials, the peak improvement relative to placebo occurs at 12 weeks of treatment.

Magnitude of response
In the pivotal monotherapy trial of moderate and severely impaired AD patients, memantine-treated patients showed a peak improvement relative to placebo of

5 SIB points (39). In combination with donepezil, the peak observed improvement in moderate-to-severe patients was 3 SIB points (40). In the reported trial involving memantine monotherapy in mild and moderate patients, effect sizes among observed cases were about 1 point (43). A one-point mean treatment effect on the ADAS cog would generally fall below the threshold of clinical detection, and memantine has not been approved by the FDA for use in AD of mild severity.

Duration of benefit
Intriguingly, mean cognitive test scores for patients begun on memantine after six months of blinded-placebo treatment were the same as for patients who had received continuous combined treatment for 12 months (42). Further studies will be required to determine whether the declining efficacy over time suggested by these results is replicated in other studies.

Tolerability
The mechanism-related adverse effects of memantine tend to be CNS-oriented, such as dizziness, headache, and hallucination. Memantine has activating effects which are evident in some patients as agitation and confusion, though overall benefits on behavior are reported (40,43).

Discontinuation
No studies of the effects of memantine discontinuation in AD have been reported.

OTHER EXISTING PRESCRIPTIVE AGENTS
No other classes of agents have been approved for treatment of AD in the United States. Small pilot studies of numerous existing drugs have been reported, but none have entered regular use. Importantly, well-conducted studies of nonsteroidal anti-inflammatory agents, prednisone, and estrogen have revealed no cognitive benefits in patients with mild and moderate AD. One 12-month study revealed that mild-moderately severe AD patients treated with atorvastatin sustained less decline in cognition relative to placebo (46). Another study suggested a cognitive response relative to placebo among AD patients treated with rosiglitazone, who lack the ε-4 allele of the apolipoprotein E risk factor gene. (47). However, further studies on these agents did not reveal clinically meaningful efficacy.

VITAMIN E AND NUTRICEUTICALS
In the 1990s many experts began to recommend high dose Vitamin E to slow progression of AD on the basis of a large clinical trial in moderately severe AD patients. (48). Treatment with Vitamin E 2000 IU daily did not provide cognitive benefit relative to placebo, and more recent studies failed to replicate the result in patients with mild cognitive impairment (49). Excess mortality for Vitamin E doses over 400 IU daily has also been reported (50). High dose vitamin E is therefore probably not appropriate for treatment of cognitive symptoms in AD. A wide range of other natural products, including Gingko biloba, has been studied, but there is little information available from appropriately conducted, double-blind placebo-controlled trials to support their use. Most do not appear to be as consistently effective on cognitive and global outcomes as currently approved prescription agents (51).

REFERENCES

1. Winblad B, Brodaty H, Gauthier S, et al. Pharmacotherapy of Alzheimer's disease: Is there a need to redefine treatment success? Int J Geriatr Psychiatry 2001; 16:653–656.
2. Geldmacher DS, Frölich L, Doody RS, et al. Realistic expectations for treatment success in Alzheimer's disease. J Nutr Health Aging 2006; 10:417–429.
3. Rainer M, Mucke HA, Kruger-Rainer C, et al. Cognitive relapse after discontinuation of drug therapy in Alzheimer's disease: cholinesterase inhibitors versus nootropics. J Neural Transm 2001; 108:1327–1333.
4. Folstein MF, Folstein SE, McHugh PR. "Mini-mental state": A practical method for grading the cognitive state of patients for the clinician. J Psychiatr Res 1975; 12:189–198.
5. Rosen WG, Mohs RC, Davis KL. A new rating scale for Alzheimer's disease. Am J Psychiatry 1984; 141:1356–1364.
6. Sahakian BJ, Coull JT. Tetrahydroaminoacridine (THA) in Alzheimer's disease: An assessment of attentional and mnemonic function using CANTAB. Acta Neurol Scand 1993; 149(supp.):29–35.
7. Foldi NS, White RE, Schaefer LA. Detecting effects of donepezil on visual selective attention using signal detection parameters in Alzheimer's disease. Int J Geriatr Psychiatry 2005; 20:485–488.
8. Rockwood K, Graham JE, Fay S, et al. Goal setting and attainment in Alzheimer's disease patients treated with donepezil. J Neurol Neurosurg Psychiatry 2002; 73:500–507.
9. Rockwood K, Black SE, Robillard A, et al. Potential treatment effects of donepezil not detected in Alzheimer's disease clinical trials: A physician survey. Int J Geriatr Psychiatry 2004; 19:954–960.
10. Morris JC. The Clinical Dementia Rating (CDR): Current version and scoring rules. Neurology 1993; 43:2412–2414.
11. Birks J. Cholinesterase inhibitors for Alzheimer's disease. Cochrane Database of Systematic Reviews 2006, Issue 1. Art. No.: CD005593. DOI: 10.1002/14651858.CD005593. (Accessed September 22, 2010).
12. Raskind MA, Peskind ER, Truyen L, et al. The cognitive benefits of galantamine are sustained for at least 36 months: A long-term extension trial. Arch Neurol 2004; 61:252–256.
13. Rogers SL, Doody RS, Pratt RD, et al. Long-term efficacy and safety of donepezil in the treatment of Alzheimer's disease: Final analysis of a US multicentre open-label study. Eur Neuropsychopharmacol 2000; 10:195–203.
14. Small GW, Kaufer D, Mendiondo MS, et al. Cognitive performance in Alzheimer's disease patients receiving rivastigmine for up to 5 years. Int J Clin Pract 2005; 59(4):473–477.
15. Panisset M, Roudier M, Saxton J, et al. Severe impairment battery. A neuropsychological test for severely demented patients. Arch Neurol 1994; 51:41–45.
16. Seltzer B, Zolnouni P, Nunez M, et al. Efficacy of donepezil in early-stage Alzheimer disease: A randomized placebo-controlled trial. Arch Neurol 2004; 61:1852–1856.
17. Feldman H, Gauthier S, Hecker J, et al. A 24-week, randomized, double-blind study of donepezil in moderate to severe Alzheimer's disease [published erratum appears in Neurology 2001; 57(11):2153]. Neurology 2001; 57:613–620.
18. Karaman Y, Erdogan F, Koseoglu E, et al. A 12-month study of the efficacy of rivastigmine in patients with advanced moderate Alzheimer's disease. Dement Geriatr Cogn Disord 2005; 19:51–56.
19. Winblad B, Kilander L, Eriksson S, et al. Donepezil in patients with severe Alzheimer's disease: Double-blind, parallel-group, placebo-controlled study. Lancet 2006; 367:1057–1065.
20. Winblad B, Engedal K, Soininen H, et al. A 1-year, randomized, placebo-controlled study of donepezil in patients with mild to moderate AD. Neurology 2001; 57:489–495.
21. AD2000 collaborative group. Long-term donepezil treatment in 565 patients with Alzheimer's disease (AD2000): Randomized double-blind trial. Lancet 2004; 363(9427):2105–2115.

22. Wilcock G, Howe I, Coles H, et al. A long-term comparison of galantamine and donepezil in the treatment of Alzheimer's disease. Drugs Aging 2003; 20:777–789.
23. Bullock R, Touchon J, Bergman H, et al. Rivastigmine and donepezil treatment in moderate to moderately-severe Alzheimer's disease over a 2-year period. Curr Med Res Opin 2005; 21:1317–1327.
24. Whitehead A, Perdomo C, Pratt RD, et al. Donepezil for the symptomatic treatment of patients with mild to moderate Alzheimer's disease: A meta-analysis of individual patient data from randomised controlled trials. Int J Geriatr Psychiatry 2004; 19: 624–633.
25. Raschetti R, Maggini M, Sorrentino GC, et al. A cohort study of effectiveness of acetycholinesterase inhibitors in Alzheimer's disease. Eur J Clin Pharmacol 2005; 61:361–368.
26. Lopez OL, Becker JT, Saxton J, et al. Alteration of a clinically meaningful outcome in the natural history of Alzheimer's disease by cholinesterase inhibition. J Am Geriatr Soc 2005; 53:83–87.
27. Gillette-Guyonnet S, Andrieu S, Cortes F, et al. Outcome of Alzheimer's disease: Potential impact of cholinesterase inhibitors. J Gerontol A Biol Sci Med Sci 2006; 61:516–520.
28. Doody RS, Geldmacher DS, Gordon B, et al. Open-label, multicenter, phase 3 extension study of the safety and efficacy of donepezil in patients with Alzheimer disease. Arch Neurol 2001; 58:427–433.
29. Mohs RC, Doody RS, Morris JC, et al. A 1-year, placebo-controlled preservation of function survival study of donepezil in AD patients [published erratum appears in Neurology 2001; 57:1942]. Neurology 2001; 57(3):481–488.
30. Karlawish JHT, Klocinski JL, Merz J, et al. Caregivers' preferences for the treatment of patients with Alzheimer's disease. Neurology 2000; 55:1008–1014.
31. Bullock R, Dengiz R. Cognitive performance in patients with Alzheimer's disease receiving cholinesterase inhibitors for up to 5 years. Int J Clin Pract 2005; 59:817–822.
32. Geldmacher DS, Provenzano G, McRae T, et al. Donepezil is associated with delayed nursing home placement in patients with Alzheimer's disease. J Am Geriatr Soc 2003; 51:937–944.
33. Bordier P, Lanusse S, Garrique S, et al. Causes of syncope in patients with Alzheimer's disease treated with donepezil. Drugs Aging 2005; 22:687–694.
34. Hager K, Calabrese P, Frolich L, et al. An observational clinical study of the efficacy and tolerability of donepezil in the treatment of Alzheimer's disease. Dement Geriatr Cogn Disord 2003; 15:189–198.
35. Boada-Rovira M, Brodaty H, Cras P, et al. Efficacy and safety of donepezil in patients with Alzheimer's disease: Results of a global, multinational, clinical experience study. Drugs Aging 2004; 21:43–53.
36. Frölich L, Gertz HJ, Heun R, et al. Donepezil for Alzheimer's disease in clinical practice–The DONALD Study. A multicenter 24-week clinical trial in Germany. Dement Geriatr Cogn Disord 2004; 18:37–43.
37. Schmidt R, Lechner A, Petrovic K. Rivastigmine in outpatient services: Experience of 114 neurologists in Austria. Int Clin Psychopharmacol 2002; 17:81–85.
38. Lipton SA. Paradigm shift in neuroprotection by NMDA receptor blockade: memantine and beyond. Nat Rev Drug Discov 2006; 5:160–170.
39. Reisberg B, Doody R, Stöffler A, et al. Memantine in moderate-to-severe Alzheimer's disease. N Engl J Med 2003; 348:1333–1341.
40. Tariot PN, Farlow MR, Grossberg GT, et al. Memantine treatment in patients with moderate to severe Alzheimer disease already receiving donepezil: A randomized controlled trial. JAMA 2004; 291:317–324.
41. Reisberg B, Ferris SH, de Leon MJ, et al. The Global Deterioration Scale for assessment of primary degenerative dementia. Am J Psychiatry 1982; 139:1136–1139.
42. Reisberg B, Doody R, Stöffler A, et al. A 24-week open-label extension study of memantine in moderate to severe Alzheimer disease. Arch Neurol 2006; 63:49–54.

43. Peskind ER, Potkin SG, Pomara N, et al. Memantine treatment in mild to moderate Alzheimer disease: A 24-week randomized, controlled trial. Am J Geriatr Psychiatry 2006; 14:704–715.
44. Winblad B, Poritis N. Memantine in severe dementia: results of the M-BEST Study (Benefit and efficacy in severely demented patients during treatment with memantine). Int J Geriatr Psychiatry 1999; 14:135–146.
45. Van Dyck CH, Schmitt FA, Olin JT, et al. A responder analysis of memantine treatment in patients with Alzheimer disease maintained on donepezil. Am J Geriatr Psychiatry 2006; 14:428–437.
46. Sparks DL, Sabbagh MN, Connor DJ, et al. Atorvastatin for the treatment of mild to moderate Alzheimer's disease. Preliminary results. Arch Neurol 2005; 62:753–757.
47. Risner ME, Saunders AM, Altman JFB, et al. Efficacy of rosiglitazone in a genetically defined population with mild-to-moderate Alzheimer's disease. Pharmacogenomics J 2006; 6:246–254.
48. Sano M, Ernesto C, Thomas RG, et al. A controlled trial of selegiline, alpha-tocopherol, or both as treatment for Alzheimer's disease. The Alzheimer's Disease Cooperative Study. N Engl J Med 1997; 336:1216–1222.
49. Petersen RC, Thomas RG, Grundman M, et al. Vitamin E and donepezil for the treatment of mild cognitive impairment. N Engl J Med 2005; 352:2379–2388.
50. Miller ER, Pastor-Barriuso R, Dalal D, et al. Meta-analysis: High dosage Vitamin E supplementation may increase all-cause mortality. Ann Intern Med 2005; 142:37–46.
51. Diamond BJ, Johnson SK, Torsney K, et al. Complementary and alternative medicines in the treatment of dementia. An evidence based review. Drugs Aging 2003; 20:981–998.
52. Rogers SL, Doody RS, Mohs RC, et al. Donepezil improves cognition and global function in Alzheimer disease: A 15-week, double-blind, Placebo-Controlled Study. Arch Intern Med 1998; 158:1021–1031.
53. Rogers SL, Farlow MR, Doody RS, et al. A 24-week double blind placebo controlled trial of donepezil in patients with Alzheimer's disease. Neurology 1998; 50:136–145.
54. Burns A, Rossor M, Hecker J, et al. The effects of donepezil in Alzheimer's disease—Results from a multinational trial. Dement Geriatr Cogn Disord 1999: 10:237–244.
55. Raskind MA, Peskind ER, Wessel T, et al. Galantamine in AD: A 6-month randomized, placebo-controlled trial with a 6-month extension. The Galantamine USA-1 Study Group. Neurology 2000; 54(12):2261–2268.
56. Tariot PN, Solomon PR, Morris JC, et al. A 5-month, randomized, placebo-controlled trial of galantamine in AD. The Galantamine USA-10 Study Group. Neurology 2000; 54(12):2269–2276.
57. Wilcock GK, Lilienfeld S, Gaens E, on behalf of the Galantamine International-1 Study Group. Efficacy and safety of galantamine in patients with mild to moderate Alzheimer's disease: Multicentre randomised controlled trial [published erratum appears in BMJ 2001; 322:405]. BMJ 2000; 321:1445–1449.
58. Corey-Bloom J, Anand R, Veach J, for the ENA 713 B352 Study Group. A randomized trial evaluating the efficacy and safety of ENA 713 (rivastigmine tartrate), a new acetylcholinesterase inhibitor, in patients with mild to moderately severe Alzheimer's disease. Int J Geriatr Psychopharmacol 1998; 1:55–65.
59. Rösler M, Anand R, Cicin-Sain A, et al. Efficacy and safety of rivastigmine in patients with Alzheimer's disease: International randomised controlled trial [published erratum appears in BMJ 2001; 322:1456]. BMJ 1999; 318(7184):633–638.

4 | Behavior management in dementia

Douglas W. Scharre

INTRODUCTION

Behavioral and neuropsychiatric symptoms are commonly encountered in Alzheimer's disease (AD) and other dementias (1–3). Up to 88% of all AD patients will exhibit some kind of behavioral disturbance, and the frequency and severity of these behaviors increase with cognitive decline (1,4). Paranoid behavior, hallucinations, and activity disturbances (restless behaviors) predict faster functional decline in AD patients, and this is independent of cognitive status (5). The behavioral manifestations of dementia including physical and verbal aggression, catastrophic reactions, and suspiciousness are very difficult for caregivers to handle and often lead earlier to nursing home placement (5).

Fortunately, most of the behaviors seen in dementia can be controlled with the use of a combination of behavioral modification techniques and pharmacotherapy. When there is successful management of the patient's behaviors, there is improved quality of life for the patient, reduced burden on the caregiver, and significantly reduced health care costs. The patients need less supervision and may avoid costly doctor visits or nursing home admissions.

Specific dementia conditions have characteristic neuropsychiatric symptoms. In AD, apathy, delusions, aggression, anxiety, depression, restless behaviors, sundowning, and sleep disturbances are the most common behavioral symptoms encountered (Table 1) (1,6). Personality changes, executive dysfunctioning, disinhibition, inappropriate laughter, self-absorption, obsessive–compulsive traits, and apathy are typical of the frontotemporal dementias (FTDs) (2). Patients with dementia with Lewy bodies often have prominent visual hallucinations (3), whereas Huntington's disease patients develop severe depression and psychotic features (7). Pseudobulbar affect or involuntary emotional expression disorder (IEED) occurs often in progressive supranuclear palsy, FTD, and some vascular dementias (8). Psychosis, depression, and acute confusional states are typical in lupus cerebritis and B12 deficiency (9). Major depression is the key manifestation of individuals with pseudodementia (10).

GENERAL PRINCIPLES OF BEHAVIORAL MANAGEMENT

For the behaviorally disturbed dementia patient, there are a number of general management principles to consider before deciding if psychotropic medications are indicated.

1. Use appropriate behavioral modification techniques described below.
2. Avoid or use anticholinergic medications with caution. Common drugs with a lot of anticholinergic properties include antihistamines, cold preparations, diphenhydramine [contained in products such as acetaminophen (Tylenol PM) and Benadryl], urinary control medications (such as tolterodine and

71

Table 1   Common Behavioral Symptoms of AD

Apathy	72%
Delusions	70%
Aggression/agitation	60%
Anxiety	48%
Psychomotor disturbance	46%
Irritability/lability	42%
Sleep/wake disturbance	42%
Depression/dysphoria	38%
Disinhibition	36%
Sundowning	18%
Hallucinations	15%
Hypersexuality	3%
Euphoria	2%
Obsessive–compulsive	2%

oxybutynin), tricyclic antidepressants (amitriptyline, doxepin), and low-potency typical antipsychotics (thioridazine).

3. Avoid benzodiazepines. They are usually confusionogenic in the demented elderly. One can build up a tolerance to them and there are withdrawal symptoms if they are suddenly stopped.
4. Avoid hazardous environmental situations that may lead to falls and broken bones.
5. Provide adequate supervision to prevent accidents, medication errors, and improper nutrition. In the hospital setting, use of a sitter for supervision needs is recommended. They can reassure, calm, and redirect the confused and irritated patient.
6. Avoid sensory deprivation by ensuring vision (glasses) and hearing (aides) is corrected to the extent possible. Ensure plenty of light to aid vision in the day and use night-lights for potentials nighttime arousals.
7. Avoid overstimulation. Too much noise, too many people, new environments, and changes in routines all increase the likelihood of behavioral disturbances in the demented elderly.
8. Educate and assist caregivers with support groups, family counseling, and social services.
9. Set goals of care and advance directives with family and patient.

When there are new behaviors or a change in behaviors the following steps should be taken:

1. Check for infection and dehydration.
2. Evaluate for any physical changes or changes in medical condition (i.e., congestive heart failure, uremia, hypothyroidism).
3. Look for adverse medication effects (i.e., medication-induced behavioral changes like depression or anxiety or sleep disturbance) and drug–drug interactions.
4. Consider stopping or changing any new drug that was added.

Identifying the key underlying behavior(s) to target provides the best chance of successful behavioral intervention. Table 2 lists the most common underlying behaviors seen in dementia patients.

Table 2 Common Underlying Behaviors in Dementia

1. Behavior due to environmental disruption
2. Psychotic behavior including suspiciousness, delusions, and hallucinations
3. Depressive symptoms including anxiety
4. Apathy and neurovegetative symptoms
5. Anxiety
6. Mood lability, disinhibition, intrusiveness, euphoria, and mania
7. Sleep disturbance
8. Eating and appetite disturbances
9. Hypersexuality
10. Aberrant motor behavior including restless activity, psychomotor agitation, pacing, and wanting-to-go behaviors
11. Obsessive–compulsive traits

BEHAVIOR MODIFICATION APPROACHES

Caregivers often have a very difficult time dealing and reacting to behavioral disturbances in demented individuals. It is hard to reason with someone who may have lost their logic, their language, and their memories. Behavioral modification techniques can help caregivers cope with and lessen disruptive behaviors (11,12).

1. Use a gentle, calm approach:
   Harsh, commanding, or loud tone of voice can intensify an unwanted behavior. Some patients feel threatened, domineered, or frightened and may react in kind. Approach the patient slowly so as not to startle them, make them feel uncomfortable, or anxious.
2. Use nonverbal communication that is nonthreatening:
   As the course of dementia progresses, less and less verbal abilities are maintained. Focus on the patient's emotional responses for communication cues as much as or more than their words. Always smile. Even an agitated patient may calm a little when everyone is smiling. If instead you look fearful or angry, they may chase you or strike out. Smiling tends to shorten and diminish disruptive behaviors. Use an open nonthreatening posture and avoid crossing arms or taking defensive stances. To help calm the patient, maintain eye contact, nod your head yes, wave hello, shrug your shoulders, and exaggerate your nonverbal movements to communicate to them you are not a threat.
3. Keep it simple:
   Speak using simple words in short phrases and talk slowly for maximum comprehension. Ask questions requiring only brief answers. Repeat frequently but allow them time to process the information or question before asking again. Break tasks into smaller steps to avoid frustration.
4. Give reassurance:
   Cognitive impairment makes the patient less confident in conducting their affairs. Give positive reinforcement for correct behaviors. When they are looking confused or anxious, reassure them that everything is going to be all right. Tell them how well they look or that they have done a great job. Adding "thank you very much for all your help" or giving other compliments may diffuse a potential volatile situation.

5. Empathize with and acknowledge their concerns:
    Although their concerns may or may not have any basis in reality, arguing
    with them seldom reduces unwanted behaviors and often exacerbates their
    anger. Do not be a stickler for the truth. You do not have to correct their
    misstatements. Instead, empathize with their predicament and acknowledge
    their concerns. Reassure them that you are on their side. Thank them for
    sharing with you their issues.
6. Don't boss:
    As the dementia progresses, patients are less and less able to make wise
    decisions on their own. Caregivers have to step in and must instruct, request,
    or tell the patient what to do next. Go to the toilet. Take your pills. Go take a
    bath. After a while patients may refuse because they do not like to be bossed.
    One of the best ways to convince a patient to do something they may not
    wish to do is to make them think that it is their choice or their idea to do
    it. Instead of bossing them to take a bath, you can inform the patient that
    you are "taking a bath but do they want to take one first?" You can also say
    "I've started the bath water and I'll take my bath right after you finish" or
    perhaps "are you going to take a bath before we go?" Emphasizing that you
    are doing the same activity reduces their feeling of being singled out. They
    may feel they had more of a choice or a say in the matter.
7. Use distraction or redirection to alter their focus:
    If the patient is about to do something beyond their abilities particularly if
    it could be dangerous to them (cook, drive), then distraction or redirection
    is useful. Bring up another topic, show them a picture, go for a walk, or
    provide them nourishment. Do something they normally enjoy doing as
    an alternative. "Can you help me?" is a phrase that is often successful in
    redirecting the patient away from another activity or from a dangerous
    situation. It is honorable to be asked to help someone else because they
    must think well of your abilities. A patient who is about to wander across
    a dangerous street might come back if you ask them to help you. "Can you
    help me?" can also be used to assist in getting the patient to a particular
    location (bathroom, kitchen). Once in the bathroom it may be much easier to
    get them to toilet or bathe.
8. Watch for utilization behaviors:
    Utilization behaviors refer to a demented patient's propensity to perform a
    task when triggered by a visual cue. This task will be done whether or not it
    is an appropriate time, place, or setting (i.e., open a front door even though
    there is a blizzard outside; getting dressed in the middle of the night; turning
    on the stove with nothing in the pot). Knowing this, caregivers should avoid
    conditions where visual stimuli will trigger actions that could be unsafe. As
    appropriate, they could place things out of sight, cover up doorknobs, hide
    clothes at night, or remove burner knobs. Utilization behaviors, however,
    can also be very helpful to distract the patient from an unwanted behavior.
    If you know that a person likes to squeeze a favorite doll, you can hand
    them this doll so that they will release whatever they are holding that you
    are trying to get away from them. Having the patient push the grocery cart
    (a utilization behavior) may keep them from wandering away or from taking
    unwanted items from the shelves.

9. Out of sight, out of mind:
   Out of sight, out of mind refers to the fact that something in plain view may frequently stimulate an unwanted behavior. Keeping certain things out of sight can be used to prevent utilization behaviors. If you do not have clothes to put on, then you are less likely to wander outside in the middle of the night. To avoid a patient consuming an entire bowl of nuts or candy in two hours, just put out a single portion. If a particular person is triggering behaviors, keep the person away. Remove or cover mirrors if the patient is responding to their reflection as if there were an intruder staring back. Keep things hidden that routinely cause certain reactions or behaviors for the patient.

10. Maintain routines to avoid disorientation:
    Keeping day-to-day activities as nearly the same as possible will help to avoid unnecessary anxiousness or agitation. A change in environment is a very common cause of disorientation and confusion. Patients may get suspicious if anything is out of place or different. Try to avoid unfamiliar environments.

11. Increase daytime activities:
    Increasing daytime activities may help keep the patient's brain stimulated. Activities can calm the patient or occupy their attention so that the caregiver can get other tasks done. Daytime stimulation decreases naps and promotes better sleep at night and may cut down on insomnia. Walking and exercise can reduce wandering and agitation (13). Increasing pleasurable activities may reduce depression. Consider daycare, home aide, and respite care to provide needed supervision and stimulation.

12. Provide an open, safe, contained environment:
    Allowing patients to pace or walk will help decrease agitated behaviors. As the disease progresses, the environment needs to be locked or the patient carefully supervised to ensure the patient's safety.

13. Avoid overstimulating environments:
    Demented patients who are already a bit restless, anxious, irritable, or delusional may exhibit increased behaviors such wanting to leave, striking out, or screaming when there is too much going on in their environment. Avoid overstimulating the patient by taking them out of the immediate environment or by altering the environment. If the patient is going to a family gathering with lots of people, it may be worthwhile to have the patient sit in a quiet room and have one or two family members at time come to visit with them where there is less commotion.

14. Watch for hyperoral behavior:
    Hyperoral behaviors are observed more commonly in frontotemporal degenerative dementias where patients use their mouth to explore both food and nonfood items. If a patient has this type of behavior, they need to be watched carefully to prevent them from ingesting inappropriate items.

15. Reduce evening and nocturnal confusion:
    Sundowning causes confusion in part due to diminished visual and sensory cues. Nighttime sleep disturbances may cause repetitive awakenings at night while it is dark. Increasing light for sundowning and adding a night-light for nighttime behaviors so that it is not totally dark in their room often helps restore calm. Regular sleep habits are a must. Avoid naps if at all possible

by increasing daytime activities. Avoid late meals, caffeine, alcohol, and excessive stimulation before bedtime.

16. Increase calming sensory stimulation:
    Music can be effective in some patients to reduce agitation and mood disturbances during bathing and eating (14). One on one social interaction may quiet verbally disruptive behavior. Pet therapy may improve socialization (15). Light therapy for 30 minutes a day for two weeks was reported to reduce restlessness in dementia subjects (16). Aromatherapy using lemon balm improved agitation and socialization in 72 severely demented residents of a nursing home (17).

GENERAL PRINCIPLES OF PHARMACOTHERAPY FOR BEHAVIORS

Many behaviors may be so persistent or severe that medications are required in addition to the behavioral modification. Unfortunately, there are very few double-blind, placebo-controlled trials that evaluate medications for the treatment of behavioral disturbances in dementia patients. Much of our data come from open-label trials or anecdotal use. As such, the suggested preferred treatment recommendations given below are based on review of the literature and personal experience. Since there are no FDA-approved agents for any of the behavioral problems seen in dementia patients, all of the drugs discussed below are for off-label use.

The potential use of polypharmacy in the treatment of behavioral disturbances is very appropriate with dementia patients. In AD, many neurotransmitters and their targets are affected. Depending on the behaviors displayed, it makes sense to apply rational pharmacotherapy to assist in the restoration of impaired serotonin, acetylcholine, dopamine, or other neural circuits/chemicals. Table 3 lists the common behavioral medications used in treating the neuropsychiatric symptoms of dementia.

General pharmacotherapy guidelines:

1. Individualize all treatments taking into account concurrent medical problems and medications.
2. All medications should start at a low dose and increase gradually.
3. For geriatric patients start medications at one-half to one-third the usual adult recommended starting dose.
4. Periodically medications should be reduced or stopped to determine ongoing need.

BEHAVIORAL DISTURBANCES AND PREFERRED PHARMACOTHERAPY APPROACHES

Aggression and Agitation Behaviors

Aggressive and combative behaviors are seen in 60% and irritability in 42% of AD patients (1). Often there is a quick onset and offset of being angry, impatient, or frustrated over something. Some trigger in the environment is usually responsible, although there may be no obvious cause. Changing the subject, redirecting focus onto something else, or moving the offending stimuli is helpful. These behaviors often result in nursing home placement for AD patients (18). Appropriate treatment may enable the patient to stay at home for a longer period.

Table 3 Common Behavioral Drugs Used to Treat Dementia Syndromes

Drugs, generic name (brand name)	Common adverse effects	Recommended target doses
Antidepressants		
Bupropion (Wellbutrin)	Agitation, seizures, restlessness, insomnia, arrhythmia	75–300 mg/day
Citalopram (Celexa)	Nausea, dry mouth, sedation	10–40 mg/day
Clomipramine (Anafranil)	Sedation, seizures, weight gain, sexual dysfunction	50–250 mg/day in two doses
Desipramine (Norpramin)	Mild anticholinergic, orthostasis	25–150 mg/day
Escitalopram (Lexapro)	Nausea, dry mouth, sedation	5–10 mg/day
Fluoxetine (Prozac)	Anxiety, insomnia, nausea, weight loss, tremor	10–40 mg/day
Fluvoxamine (Luvox)	Nausea, insomnia, sedation	50–300 mg/day in two doses
Mirtazapine (Remeron)	Sedation, weight gain, dry mouth	15–30 mg/day
Nortriptyline (Pamelor)	Mild anticholinergic, sedation, orthostasis	25–100 mg/day; check plasma levels
Paroxetine (Paxil)	Insomnia, nausea, anxiety	10–40 mg/day
Sertraline (Zoloft)	Insomnia, diarrhea, tremor	50–200 mg/day
Trazodone (Desyrel)	Sedation, mild orthostasis	50–300 mg/day
Venlafaxine (Effexor)	Nausea, sedation	37.5–150 XR mg/day
Antipsychotics		
Aripiprazole (Abilify)	Activation, sedation	5–15 mg/day
Clozapine (Clozaril)	Agranulocytosis, orthostasis, anticholinergic, sedation, weight gain, seizures	6.25–100 mg/day in one or two doses; WBC w/diff q week
Haloperidol (Haldol)	Parkinsonism, sedation, falling, dyskinesia	0.25–2 mg/day; increase gradually
Olanzapine (Zyprexa)	Orthostasis, anticholinergic, sedation, weight gain	2.5–10 mg/day
Quetiapine (Seroquel)	Sedation, orthostasis, weight gain	12.5–200 mg/day in two doses
Risperidone (Risperdal)	Sedation, Parkinsonism, weight gain	0.5–2 mg/day in two doses
Ziprasidone (Geodon)	QT prolongation, sedation, Parkinsonism, orthostasis	20–160 mg/day
Miscellaneous		
Buspirone (Buspar)	Dizziness, nausea, headache	10–60 mg/day in divided doses
Carbamazepine (Tegretol)	Cognitive impairment, ataxia, nausea, leukopenia	200–800 mg/day in three divided doses
Cimetidine (Tagamet)	Headache, diarrhea	100–300 mg qid
Donepezil (Aricept)	Nausea, vomiting, diarrhea, anorexia	5–10 mg once daily
Gabapentin (Neurontin)	Sedation, ataxia, confusion	100–600 mg/day in two divided doses
Galantamine (Razadyne)	Nausea, vomiting, diarrhea, anorexia	16–24 mg/day in two divided doses or extended-release (ER) 16–24 mg once daily
Lamotrigine (Lamictal)	Rash, hepatic/renal failure, arthritis	50–500 mg/day in two divided doses
Lorazepam (Ativan)	Confusion, sedation, disinhibition, ataxia	0.5–2 mg/day in divided doses

(Continued)

Table 3   Common Behavioral Drugs Used to Treat Dementia Syndromes (*Continued*)

Drugs, generic name (brand name)	Common adverse effects	Recommended target doses
Megestrol acetate (Megace)	Thrombophlebitis, pulmonary embolism, glucose intolerance	400–800 mg/day in two divided doses
Melatonin or Ramelteon (Rozerem)	Sleepiness	8 mg/day before bed
Memantine (Namenda)	Headache, dizziness, agitation	10 mg twice a day
Propranolol (Inderal)	Bradycardia, hypotension	40–320 mg/day
Rivastigmine (Exelon)	Nausea, vomiting, diarrhea, anorexia	6–12 mg/day in two divided doses or one 9.5 mg/24 hour patch daily
Valproate (Depakote)	Nausea, sedation, rare hepatotoxicity, pancreatitis	125–1000 mg/day in three divided doses
Zolpidem (Ambien)	Daytime drowsiness, dizziness, headache	5 mg/day

Often the most successful way to decrease aggressive outbursts is to look for the underlying behavioral symptoms (Table 2) that led to the agitation and to target treatment to those underlying behaviors. Aggression is not on the list in Table 2 as it is usually the end result of one or more of the different types of underlying behaviors. Environmental disruption can lead to reactive aggression by the patient who is being bossed by others or being told what to do. Psychosis, delusional beliefs, or suspicious often results in agitation. Anxiousness or fear can lead to aggression. The excessively restless patient, who needs to keep moving, may strike out at anyone who gets in their way. Intrusive or disinhibited patients can encroach on others to such an extent that it draws out a fight.

Treatment of Aggressive and Agitated Behaviors in Dementia

There have been numerous pharmacotherapy trials testing if a specific drug reduced aggression in dementia subjects (Table 4). Double-blind controlled trials have shown significance in reducing aggression with the use of citalopram (19,20), trazodone (21), haloperidol (21–25), risperidone (20,23,24,26–31), quetiapine (31–33), olanzapine (25,30,34–36), aripiprazole (37,38), valproate (39), carbamazepine (40–42), lorazepam (36), memantine (43,44), and cyproterone (an antiandrogen agent) (45). Open-label trials with gabapentin (46), trazodone (47,48), risperidone (49,50) quetiapine (51,52), clozapine (53), ziprasidone (54–56), valproate (57–59), carbamazepine (60,61), topiramate (62), clonazepam (63), buspirone (64), rivastigmine (65,66), and propranolol (67,68) have also shown benefit. However, two double-blind, placebo-controlled study of divalproex sodium in AD subjects found no reduction in agitation or other behaviors compared with placebo (69,70). One placebo-controlled study using haloperidol or fluoxetine and another using quetiapine or rivastigmine found no differences in agitation versus placebo (71,72). Another study in AD outpatients comparing placebo, haloperidol, trazodone, and behavior management techniques showed no differences in agitated behavior between the groups (73).

With all these treatments that have shown efficacy, it is hard for the practitioner to decide which agent may have the best chance of success in a specific

Table 4 Studies for the Treatment of Aggression and Agitation in Dementia

Study	Subjects	Agents	Design	Results
Pollock et al., 2002 (19)	N = 85 inpatient dementia	Citalopram 20 mg/day	DBPC	→ Agitation, ↓ lability, ↓ psychosis
Pollock et al., 2007 (20)	N = 103 inpatient dementia	Citalopram or risperidone	DB	→ Agitation and psychosis with both agents
Sultzer et al., 1997 (21)	N = 28 dementia	Trazodone 50–250 mg or haloperidol 1–5 mg	DB	→ Agitation with both agents
Kitamura et al., 2006 (47)	N = 13 AD with aggression	Trazodone various doses	Retrospective chart review	6 of 13 ↓ aggression; 9 of 13 ↓ overall behaviors
Lopez-Pousa et al., 2008 (48)	N = 24 AD	Trazodone various doses	Open label	↓ Irritability, no change in overall behavior score
Devanand et al., 1998 (22)	N = 71 AD outpatients	Haloperidol 0.5–0.75 mg or haloperidol 2–3 mg or placebo	DBPC	↓ Agitation and psychosis in haloperidol high dose
De Deyn et al., 1999 (23)	N = 344 dementia	Risperidone 0.5–4 mg or haloperidol 0.5–4 mg	DB	→ Aggression with risperidone
Chan et al., 2001 (24)	N = 58 AD or vascular dementia	Risperidone 0.5–2 mg (mean 0.85 mg) or haloperidol 0.5–2 mg	DB 12 wk	Improved diurnal rhythm, → activity disturbances, and → agitation in both groups
Suh et al., 2006 (26)	N = 114 dementia nursing home with behaviors	Risperidone 0.5–1.5 mg or haloperidol 0.5–1.5 mg	DB	→ Agitation, wandering, and anxiety with risperidone
Katz et al., 1999 (27)	N = 625 AD and/or vascular dementia	Risperidone 0.5, 1.0, or 2.0 mg or placebo	DBPC	→ Aggression and psychosis
Brodaty et al., 2003 (28)	N = 345 nursing home dementia	Risperidone 0.5–2 mg or placebo	PC	→ Aggression and psychosis
Holmes et al., 2007 (29)	N = 28 AD	Risperidone 0.5–1 mg or rivastigmine 3 mg bid	DB	↓ Agitation with risperidone
Lavretsky et al., 1998 (49)	N = 15 dementia with agitation	Risperidone (variable dose, modal 0.5 mg)	Open label	↓ Agitation in all 15
Onor et al., 2007 (50)	N = 135 AD	Risperidone 1 mg (mean)	Open 12-wk study	↓ Agitation, psychosis, and anxiety

(Continued)

Table 4 Studies for the Treatment of Aggression and Agitation in Dementia (*Continued*)

Study	Subjects	Agents	Design	Results
Schneider et al., 2006 (30)	N = 421 AD with psychosis or agitation	Olanzapine, quetiapine, risperidone, or placebo	DBPC	Longer time to treatment discontinuation for lack of efficacy for olanzapine and risperidone
Rainer et al., 2007 (31)	N = 72 dementia	Quetiapine 77 mg (mean) or risperidol 0.9 mg (mean)	Rater blinded	↓ Agitation with both
Zhong et al., 2007 (32)	N = 333 nursing home dementia	Quetiapine 100 or 200 mg or placebo	DBPC	↓ Agitation with quetiapine 200 mg/day
Tariot et al., 2006 (33)	N = 284 AD with psychosis	Quetiapine 97 mg (mean) or haloperidol 2 mg (mean) or placebo	DBPC	↓ Agitation with quetiapine vs. placebo; ↓ psychosis in all groups but not significant
Scharre et al., 2002 (51)	N = 10 AD	Quetiapine 50–150 mg range	Open 12 wk	↓ Aggression, delusions, overall behaviors
Onor et al., 2006 (52)	N = 41 (20 AD, 6 vascular, 6 mixed, 5 Lewy)	Quetiapine	Open	↓ Aggression, psychosis, sleep disturbance
Street et al., 2000 (34)	N = 206 Nursing home AD	Olanzapine 5, 10, 15 mg or placebo	DBPC	↓ Agitation and psychosis for 5 and 10 mg
De Deyn et al., 2004 (35)	N = 652 AD with psychosis	Olanzapine 1, 2.5, 5, 7.5 mg or placebo	DBPC	↓ Psychosis and overall behaviors for 7.5 mg
Meehan et al., 2002 (36)	N = 272 dementia with agitation	IM Olanzapine 2.5 or 5 mg, IM lorazepam 1 mg or IM placebo	DBPC	↓ Agitation for all groups vs. placebo
Verhey et al., 2006 (25)	N = 58 dementia outpatients with agitation	Olanzapine 4.71 mg (average) or haloperidol 1.75 mg (average)	DB	↓ Agitation for both groups
Mintzer et al., 2007 (37)	N = 487 AD with psychosis, institutionalized	Aripiprazole 2, 5, or 10 mg/day, and placebo	DBPC	↓ Psychosis and aggression at 10 mg/day; ↓ aggression at 5 mg; no effect at 2 mg
Streim et al., 2008 (38)	N = 265 AD with psychosis, institutionalized	Aripiprazole 2–15 mg/day variable and placebo	DBPC	↓ Agitation, anxiety, depression; no effect on psychosis

Study	Sample	Drug/dose	Design	Outcome
Lee et al., 2007 (53)	N = 16 dementia with agitation	Clozapine (variable dose, mean 44.6 mg)	Retrospective chart review	62.5% much improved agitation
Cole et al., 2005 (54)	N = 4 dementia with agitation and psychosis	Ziprasidone 20–160 mg	Open	↓ Psychosis and agitation
Rocha et al., 2006 (55)	N = 25 dementia	Ziprasidone	Open 7-wk study	↓ Behavioral symptoms of dementia
Rais et al., 2010 (56)	N = 14 dementia with agitation or psychosis	IM ziprasidone 10 mg once or twice	Open	↓ Psychosis and agitation
Porsteinsson et al., 2001 (39)	N = 56 nursing home dementia with agitation	Divalproex sodium (variable dose) or placebo	SBPC	↓ Agitation
Lott et al., 1995 (57)	N = 10 nursing home dementia with agitation	Valproate 375–750 mg	Open	↓ Agitation by 50% in 8 out of 10
Porsteinsson et al., 2003 (58)	N = 46 Nursing home dementia with agitation	Divalproex sodium (variable dose)	Open	↓ Agitation
Forester et al., 2007 (59)	N = 15 dementia	Divalproex sodium 656 mg (mean) alone or with antipsychotic	Open	↓ Aggressive behaviors and disinhibition
Tariot et al., 2005 (69)	N = 153 Nursing home AD with agitation	Divalproex sodium 800 mg (mean) or placebo	DBPC	No significant change in agitation from placebo
Herrmann 2007 (70)	N = 14 AD with aggression	Valproate or placebo	DBPC 6-wk crossover study	Agitation and aggression worsened with valproate
Tariot et al., 1994 (40)	N = 25 nursing home dementia with agitation	Carbamazepine 300 mg (modal dose) or placebo	PC	↓ Agitation
Tariot et al., 1998 (41)	N = 51 nursing home dementia with agitation	Carbamazepine (variable dose) or placebo	SBPC	↓ Agitation
Olin et al., 2001 (42)	N = 21 AD with agitation	Carbamazepine 400 mg or placebo	DBPC	↓ Hostility
Gleason et al., 1990 (60)	N = 9 AD	Carbamazepine	Open	↓ Agitation in 5 out of 9
Lemke, 1995 (61)	N = 15 dementia with agitation	Carbamazepine 246 mg (mean)	Open	↓ Agitation, emotional lability and impulsivity

(Continued)

Table 4 Studies for the Treatment of Aggression and Agitation in Dementia (*Continued*)

Study	Subjects	Agents	Design	Results
Hawkins et al., 2000 (46)	N = 24 Nursing home dementia with agitation	Gabapentin (variable dose)	Retrospective chart review	17 out of 22 were much or greatly improved, 2 discontinued (sedation)
Cummings et al., 2005 (65)	N = 173 Nursing home AD	Rivastigmine 3–12 mg	Open	→ Delusions, hallucinations, agitation, apathy, lability, aberrant motor behaviors, sleep disturbance, eating changes
Gauthier et al., 2007 (66)	N = 2119 AD	Rivastigmine	Open	Subjects improved anxiety in 62%, apathy in 63%, and agitation in 56%
Gauthier et al., 2005 (43)	N = 252 AD	Memantine	DBPC	→ Delusions, agitation
Cummings et al., 2006 (44)	N = 404 AD	Memantine + donepezil vs. donepezil alone	DBPC	→ Lability, agitation, appetite/eating change
Huertas et al., 2007 (45)	N = 24 AD with aggression	Cyproterone 100 mg or haloperidol 2 mg	DB	→ Aggression with cyproterone
Fhager et al., 2003 (62)	N = 15 dementia and aggression	Topiramate 75 mg (median) alone or with antipsychotic	Retrospective study	→ Agitation with both groups
Calkin et al., 1997 (63)	N = 21 with 50% dementia inpatients	Clonazepam 1.2 mg (mean)	Retrospective study	→ Agitation and total behavioral scores
Weiler et al., 1988 (67)	N = 6 dementia	Propranolol 80–560 mg	Open	→ Agitation
Shankle et al., 1995 (67)	N = 12 dementia	Propranolol 10–80 mg	Open	→ Agitation
Auchus et al., 1997 (71)	N = 15 AD with agitation	Haloperidol, fluoxetine, or placebo	PC	No differences in agitation vs. placebo
Ballard et al., 2005 (72)	N = 93 AD in nursing homes	Quetiapine 50–100 mg or rivastigmine 6–9 mg or palcebo	DBPC 26-week study	No differences in agitation vs. placebo
Teri et al., 2000 (73)	N = 149 AD outpatients with agitation	Haloperidol, trazodone, behavior modification, or placebo	PC	No differences in agitation vs. placebo

AD, Alzheimer's disease; DB, double blind; PC, placebo control; SB, dingle blind.

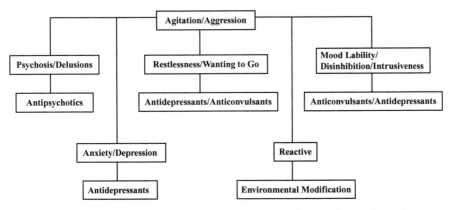

Figure 1 Preferred approaches for agitation and aggression: first decide upon the main underlying symptoms of the agitation and aggression and then try the suggested behavioral pharmacotherapy or management.

individual. It is recommended that instead of just guessing, the chance of success is far better if treatment is targeted to the individual's specific underlying behaviors (Fig. 1) leading to their agitation. That is in patients with aggression due to delusions and psychosis, atypical antipsychotics are preferred. If agitation is associated with restlessness or wanting to go behaviors, then antidepressants or possibly anticonvulsants should be considered. When disinhibition or intrusiveness is the cause of the aggression, try anticonvulsants before antidepressants. When anxiety, dysphoria, or depression seems to be the trigger for aggression, antidepressants are the suggested first-line treatments (74). Finally for reactive agitation, modifying the environment, which is often the culprit, is the best treatment. The preferred approaches to pharmacotherapy of the underlying behaviors are described in detail below.

Psychotic Behaviors

Delusions (false fixed beliefs) occur in up to 70% of AD patients (75). The most common delusions include people stealing things, suspiciousness and paranoia, unwelcome visitors, one's house is not one's home, the spouse is an impostor, the delusion of abandonment, the delusion of infidelity, somatic delusions, misidentification of people, the image in mirror is not the patient, and television characters being real. Hallucinations can be seen in AD patients and are mostly visual. They occur in 12% to 15% of AD patients (1). Patients with dementia with Lewy bodies have a much higher frequency of visual hallucinations and this is one criterion for the diagnosis of that disorder (3).

Treatment of Psychotic Behaviors in Dementia

Treatment studies targeting psychotic behaviors in dementia have mostly used typical and atypical antipsychotic medications. However, other agents are also being evaluated. Suggested preferred treatments for psychosis are listed in Table 5 and specific studies are listed in Table 6 (76). Atypical antipsychotic agents are generally preferred over typical antipsychotic drugs due to tolerance issues, and low-potency neuroleptics are generally avoided because of their anticholinergic

Table 5 Suggested Preferred Treatments for Psychosis in Dementia

Psychosis: First-line suggested preferred treatments
1. Quetiapine[a], risperidone[a], ziprasidone
2. Olanzapine[a], aripiprazole[a]

Psychosis: Second-line suggested preferred treatments
1. Haloperidol[a]
2. Clozapine
3. Cholinesterase inhibitors[a], memantine[a]

Psychosis: Avoid
1. Thioridazine and other typical antipsychotics

[a]Positive double-blind studies.

properties. Antipsychotics as a group are not FDA approved for agitation or psychosis associated with dementia, and in fact there is some concern regarding adverse effects offsetting their advantages (30). However, their advantages are understated since most of the placebo-controlled studies using antipsychotics are limited by selection bias as most moderate to severe psychotic patients will generally not be willing to join a study and to take the chance on a placebo.

Positive double-blind and/or placebo-controlled studies for reduction of psychotic behaviors with haloperidol (22), risperidone (27,28,30), quetiapine (32), olanzapine (30,34,35,77,78), and aripiprazole (37,79) have been reported. Aripiprazole was shown not to be effective for psychosis or behavioral symptoms in AD subjects in some studies (38,79,80), and negative results have been reported with quetiapine and risperidone (81–83). One double-blind comparative study between risperidone and haloperidol indicated a better response with risperidone (23). A double-blind comparative study between citalopram and risperidone showed no difference in reduction of agitation or psychosis (20). A double-blind, placebo-controlled trial comparing quetiapine and haloperidol showed reduced psychosis in all groups, but there were no significant differences between groups (33). Positive open-label studies showed reduction in psychosis with risperidone in AD subjects, with ziprasidone in dementia cases, and with quetiapine in AD individuals, in a mixed dementia cohort and in Lewy body dementia (50–52,54,56,84).

Use of a particular agent is usually based on side effect profiles and dosing considerations. Of my first-line suggested medications, quetiapine, risperidone, and ziprasidone have very little anticholinergic properties. All agents with anticholinergic characteristics can increase confusion in dementia patients, and they will directly counter some of the benefits of cholinesterase inhibitors (donepezil, rivastigmine, galantamine). Quetiapine, risperidone, and ziprasidone all have low strength options allowing individual flexibility in dosing. Ziprasidone also has an intramuscular formulation with low sedative qualities that is very useful for out-of-control patients. Olanzapine has a bit more anticholinergic side effects than my top three choices, and aripiprazole can be activating. Quetiapine may be sedating at its lowest doses, and risperidone can increase the risk of extrapyramidal symptoms.

I have included haloperidol as a second-line suggested treatment since it comes in an intramuscular form and is very inexpensive. Clozapine is useful in treatment refractory cases with moderate to severe psychosis especially

Table 6 Studies for the Treatment of Psychosis in Dementia

Study	Subjects	Agents	Design	Results
Devanand et al., 1998 (22)	N = 71 AD outpatients	Haloperidol 0.5–0.75 mg or haloperidol 2–3 mg or placebo	DBPC	→ Agitation and psychosis in haloperidol high dose
Katz et al., 1999 (27)	N = 625 AD and/or vascular dementia	Risperidone 0.5, 1.0, or 2.0 mg or placebo	DBPC	→ Aggression and psychosis
Brodaty et al., 2003 (28)	N = 345 nursing home dementia	Risperidone 0.5–2 mg or placebo	PC	→ Aggression and psychosis
Mintzer et al., 2006 (83)	N = 473 nursing home AD	Risperidone 1–1.5 mg or placebo	DBPC 8-wk	→ Psychosis for both with no significant difference
Schneider et al., 2006 (30)	N = 421 AD with psychosis or agitation	Olanzapine, quetiapine, risperidone, or placebo	DBPC	Longer time to treatment discontinuation for lack of efficacy for olanzapine and risperidone
Onor et al., 2007 (50)	N = 135 AD	Risperidone 1 mg (mean)	Open 12-wk study	→ Agitation, psychosis, and anxiety
Zhong et al., 2007 (32)	N = 333 nursing home dementia	Quetiapine 100 or 200 mg or placebo	DBPC	→ Agitation with quetiapine 200 mg/day
Tariot et al., 2006 (33)	N = 284 AD with psychosis	Quetiapine 97 mg (mean) or haloperidol 2 mg (mean) or placebo	DBPC	→ Agitation with quetiapine vs. placebo; ↓ psychosis in all groups but not significant
Scharre et al., 2002 (51)	N = 10 AD	Quetiapine 50–150 mg range	Open 12-week	→ aggression, delusions, overall behaviors
Fernandez et al., 2002 (84)	N = 11 Lewy body dementia	Quetiapine	Retrospective chart review	10/11 with partial/complete psychosis resolution
Onor et al., 2006 (52)	N = 41 (20 AD, 6 vascular, 6 mixed, 5 Lewy)	Quetiapine	Open	→ Aggression, psychosis, sleep disturbance
Kurlan et al., 2007 (81)	N = 40 (23 = Lewy body dementia, 8 = Parkinson's dementia, 9 = AD)	Quetiapine 120 mg median dose	DBPC	No differences in agitation or psychosis from placebo

(Continued)

Table 6 Studies for the Treatment of Psychosis in Dementia (*Continued*)

Study	Subjects	Agents	Design	Results
Paleacu et al., 2008 (82)	N = 40 AD	Quetiapine 200 mg average	DBPC 6-wk trial	No differences in behaviors from placebo
Street et al., 2000 (34)	N = 206 Nursing home AD	Olanzapine 5, 10, 15 mg, or placebo	DBPC	↓ Psychosis and agitation for 5 and 10 mg
Clark et al., 2001 (77)	N = 165 Nursing home AD with no psychosis	Olanzapine 5, 10, 15 mg, or placebo	DBPC post hoc subgroup analysis	Attenuation of the emergence of psychosis
Cummings et al., 2002 (78)	N = 29 Dementia with Lewy bodies	Olanzapine 5, 10, 15 mg, or placebo	DBPC post hoc subgroup analysis	↓ Psychosis for 5 and 10 mg groups
De Deyn et al., 2004 (35)	N = 652 AD with psychosis	Olanzapine 1, 2.5, 5, 7.5 mg or placebo	DBPC	↓ Psychosis and overall behaviors for 7.5 mg
Mintzer et al., 2007 (37)	N = 487 AD with psychosis, institutionalized	Aripiprazole 2, 5, or 10 mg/day, and placebo	DBPC	↓ Psychosis and aggression at 10 mg/day; ↓ aggression at 5 mg; no effect at 2 mg
De Deyn et al., 2005 (79)	N = 208 AD with psychosis, outpatients	Aripiprazole 2–15 mg/day variable, and placebo	DBPC	↓ Psychosis on one scale but not another vs. placebo
Hamuro A 2007 (80)	N = 10 (7 AD, 2 vascular, 1 FTD)	Aripiprazole minimum of 3 mg	Open	No effect on behavioral symptoms
Streim et al., 2008 (38)	N = 265 AD with psychosis, institutionalized	Aripiprazole 2–15 mg/day variable and placebo	DBPC	↓ Agitation, anxiety, depression; no effect on psychosis
De Deyn et al., 1999 (23)	N = 344 dementia	Risperidone 0.5–4 mg or haloperidol 0.5–4 mg	DB	↓Aggression with risperidone
Pollock et al., 2007 (20)	N = 103 inpatient dementia	Citalopram or risperidone	DB	↓ Agitation and psychosis with both agents
Cole et al., 2005 (54)	N = 4 dementia with agitation and psychosis	Ziprasidone 20–160 mg	Open	↓ Psychosis and agitation
Rais et al., 2010 (56)	N = 14 dementia with agitation or psychosis	IM ziprasidone 10 mg once or twice	Open	↓ Psychosis and agitation

Study	Population	Drug	Design	Outcome
Tanaka et al., 2005 (85)	N = 2 Lewy body with visual hallucinations	Paroxetine	Open	↓ Visual hallucinations
Cummings et al., 2006 (86)	N = 120 AD with severe behaviors	Donepezil	Open	Total or partial resolution of depressions and delusions
Cummings et al., 2005 (65)	N = 173 Nursing home AD	Rivastigmine 3–12 mg	Open	↓ Delusions, hallucinations, agitation, apathy, lability, aberrant motor behaviors, sleep disturbance, eating changes
Monsch et al., 2004 (87)	N = 124 AD	Galantamine 8–24 mg	Open	30% improvement in anxiety, aberrant motor behaviors, delusions, euphoria, sleep disturbance
Tangwongchai et al., 2008 (88)	N = 75 AD and mixed dementia	Galantamine 16–24 mg	Open	↓ Delusions, anxiety, phobias, sleep disturbance
Erkinjuntti et al., 2002 (89)	N = 592 Vascular and AD/vascular mixed	Galantamine 24 mg	DBPC 6-mo	↓ Anxiety, apathy, delusions compared with placebo
Litvinenko et al., 2008 (90)	N = 41 Parkinson's disease dementia	Galantamine 16 mg	PC	↓ Hallucinations, anxiety, apathy, sleep disturbance
Edwards et al., 2007 (91)	N = 50 Lewy body dementia	Galantamine 16–24 mg	Open 24-wk	↓ Visual hallucinations, sleep disturbance
Gauthier et al., 2005 (43)	N = 252 AD	Memantine	DBPC	↓ Delusions, agitation

AD, Alzheimer's disease; DB, double blind; FTD, frontotemporal dementia; PC, placebo control.

if the patient has Parkinsonism or tardive dyskinesia. Paroxetine was found useful for the visual hallucinations seen in dementia with Lewy bodies (85). The cholinesterase inhibitors, donepezil, rivastigmine, and galantamine have shown some propensity to reduce psychosis in AD (65,86–89), and galantamine may reduce hallucinations in those with vascular dementia, Parkinson's disease dementia, and in dementia with Lewy bodies (89–91). Memantine may also reduce delusions (43).

Side effects of antipsychotics, most commonly seen with the typical agents (Table 3), include Parkinsonism, tardive dyskinesia, anticholinergic effects, orthostasis, akathisia, gait disturbance, sedation, and weight gain (92). Mortality incidence with olanzapine was significantly higher than with placebo in olanzapine dementia clinical trials (93). A meta-analysis of randomized placebo-controlled trials of atypical antipsychotic drug treatments for dementia found a significantly higher risk of death with these medications (94), but this was similar to the risk with typical antipsychotics (95). QT prolongation and possible arrhythmias with the use of ziprasidone initially were of concern but are rarely seen. Monitoring of those at high risk or QT prolongation is suggested (96). Weight gain, elevated glucose, and hypertriglyceridemia are reported with the atypical antipsychotics but appear to be most prevalent with the use of olanzapine (30,97). Thioridazine and other typical antipsychotics are to be avoided because their effective doses often cause undesirable side effects (98).

Depression

A depressed mood and a loss of interest or pleasure in activities characterize depression (99). Symptoms may include sadness, crying, hopelessness, helplessness, worthlessness, guilt, and suicidal ideation. Patients with depression enjoy life less. Neurovegetative dysfunction is common with fatigue, significant weight changes, sleep disturbances, and decreased libido as examples. Psychomotor activation or retardation, cognitive disturbances, impaired attention, poor concentration, and even dementia may occur.

Pseudodementia, dementia due solely to the depression condition, is uncommon but is in the differential of patients with cognitive disturbances (10). A subcortical pattern of impairment on mental status testing is seen typically with frontal subcortical deficits (6). The cognitive impairments will clear as the depression is treated.

Of course, many dementia conditions may also show features of depression due to the involvement of specific neuroanatomical circuits or neurotransmitter systems. The locus ceruleus, substantia nigra, limbic regions, frontal circuits, and subcortical areas are some examples where damage has been associated with increased symptoms of depression (100). Depression is very common in Huntington's disease with its subcortical and basal ganglia pathology (7). Severe small vessel vascular disease causing dementia heavily damages subcortical white matter and basal ganglia regions and is often associated with depression. In AD, depression is reported in 14% to 85% depending on the study and how investigators defined depression (1,101,102). However, major depressive disorder occurs fairly infrequently in AD. Neurotransmitter deficiencies particularly serotonin and norepinephrine are related to depressive symptoms and treatments are often

Table 7 Suggested Preferred Treatments for Depression and Dysphoria in Dementia

Depression: First-line suggested preferred treatments
1. Sertraline[a], citalopram[a], escitalopram
2. Paroxetine[a], fluvoxamine[a], fluoxetine[a]

Depression: Second-line suggested preferred treatments
1. Venlafaxine, bupropion, mirtazapine
2. Trazodone[a]
3. Lamotrigine
4. Clomipramine[a], nortriptyline, desipramine

Depression: Avoid
1. Tertiary tricyclic antidepressants

[a]Positive double-blind studies.

directed at these neurochemicals. Caregiver distress over the symptoms of depression can be significant. One study showed that 70% of caregivers were moderate to highly distressed with the patient's depressive symptoms (103).

Treatment of Depression and Dysphoria Behaviors in Dementia

Antidepressants are the mainstays of treatment for depression in dementia. Suggested preferred treatments for depression and dysphoria are listed in Table 7 and specific studies are listed in Table 8. There are several studies in the literature using selective-serotonin reuptake inhibitors (SSRIs) (citalopram, escitalopram, sertraline, paroxetine, fluoxetine, fluvoxamine, mirtazapine, and trazodone) that found them to be beneficial for depression in dementia patients (104–123). Only very few studies using SSRIs in AD have not shown benefit for depression (124–126). SSRIs have gained the most popularity as first-line treatments for the depression symptoms seen in dementia due to their favorable side effect profile. They are very effective agents for depression, have low anticholinergic properties in general, minimal effects on cognition, and typically do not have a lot of sedative properties (109,110,127). The choice of SSRI is usually based on matching their side effect profile to the patient. Paroxetine and fluvoxamine are slightly more sedating, fluoxetine is more energizing, and sertraline and citalopram are in-between. Paroxetine has mild anticholinergic properties and has been noted to impair cognition without efficacy in a double-blind randomized controlled trial in FTD subjects (128). For most AD patients, I will use either sertraline or citalopram before the others to avoid insomnia, sedation, and anticholinergic effects.

Alternative treatment choices include venlafaxine, bupropion, and mirtazapine all of which block serotonin and norepinephrine reuptake. Bupropion blocks dopamine reuptake as well. Venlafaxine can increase blood pressure and may have less tolerability in the frail elderly than sertraline (112). Bupropion lowers seizure threshold. Mirtazapine may be useful in patients who are losing weight and have insomnia (121). Trazodone can help with insomnia, although it may not be as effective as other antidepressants for depression symptoms (123). Three studies using tricyclic antidepressants (clomipramine, moclobemide, and maprotiline) in dementia patients with depression showed benefit (129–131) but

Table 8 Studies for the Treatment of Depression in Dementia

Study	Subjects	Agents	Design	Results
Nyth et al., 1990 (104)	N = 98 AD, Vascular dementia	Citalopram 10–30 mg/day	DB and open	↑ Mood, ↓ anxiety, irritability for AD only
Nyth et al., 1992 (105)	N = 29 dementia	Citalopram 10–20 mg	DBPC	→ Depressive symptoms
Karlsson et al., 2000 (106)	N = 336 demented and nondemented	Citalopram 20–40 mg; mianserin 30–60 mg	DB	→ Depression with both agents
Rao et al., 2006 (107)	N = AD with depression	Escitalopram	Open	→ Depression
Lyketsos et al., 2000 (108)	N = 22 AD	Sertraline	DBPC	→ Depression
Lyketsos et al., 2003 (109,110)	N = 44 AD and MDD	Sertraline, mean dose 95 mg/day	DBPC	→ Depression and behavior disturbance
Finkel et al., 2004 (111)	N = 109 AD	Sertraline or placebo both with donepezil	DBPC	→ Dysphoria, anxiety, irritability, aggression
Magai et al., 2000 (124)	N = 31 severe AD	Sertraline	DBPC	No benefit
Oslin et al., 2003 (112)	N = 34 dementia and 18 not	Sertraline up to 100 mg/day; venlafaxine up to 150 mg/day	DB	No difference in efficacy; venlafaxine less safe and well tolerated
Volicer et al., 1994 (113)	N = 10 AD with depression	Sertraline various doses	Open label	8 out of 10 ↓ depression, 5 out of 6 ↓ food refusal
Burke et al., 1997 (114)	N = 20 dementia (12 AD)	Sertraline 50 mg; one paroxetine	Retrospective	Moderate to markedly improved
Katona et al., 1998 (115)	N = 198 dementia	Paroxetine 20–40 mg; imipramine 50–100 mg	DB	→ Depression for both Paroxetine and imipramine
Moretti et al., 2003 (116)	N = 16 FTD	Paroxetine 20 mg; piracetam 1200 mg	Open	↓Weeping, depression, social dysdecorum, agitation with paroxetine
Taragano et al., 1997 (117)	N = 37 AD	Fluoxetine; amitriptyline	DB	→ Depression with both agents
Petracca et al., 2001 (125)	N = 41 AD	Fluoxetine up to 40 mg/day	DBPC	No benefit
Sobow et al., 2001 (118)	N = 35 AD	19 on fluoxetine; 16 on tianeptine	Retrospective	→ Depression with both agents
Swartz et al., 1997 (119)	N = 11 FTD	Fluoxetine, sertraline, or paroxetine	Open	→ Depression, compulsions, and disinhibition in at least half

Study	Population	Drug/Dose	Design	Outcome
Olafsson et al., 1992 (120)	N = 46 dementia	Fluvoxamine 150 mg	DBPC	Trends for ↑ mood, ↓ irritability, fear, anxiety, restlessness
de Vasconcelos et al., 2007 (126)	N = 31 dementia	Venlafaxine flexible dose	DBPC	No benefit
Raji et al., 2001 (121)	N = 3 dementia and depression	Mirtazapine	Open	→ Depression, weight loss, sleep disturbances, anxiety
Lebert et al., 2004 (122)	N = 26 FTD	Trazodone	DBPC	→ Irritability, agitation, dysphoria, eating disorders
Lebert et al., 1994 (123)	N = 13 AD	Trazodone 25 mg tid	Open	→ Irritability, anxiety, restlessness, affective disturbance
Petracca et al., 1996 (129)	N = 24 AD	Clomipramine 25–100 mg/day	DBPC	→ Depression
Roth et al., 1996 (130)	N = 520 dementia and 174 depression	Moclobemide 400 mg/day max	RCT	→ Depression in dementia group
Fuchs et al., 1993 (131)	N = 127 dementia	Maprotiline 25 mg qd to tid	DBPC	→ Depression (GDS score)
Reifler et al., 1989 (132)	N = 28 AD	Imipramine 83 mg mean dose	DBPC	No benefit over placebo
Tekin et al., 1998 (134)	N = 11 AD	Lamotrigine 300 mg/day	Open	→ Depressed mood
Cummings et al., 2006 (86)	N = 120 AD with severe behaviors	Donepezil	Open	Total or partial resolution of depressions and delusions
Belzie 1996 (135)	N = 9 AIDS dementia	Risperidone 0.5–1 mg bid	Open	6 out of 9 had brighter mood and less agitation
Yoon et al., 2003 (136)	N = 48 AD	Risperidone 1 mg average dose/day	Open 8-wk study	→ Restlessness, sleep disturbances, and depression
Fontaine et al., 2003 (137)	N = 39 dementia	Olanzapine avg dose 6.7 mg vs. risperidone avg dose 1.5 mg	DB 15-day study	Both drugs ↓ depression and anxiety
Streim et al., 2008 (38)	N = 265 AD with psychosis, institutionalized	Aripiprazole 2–15 mg/day variable and placebo	DBPC	→ Agitation, anxiety, depression; no effect on psychosis

AD, Alzheimer's disease; avg, average; DB, double blind; FTD, frontotemporal dementia; MDD, major depressive disorder; PC, placebo control; RCT, randomized controlled trial.

one using imipramine showed no benefit over placebo (132). These and other tricyclics like nortriptyline and desipramine have more anticholinergic properties than the newer antidepressants listed earlier but they have less than many other tricyclic antidepressants like amitriptyline. The tricyclics can worsen cognition and cause dry mouth, sedation, orthostasis and constipation (132,133). In one small open-label study, lamotrigine was found to improve depressed mood in AD (134). In another report, donepezil showed clinically meaningful treatment effects for mood in AD subjects with severe behaviors (86). While atypical antipsychotics in some studies have reduced affective disturbances and depression (38,135–137), they are not recommended if depression is the only target symptom as SSRIs in general have improved tolerability.

Apathy

Apathy is one of the most common behavioral symptoms seen in AD patients (1). It is more common than depression. Apathy often is encountered early in AD but increases in frequency as the disease progresses. Apathy can become very severe in frontal lobe dementia, head trauma, anterior communicating artery aneurysms, and hypothalamic damage (138). All of these conditions may be associated with a dementia and they are more likely than AD patients are to receive treatment for apathy. Dorsolateral hypoperfusion on functional imaging correlated with the degree of apathy in frontal lobe dementia patients in one study (139). Apathy is characterized by a lack of motivation, social withdrawal, and little interest in any activities. Apathy is often misrepresented and the patient is described as being depressed by their caregivers. However the lack of sadness, hopelessness, crying and depressed mood distinguishes apathy from depression.

Treatment of Apathy Behaviors in Dementia

There is a lack of studies and data regarding treatment for apathy in dementia (140). Suggested preferred treatments for apathy are listed in Table 9 and specific studies are listed in Table 10. Most of the time apathy is not treated in AD, as it is usually not severe. The cholinesterase inhibitors tacrine, donepezil, and rivastigmine showed significant improvement of apathy in AD studies (65,66,141,142). Galantamine reduces apathy in patients with vascular dementia mixed with AD/vascular dementia and in a cohort of Parkinson's disease dementia subjects (89,90). Since antidepressants often help apathy when it is associated with depression, they may be useful to try when apathy is the only symptom. Fluoxetine is the most activating SSRI and possibly may help. Bupropion and to a lesser extent

Table 9 Suggested Preferred Treatments for Apathy in Dementia

Apathy: First-line suggested preferred treatments
1. Donepezil[a], galantamine[a], and the other cholinesterase inhibitors
2. Fluoxetine, bupropion, sertraline, and the other antidepressants

Apathy: Second-line suggested preferred treatments
1. Methylphenidate, amphetamine, modafinil, and other psychostimulants
2. Amantadine, carbidopa/levodopa, bromocriptine
3. Risperidone, olanzapine, and other atypical antipsychotics
4. Valproate

[a]Positive double-blind studies.

Table 10 Studies for the Treatment of Apathy in Dementia

Study	Subjects	Agents	Design	Results
Kaufer et al., 1998 (141)	N = 40 AD	Tacrine 80–160 mg	Open	→ Apathy, aberrant motor behaviors, disinhibition, anxiety
Gauthier et al., 2002 (142)	N = 290 AD	Donepezil	DBPC	→ Apathy, anxiety, irritability, depression
Cummings et al., 2005 (65)	N = 173 Nursing home AD	Rivastigmine 3–12 mg	Open	→ Delusions, hallucinations, agitation, apathy, lability, aberrant motor behaviors, sleep disturbance, eating changes
Gauthier et al., 2007 (66)	N = 2119 AD	Rivastigmine	Open	Subjects improved anxiety in 62%, apathy in 63%, and agitation in 56%
Erkinjuntti et al., 2002 (89)	N = 592 Vascular and AD/vascular mixed	Galantamine 24 mg	DBPC 6-mo	→ Anxiety, apathy, delusions compared with placebo
Litvinenko et al., 2008 (90)	N = 41 Parkinson disease dementia	Galantamine 16 mg	PC	→ Hallucinations, anxiety, apathy, sleep disturbance
Padala et al., 2007 (144)	N = 1 dementia	Modafinil 200 mg	Open	→ Apathy
Negron et al., 2000 (145)	N = 50 AD	Risperidone	Chart review	↑ Initiative, drive, ↓negative symptoms
Rankin et al., 2005 (146)	N = 14 AD	Olanzapine	Open 8-wk study	→ Apathy, anxiety, and irritability
Sival et al., 2004 (147)	N = 29 dementia	Sodium valproate average 611 mg/day	Open 12-wk study	→ Apathy, nonsocial behaviors, loss of decorum

AD, Alzheimer's disease; DB, double blind; PC, placebo control.

sertraline have the most dopaminergic promoting action of any of the antidepressants and may be worth a try. Apathy has been treated successfully in a variety of other brain conditions (143). The most common agents tried have been the psychostimulants (methylphenidate and amphetamines) and the dopaminergic agents (amantadine, carbidopa/levodopa, bromocriptine, and bupropion). The newer longer acting extended-release methylphenidate and amphetamine products may provide more sustained assistance. Modafinil, a vigilance-promoting agent showed benefit in reducing apathy in one dementia patient (144). Atypical antipsychotics typically help negative symptoms that include diminished initiative, drive, and motivation (145,146). However, due to their potential adverse effects, I would not use them if apathy was the only symptom being treated. In one 12-week study of aggressive dementia subjects, sodium valproate not only reduced aggression and suspiciousness but also reduced apathy, non-social behaviors, and loss of decorum (147).

Anxiety
Anxiety is seen in 48% of AD patients and is most common in the early to middle stages (1). Worry, nervousness, fidgety, fear, or somatic complaints are typical. Anxiety regarding upcoming events (Godot syndrome) is occasionally seen. Patients if told of an upcoming appointment, may repeatedly ask when the appointment is and may prepare for the appointment hours before they need to ready themselves. Fear of being left alone or other phobias are also typically seen. Early in the course of dementia, anxiety can be caused by the loss of ability to join in conversations as readily or the concern they will embarrass themselves out in public. Worries are often exacerbated by memory loss, and the demented patients need constant reassurance that things are all right since they forget they have been reassured before. Anxiety can also be a manifestation of depression or of psychomotor agitation. It can lead to irritability or aggression.

Treatment of Anxiety Behaviors in Dementia
Anxiety often coexists with depression. Suggested preferred treatments for anxiety in dementia are listed in Table 11 and specific studies are listed in Table 12. SSRIs in general are very good antianxiolytic agents. The studies in AD patients

Table 11   Suggested Preferred Treatments for Anxiety in Dementia

---

Anxiety: First-line suggested preferred treatments
1. SSRIs[a]
2. Trazodone

Anxiety: Second-line suggested preferred treatments
1. Valproate[a]
2. Gabapentin
3. Buspirone
4. Donepezil[a], galantamine[a], rivastigmine
5. Propranolol and other beta-blockers
6. Olanzapine[a], risperidone[a], other atypical antipsychotics

Anxiety: Avoid
1. Benzodiazepines

---

[a]Positive double-blind studies.

Table 12 Studies for the Treatment of Anxiety in Dementia

Study	Subjects	Agents	Design	Results
Nyth et al., 1990 (104)	N = 98 AD, vascular dementia	Citalopram, 10–30 mg/day	DB and open	↑ Mood, ↓ anxiety, irritability for AD only
Finkel et al., 2004 (111)	N = 109 AD	Sertraline + donepezil placebo + donepezil	DBPC	→ Dysphoria, anxiety, irritability, aggression
Katona et al., 1998 (115)	N = 198 dementia	Paroxetine 20–40 mg; imipramine 50–100 mg	DB	→ Depression for both paroxetine and imipramine
Olafsson et al., 1992 (120)	N = 46 dementia	Fluvoxamine, 150 mg	DBPC	Trends for ↑ mood, ↓ irritability, fear, anxiety, restlessness
Raji et al., 2001 (121)	N = 3 dementia and depression	Mirtazapine	Open	→ Depression, weight loss, sleep disturbances, anxiety
Lebert et al., 1994 (123)	N = 13 AD	Trazodone, 25 mg tid	Open	→ Irritability, anxiety, restlessness, affective disturbance
Sival et al., 2002 (149)	N = 42 dementia	Valproate	DBPC	→ Anxious behaviors, no help in aggression
Moretti et al., 2003 (150)	N = 20 AD	Gabapentin 980 mg average dose/day	Open	→ Sleep disturbances, anxiety, aggression
Kunik et al., 1994 (151)	N = 12 dementia	Buspirone	Single-blind	→ Agitation, anxiety
Colenda 1988 (152)	N = 1 dementia	Buspirone	Open	→ Agitation, anxiety
Kaufer et al., 1998 (141)	N = 40 AD	Tacrine 80–160 mg	Open	→ Apathy, aberrant motor behaviors, disinhibition, anxiety
Gauthier et al., 2002 (142)	N = 290 AD	Donepezil	DBPC	→ Apathy, anxiety, irritability, depression
Gauthier et al., 2007 (66)	N = 2119 AD	Rivastigmine	Open	Subjects improved anxiety in 62%, apathy in 63%, and agitation in 56%
Tariot et al., 2000 (153); Cummings et al., 2004 (154)	N = 978 AD	Galantamine 8–24 mg	DBPC	→ Aberrant motor behaviors, anxiety, disinhibition, hallucinations
Herrmann et al., 2005 (155)	N = 2033 AD	Galantamine 16–32 mg (N = 1347) or placebo (N = 686)	Post hoc analysis of three DBPC trials	→ Anxiety, disinhibition, aberrant motor behaviors, and agitation

(Continued)

Table 12 Studies for the Treatment of Anxiety in Dementia (*Continued*)

Study	Subjects	Agents	Design	Results
Monsch et al., 2004 (87)	N = 124 AD	Galantamine 8–24 mg	Open	30% improvement in anxiety, aberrant motor behaviors, delusions, euphoria, sleep disturbance
Tangwongchai et al., 2008 (88)	N = 75 AD and mixed dementia	Galantamine 16–24 mg	Open	→ Delusions, anxiety, phobias, sleep disturbance
Erkinjuntti et al., 2002 (89)	N = 592 Vascular and AD/vascular mixed	Galantamine 24 mg	DBPC 6-mo	→ Anxiety, apathy, delusions compared with placebo
Litvinenko et al., 2008 (90)	N = 41 Parkinson's disease dementia	Galantamine 16 mg	PC	→ Hallucinations, anxiety, apathy, sleep disturbance
Suh et al., 2006 (26)	N = 114 dementia nursing home with behaviors	Risperidone 0.5–1.5 mg or haloperidol 0.5–1.5 mg	DB	→ Agitation, wandering, and anxiety with risperidone
Onor et al., 2007 (50)	N = 135 AD	Risperidone 1 mg (mean)	Open 12-week study	→ Agitation, psychosis, and anxiety
Mintzer et al., 2001 (157)	N = 120 AD	Olanzapine 5, 10, and 15 mg/day	DBPC post hoc analysis	→ Anxiety only in the 5 mg/day dose vs. placebo
Fontaine et al., 2003 (137)	N = 39 dementia	Olanzapine avg dose 6.7 mg vs. risperidone avg dose 1.5 mg	DB 15-day study	Both drugs ↓ depression and anxiety
De Deyn et al., 2004 (35)	N = 652 AD with psychosis	Olanzapine 1, 2.5, 5, and 7.5 mg/day	DBPC 10-wk study	→ Anxiety in the 5 and 7.5 mg doses
Street et al., 2001 (158)	N = 91 nursing home AD	Olanzapine 7 mg/day average dose	Open	→ Anxiety, disinhibition, and irritability/lability
Moretti et al., 2004 (159)	N = 94 subcortical vascular dementia and aggression	Olanzapine 2.5–5 mg/day vs. bromazepam 0.25%	Open matched study	→ Anxiety rating with olanzapine compared with bromazepam
Rankin et al., 2005 (146)	N = 14 AD	Olanzapine	Open 8-wk study	→ Apathy, anxiety, and irritability
Fujikawa et al., 2004 (160)	N = 16 AD	Quetiapine 77 mg average dose/day	Open 8-wk study	→ Restlessness, sleep disturbances, and anxiety

AD, Alzheimer's disease; DB, double blind; PC, placebo control.

with depression show that the SSRIs improve anxiety and depression symptoms (104,111,115,120,121). They may help if anxiety is the only symptom; however, clinical studies looking only at anxiety are lacking. The efficacy and favorable tolerance profile of SSRIs make them the first choice in dementia. Trazodone may also help with anxiety (123).

Second-line treatments include valproate, which may be helpful for symptoms of anxiety in dementia (148,149). Valproate works particularly well if anxiety is mixed with mood lability. Gabapentin has few adverse effects and may improve anxiety and agitation symptoms (150). There have also been a few studies showing a reduction in anxiety with the use of buspirone (151,152). Buspirone has some serotonergic properties and has very few side effects. It may also help with agitation. However, buspirone can take several weeks to show effectiveness and, in my experience, that effect often wanes after several months in dementia patients. I have not found it overly useful, but there are some patients whom it may help. Studies with the cholinesterase inhibitors including donepezil, rivastigmine, and galantamine have all shown significant reduction in anxiety symptoms in AD patients and also with galantamine in vascular dementia and Parkinson's disease dementia (66,87–90,141,142,153–155). These agents may be helpful for anxious AD patients even if they have very low cognitive functioning when the use of cholinesterase inhibitors may be debated. Propranolol has some antianxiolytic properties and has been used for anxiety and irritability in AD patients even though it has only been studied for the prevention of aggression, rage, and violence in dementia patients (67,68,156). Beta-blockers need to be used with caution in those with diabetes, chronic obstructive pulmonary disease, asthma, hypotension, or bradycardia. Atypical antipsychotics including risperidone, olanzapine, and quetiapine may be helpful for anxiety symptoms as well (26,35,50,137,146,157–160). However, atypical antipsychotics should be used as a last resort for anxiety symptoms unless the patient has significant psychotic behaviors along with the anxiety. Try to completely avoid benzodiazepines in the demented elderly. The only exception may be the use of short-acting benzodiazepines (i.e., lorazepam) to sedate the patient with acute, severe aggression. Even so, in those cases, intramuscular antipsychotic medications may be better due to improved tolerability. Controlled studies using benzodiazepines in dementia are lacking. Although these agents have antianxiolytic properties, they often have too many side effects to be given on a regular basis in this population. They may cause confusion, impaired concentration, diminished attention and reaction time, memory loss (verbal and visual), functional difficulties, depression, sedation, falls, and institutionalization (161,162). Occasionally, they can cause aggression and disinhibition (163). Tolerance can build up over time and reduce effectiveness. Dependency occurs easily, and severe, life-threatening withdrawal symptoms may occur if the drugs are suddenly stopped. It is very useful to slowly taper and discontinue all benzodiazepines in demented patients, as this will tend to improve their memory scores and cognitive abilities (163).

Mood Lability, Disinhibition, Intrusiveness, Euphoria, and Mania

Mood lability is common in AD and in FTDs. Pseudobulbar affect and extreme emotional lability with pathological crying and inappropriate laughter is also referred to as intermittent emotional expression disorder (IEED) (8). It can occur in progressive supranuclear palsy, FTDs, traumatic dementias, AD, and in some cases of vascular dementias (8,164).

Disinhibition is seen in 36% of AD patients but is not typically severe (1). Many times the disinhibited behavior is an acceptable behavior, but it is done at an inappropriate time or place. Undressing in a dining room full of people to adjust a diaper is one example. The patient is self-absorbed and not thinking about how this may be offensive to others. Using poor judgment and being impulsive will often led to disinhibited behaviors. Symptoms of intrusiveness also go hand in hand with disinhibition. Intrusive behaviors are often seen in conditions affecting the frontal lobes and are fairly common in AD and are even more so in FTDs. Orbitofrontal hypoperfusion on functional imaging correlated with the degree of disinhibition in frontal lobe dementia patients in one study (139).

Euphoria and mania are rare in AD occurring in about 2%. They are more often seen in FTDs. Treatments are usually not given to those with just elevated moods. Secondary mania symptoms with decreased need for sleep, racing thoughts, easy distractibility, hyperverbalness, pressured speech, and psychomotor agitation should be treated and causes explored.

Treatment of Mood Lability, Disinhibition, Intrusiveness, Euphoria, and Manic Behaviors in Dementia

Suggested preferred treatments for mood lability, disinhibition, intrusiveness, euphoria, and mania in dementia are listed in Table 13 and specific studies are listed in Table 14. Anticonvulsants with their proven mood-stabilizing properties seem to do very well with all of these symptoms (165). Although valproate is one of the best-tolerated anticonvulsants with mood-stabilizing properties, studies are few in its use for the treatment of mood lability, disinhibition, intrusiveness, or mania in dementia patients (59,166). Nevertheless, in my experience, individuals with significant mood lability especially those who have a quick onset or offset of their mood or anger are often helped with valproate. Doses of valproate often do not have to be very high to be effective for these symptoms in AD patients. Usually 250 to 1000 mg/day in two or three divided doses is enough. At these doses, valproate has minimal effect on cognitive abilities and low sedation potential. It

Table 13 Suggested Preferred Treatments for Mood Lability, Disinhibition, Intrusiveness, Euphoria, and Mania in Dementia

Mood lability, disinhibition, intrusiveness, euphoria, and mania: First-line suggested preferred treatments
1. Valproate

Mood lability, disinhibition, intrusiveness, euphoria, and mania: Second-line suggested preferred treatments
1. Citalopram[a] and other SSRIs
2. Gabapentin, lamotrigine, carbamazepine, and other anticonvulsants
3. Galantamine[a], memantine[a], rivastigmine
4. Olanzapine[a] and other atypical antipsychotics
5. Buspirone

Mood lability, disinhibition, intrusiveness, euphoria, and mania: Avoid
1. Lithium

[a]Positive double-blind studies.

Table 14 Studies for the Treatment of Mood Lability, Disinhibition, Intrusiveness, Euphoria, and Mania in Dementia

Study	Subjects	Agents	Design	Results
Swartz et al., 1997 (119)	N = 11 FTD	Fluoxetine, sertraline, or paroxetine	Open	→ Disinhibition, compulsions, and depression in at least half
Moretti et al., 2003 (116)	N = 16 FTD	Paroxetine 20 mg; piracetam 1200 mg	Open	→ Social dysdecorum, weeping, depression, agitation with paroxetine
Pollock et al., 2002 (19)	N = 85 dementia	Citalopram, perphenazine, placebo	DBPC	→ Lability/tension and aggression factors with citalopram vs. placebo
Tiller et al., 1988 (171)	N = 1 vascular dementia	Buspirone	Open	→ Disinhibition
Haas et al., 1997 (166)	N = 12 dementia	Divalproex 750–1500 mg	Open	→ Disruptive behaviors, improved emotional control
Forester et al., 2007 (59)	N = 15 dementia	Divalproex sodium 656 mg (mean) alone or with antipsychotic	Open	→ Aggressive behaviors and disinhibition
Lemke, 1995 (61)	N = 15 dementia with agitation	Carbamazepine 246 mg (mean)	Open	→ Agitation, emotional lability, and impulsivity
Miller 2001 (168)	N = 1 vascular dementia	Gabapentin	Open	→ Lability, sexual inappropriateness, agitation
Devarajan et al., 2000 (169)	N = 1 FTD	Lamotrigine 100 mg/day	Open	→ Disinhibition and aggression
Ng et al., 2009 (170)	N = 5 dementia	Lamotrigine 100–300 mg	Retrospective chart review	→ Mania-like symptoms
Kaufer et al., 1998 (141)	N = 40 AD	Tacrine 80–160 mg	Open	→ Apathy, aberrant motor behaviors, disinhibition, anxiety
Cummings et al., 2005 (65)	N = 173 Nursing home AD	Rivastigmine 3–12 mg	Open	→ Delusions, hallucinations, agitation, apathy, lability, aberrant motor behaviors, sleep disturbance, eating changes
Tariot et al., 2000 (153)	N = 978 AD	Galantamine 8–24 mg	DBPC	→ Aberrant motor behaviors, anxiety, disinhibition, hallucinations

(Continued)

Table 14 Studies for the Treatment of Mood Lability, Disinhibition, Intrusiveness, Euphoria, and Mania in Dementia (*Continued*)

Study	Subjects	Agents	Design	Results
Herrmann et al., 2005 (155)	N = 2033 AD	Galantamine 16–32 mg (N = 1347) or placebo (N = 686)	Post hoc analysis of three DBPC trials	↓ Anxiety, disinhibition, aberrant motor behaviors, and agitation
Monsch et al., 2004 (87)	N = 124 AD	Galantamine 8–24 mg	Open	30% improvement in anxiety, aberrant motor behaviors, delusions, euphoria, sleep disturbance
Cummings et al., 2006 (44)	N = 404 AD	Memantine + donepezil vs. donepezil alone	DBPC	↓ Lability, agitation, appetite/eating change
Street et al., 2001 (158)	N = 91 Nursing home AD	Olanzapine 7 mg/day average dose	Open	↓ Anxiety, disinhibition, and irritability/lability
De Deyn et al., 2004 (35)	N = 652 AD with psychosis	Olanzapine 1, 2.5, 5, and 7.5 mg/day	DBPC 10-wk study	↓ Euphoria/elation in the 5 mg dose only

AD, Alzheimer's disease; DB, double blind; PC, placebo control; FTD, frontotemporal dementia.

also has the added benefit of a tendency to increase weight, which is often needed in dementia patients. Sprinkle formulation (125 mg sprinkles) can be used when the patient has difficulty with swallowing pills or refuses medications. It is an extended-release formulation that can be sprinkled on food for ingestion.

SSRIs are also potentially good choices for mood lability, social dysdecorum, disinhibition, or intrusiveness especially in frontotemporal patients (116,119). Serotonin pathways may be involved. Citalopram was significantly more effective than placebo in hospitalized dementia patients in controlling their behavioral disturbances including lability and agitation factors (19). The SSRIs may precipitate mania in certain individuals and should be used with caution in patients with euphoria or mania. If mania develops or if the patient becomes severely disinhibited and intrusive, atypical antipsychotics or more sedating anticonvulsants (i.e., carbamazepine) may be of more utility (167).

Carbamazepine in an open-label study has shown improved emotional lability and impulsivity in dementia patients (61). Single case reports describe benefits with the anticonvulsants gabapentin for reduction of mood lability and lamotrigine for reduction of disinhibition and aggression where other psychotropic agents failed (168,169). Reduction of manic-like symptoms in dementia patients by lamotrigine is noted in another study (170). There is some data showing significant reductions in mood lability, disinhibition, or euphoria symptoms when using the cholinesterase inhibitors including rivastigmine and galantamine (65,87,141,153,155). Mood lability may also be less with memantine use (44). Olanzapine and perhaps other atypical antipsychotics may also be helpful for disinhibition, mood lability, and euphoria (35,158). In one patient buspirone was shown to reduce disinhibition (171).

Try to avoid lithium in the demented elderly population. Lithium has a narrow therapeutic window and has a high chance of causing adverse events.

Sleep Disturbances

Diurnal rhythm disturbance (reversal of sleep–wake cycle) is seen in about 42% of AD patients and consists of repetitive wakenings during the night to near complete day/night sleep pattern reversal (172,173). These symptoms are seen with increasing frequency as the disease progresses. It is particularly bothersome and exhausting to caregivers who have to be wary about the patient's safety while they are up all night. Falls in the dark, wandering out of the house, and turning on the stove are all safety concerns. Although patients will catch up on their sleep the next day, this may be impossible for the caregivers. There are multiple factors that can lead to sleep disturbances ranging from medications and mood state to the brain impairment from the dementia itself. Pain or distress associated with general medical conditions should also be considered.

Insomnia is common in the elderly and is often due to reduced sleep efficiency seen with aging. There is diminished rapid eye movement sleep, decreased deep sleep, and increased nocturnal awakenings (172,173). In dementia patients, insomnia can be seen in isolation or associated with anxiety or dysphoria.

Increased confusion in the evening or at night (sundowning) is seen in 18% of AD patients. When the sun sets, there is a loss of visual sensory stimuli due to diminished light. This may be superimposed on the individuals' hearing loss and perceptual loss (i.e., peripheral neuropathy) leading to an overall impairment in sensory stimuli. Fatigue in the evening as well as disturbed circadian rhythms

Table 15 Suggested Preferred Treatments for Sleep Disturbances in Dementia

Sleep disturbances: First-line suggested preferred treatments
1. Trazodone
2. Zolpidem

Sleep disturbances: Second-line suggested preferred treatments
1. Mirtazapine and nortriptyline if accompanied with depression
2. Quetiapine, risperidone[a], and olanzapine if accompanied with psychosis
3. Valproate if accompanied with excessive restlessness, psychomotor activity
   disturbance, intrusiveness, disinhibition, or mania
4. Gabapentin
5. Melatonin[a]

Sleep Disturbances: Avoid
1. Barbiturates
2. Benzodiazepines
3. Hydroxyzine
4. Diphenhydramine

[a]Positive double-blind studies.

may also play a part (174). All of these factors enhance the possibility of disorientation, inability to recognize surroundings, confusion and agitation. Wanting to leave, wandering, restless activities and yelling are not uncommon.

Treatment of Sleep Disturbances in Dementia

Many of the usual treatments for sleep disturbances (sedative/hypnotics) are not well suited for dementia patients. Many cause cognitive impairment. Most are not intended for long-term use and dementia patients often need long-term treatment of their sleep disturbances. Suggested preferred treatments for sleep disturbances in dementia are listed in Table 15 and specific studies are listed in Table 16. Trazodone, an antidepressant with sedative properties, is ideally suited for dementia patients (123). It can be given for the long term and has very little anticholinergic effects to cause memory loss. At higher doses it can cause orthostasis. Trazodone appears to revert back to normal the reversal of the sleep–wake cycle in patients with AD and other conditions (175). It has been very helpful for insomnia (176). It does not appear to have a hangover effect in clinical use. As trazodone is also an antidepressant, it is particularly useful in sleep disturbances associated with depression, anxiety, and irritability (177). Zolpidem also has helped sleep disturbance associated with dementia (178). It is well tolerated and does not seem to have the tolerance or withdrawal symptoms seen with benzodiazepines.

When a patient has disrupted sleep in combination with other behaviors that need treatment, one should consider using a more sedating agent for the nonsleep disturbance behavior to treat both problems with one medication. In patients with significant depression, something stronger than trazodone for the depression may be desired. Mirtazapine and nortriptyline both have sleep-promoting effects and could be considered. However, nortriptyline has mild anticholinergic properties that may be problematic in dementia. It is not unusual to treat patients with insomnia and depression with both trazodone and another SSRI. In patients with delusions and suspiciousness, sleep-promoting atypical antipsychotics like quetiapine or olanzapine may be the best choice. Several

Table 16 Studies for the Treatment of Sleep Disturbances in Dementia

Study	Subjects	Agents	Design	Results
Lebert et al., 1994 (123)	N = 13 AD	Trazodone, 25 mg tid	Open	↓ Irritability, anxiety, restlessness, affective disturbance
Shelton et al., 1997 (178)	N = 2 AD	Zolpidem 10–15 mg/night	Open	↓ Insomnia, ↓ nighttime wandering
McCarten et al., 1995 (191)	N = 7 AD	Triazolam 0.125 mg qhs	Open	No help with disturbed sleep
Chan et al., 2001 (24)	N = 58 AD or vascular dementia	Risperidone 0.5–2 mg (mean 0.85 mg) or haloperidol 0.5–2 mg	DB 12-wk	Improved diurnal rhythm, ↓ activity disturbances, and ↓ agitation in both groups
Yoon et al., 2003 (136)	N = 48 AD	Risperidone 1 mg average dose/day	Open 8-wk study	↓ Restlessness, sleep disturbances, and depression
Fujikawa et al., 2004 (160)	N = 16 AD	Quetiapine 77 mg average dose/day	Open 8-wk study	↓ Restlessness, sleep disturbances, and anxiety
Onor et al., 2006 (52)	N = 41 (20 AD, 6 vascular, 6 mixed, 5 Lewy)	Quetiapine	Open	↓ Aggression, psychosis, sleep disturbance
Wirz-Justice et al., 2000 (179)	N = 1 AD	Clozapine	Open	Improvement of sleep/wake cycle disturbance
Moretti et al., 2003 (150)	N = 20 AD	Gabapentin 980 mg average dose/day	Open	↓ Sleep disturbances, anxiety, aggression
Asayama et al., 2003 (183)	N = 18 AD	Melatonin 3 mg qhs for 4 weeks	DBPC	↓ Actigraph activity at night, prolonged sleep time
Serfaty et al., 2002 (188)	N = 25 dementia	Melatonin 6 mg qhs	DBPC 7 wk	No effect on total sleep, awakenings, or efficiency
Singer et al., 2003 (189)	N = 157 AD	Melatonin 2.5 or 10 mg qhs	DBPC	No sleep benefits
Gehrman et al., 2009 (190)	N = 41 institutionalized AD	Melatonin 8.5 mg immediate and 1.5 mg sustained-release	DBPC 10 days	No effect on sleep, circadian rhythm, or agitation
Jean-Louis et al., 1998 (184)	N = 2 AD	Melatonin	Open	↓ Daytime sleepiness in one; ↓ cognitive impairment in one
Brusco et al., 1998 (185)	N = 1 AD	Melatonin	Open	Substantial improvement of sleep quality

(Continued)

Table 16 Studies for the Treatment of Sleep Disturbances in Dementia (*Continued*)

Study	Subjects	Agents	Design	Results
Brusco et al., 1999 (186)	N = 14 AD	Melatonin, 9 mg	Open	↑ Sleep, ↓ agitated behavior at night
Cardinali et al., 2002 (187)	N = 45 AD	Melatonin, 6 mg/day	Open	↑ Seep, ↓ sundowning
Cummings et al., 2005 (65)	N = 173 Nursing home AD	Rivastigmine 3–12 mg	Open	↓ Delusions, hallucinations, agitation, apathy, lability, aberrant motor behaviors, sleep disturbance, eating changes
Monsch et al., 2004 (87)	N = 124 AD	Galantamine 8–24 mg	Open	>30% improvement in anxiety, aberrant motor behaviors, delusions, euphoria, sleep disturbance
Tangwongchai et al., 2008 (88)	N = 75 AD and mixed dementia	Galantamine 16–24 mg	Open	↓ Delusions, anxiety, phobias, sleep disturbance
Litvinenko et al., 2008 (90)	N = 41 Parkinson disease dementia	Galantamine 16 mg	PC	↓ Hallucinations, anxiety, apathy, sleep disturbance
Edwards et al., 2007 (91)	N = 50 Lewy body dementia	Galantamine 16–24 mg	Open 24 wk	↓ Visual hallucinations, sleep disturbance

AD, Alzheimer's disease; DB, double blind; PC, placebo control.

antipsychotic agents have been shown to improve diurnal rhythm disturbances, but it is not recommended to use antipsychotics solely to help with sleep due to their adverse safety profile and the availability of other sleep-promoting agents (24,52,136,160,179). Valproate may help with insomnia and could be tried in patients with excessive restlessness, psychomotor activity disturbance, intrusiveness, disinhibition, or mania.

Second-line treatments for sleep disturbances can include gabapentin, which is well tolerated and has been shown beneficial for sleep disturbances in AD subjects (150). Melatonin, in some studies, has been useful for insomnia in the elderly (180,181). It may also be useful in helping with the disrupted circadian sleep–wake rhythm and the chronobiological changes of aging seen with dementia patients. There is some evidence that AD patients with sleep–wake cycle disturbances also have melatonin secretion rhythm disorders (182). Indeed, a few case reports and one small placebo-controlled study have shown some sleep benefit in AD patients using melatonin (183–187). However, larger placebo-controlled studies using melatonin showed no benefit for sleep (188–190). Melatonin, therefore, may offer little to no benefit for sleep disturbances in AD subjects. Rivastigmine use resulted in less sleep disturbances in one open-label nursing home study (65). Galantamine was shown to reduce sleep disturbances in AD, Parkinson's disease dementia, and dementia with Lewy body patients (87,88,90,91).

Less desirable treatments for sleep issues in dementia patients include the short-acting benzodiazepines (i.e., lorazepam, oxazepam) due to their potential significant adverse effects. These agents should only be used rarely and only for short periods of time as they generally are not useful for the long-term sleep disrupted symptoms seen in AD and other dementia patients (191). Other agents to try to avoid in the demented elderly include antihistamines used for sleep. Some of these include hydroxyzine (Vistaril), diphenhydramine (Benadryl), and diphenhydramine with acetaminophen (Tylenol PM). Most cause a sleepy hangover effect and all have significant anticholinergic properties that can increase confusion and counteract to some degree the effect of cholinesterase inhibitors in the AD patients. Barbiturates and long-acting hypnotics/benzodiazepines are very sedating and can stay in the system for many weeks sometimes causing a dementia syndrome by itself. They should be avoided in the demented elderly.

Eating Disturbances

Diminished appetite and weight loss are common in the middle and later stages of AD. Patients still living by themselves may not prepare meals as well, may skip meals, or forget to eat if there is nothing to cue them. They will lose weight, and this is an important sign of the need for increased supervision. In the later stages of the disease, apraxia becomes severe and patients need help in feeding and may eventually have trouble even in swallowing. Behavioral disturbances including depression, psychosis, restless activity, and pacing may be responsible for weight loss as well. Someone may be so restless that they cannot sit long enough to eat and will lose weight even though there is no disturbance in their appetite. Food refusal may be observed if the patient thinks that it has been poisoned. Medication side effects and gastrointestinal conditions may also lead to poor appetite.

Hyperoral behaviors can be seen in dementia patients (6). This is observed more commonly in frontotemporal degenerative dementias where patients use their mouth to explore both food and nonfood items. This may lead to an increase

Table 17 Suggested Preferred Treatments for Eating and Appetite Disturbances in Dementia

---

Anorexia eating disturbances: First-line suggested preferred treatments
1. Megestrol acetate

Anorexia eating disturbances: Second-line suggested preferred treatments
1. Mirtazapine
2. Valproate

Hyperphagia eating disturbances: First-line suggested preferred treatments
1. Fluvoxamine
2. Trazodone[a]
3. SSRIs

Hyperphagia eating disturbances: Second-line suggested preferred treatments
1. Clomipramine

---

[a]Positive randomized trial.

in eating and significant weight gain. Obsessive–compulsive behaviors in dementia patients, frequently noted in individuals with FTD, may also result in obesity due to specific cravings, food fetishes, and hyperphagia. Classically, these patients also have the habit of eating off other people's plates without asking.

Treatment of Eating Disturbances in Dementia

Anorexia with weight loss is very common in AD and other dementias and can be predictive of mortality (192). Supervision or assistance with eating, nutritional educational programs for caregivers, and nutritional supplements are the mainstays of treatment (193). Suggested preferred treatments for eating disturbances in dementia are listed in Table 17 and specific studies are listed in Table 18. Megestrol acetate has been used for the treatment of anorexia associated with AIDS and cancer and may be helpful in dementia-related weight loss (194). Data are

Table 18 Studies for the Treatment of Eating and Appetite Disturbances in Dementia

Study	Subjects	Agents	Design	Results
Volicer et al., 1994 (113)	N = 10 AD with depression	Sertraline various doses	Open label	8 out of 10 ↓ depression, 5 out of 6 ↓ food refusal
Lebert et al., 2004 (122)	N = 26 FTD	Trazodone	DBPC	↓ Irritability, agitation, dysphoria, eating disorders
Cummings et al., 2005 (65)	N = 173 Nursing home AD	Rivastigmine 3–12 mg	Open	↓ Delusions, hallucinations, agitation, apathy, lability, aberrant motor behaviors, sleep disturbance, eating changes
Cummings et al., 2006 (44)	N = 404 AD	Memantine + donepezil vs. donepezil alone	DBPC	↓ Lability, agitation, appetite/eating change

AD, Alzheimer's disease; DB, double blind; FTD, frontotemporal dementia; PC, placebo control.

lacking regarding its use in dementia. In my own practice, I have had good results in weight gain for demented patients using megestrol acetate. Occasionally, I am successful using 40 mg po bid, but typically I have to use the oral solution with doses of 300 to 400 mg bid [7 (5) to 10 mL bid of the 40 mg/mL oral solution]. Since megestrol acetate is a progesterone derivative, care must be used in those patients with limited ambulation abilities due to its potential risk for thrombophlebitis and pulmonary embolism. Sertraline has shown to reduce food refusal in advanced AD patients (113). Mirtazapine and valproate both can commonly cause weight gain. These may be good choices to consider second line in those demented patients losing weight whom otherwise might benefit from either of those agents.

The hyperphagia sometimes seen in demented patients may be the result of obsessive–compulsive traits. Fluvoxamine or one of the other SSRIs, used in high doses, may be helpful. One randomized controlled trial found trazodone to be useful (122). Rivastigmine and memantine have also been shown to reduce abnormal appetite and eating behaviors (44,65). Clomipramine, in my experience, may also work well for hyperphagia, but I consider it second line since clomipramine is a tricyclic antidepressant and therefore has more sedative and anticholinergic properties that can impair memory function.

Hypersexual Disturbances

Hypersexuality is unusual but can be persistent and problematic (102). It is seen in about 3% of AD patients and often occurs in the later stages of the disease. Frequent verbal sexual comments, fondling, and sexual aggressiveness can be seen. Hypersexuality should be differentiated from symptoms such as hand holding, hugging, and brief kisses, which are common behaviors and, if excessive, are often due to impulsivity or disinhibition and are not thought to be hypersexual in nature. As a rule, decreased sexual interests are the norm for most dementia patients (102).

Treatment of Hypersexual Disturbances in Dementia

Many treatments have been tried for hypersexuality symptoms in the nursing home population (195). Usually redirection, separation, and closer supervision are successful. Offering privacy for self-stimulating behaviors may help. Suggested preferred pharmacotherapies for hypersexual disturbances in dementia are listed in Table 19 and specific studies are listed in Table 20. There are some studies suggesting that SSRIs may help with hypersexuality in dementia (196–198). SSRIs

Table 19 Suggested Preferred Treatments for Hypersexual Disturbances in Dementia

Hypersexual disturbances: First-line suggested preferred treatments
1. SSRIs
2. Cimetidine
Hypersexual disturbances: Second-line suggested preferred treatments
1. Clomipramine
2. Gabapentin
5. Quetiapine, haloperidol
6. Leuprolide acetate, medroxyprogesterone acetate, estrogen

Table 20   Studies for the Treatment of Hypersexual Disturbances in Dementia

Study	Subjects	Agents	Design	Results
Anneser et al., 2007 (196)	$N = 1$ ALS-FTD	Sertraline	Open	→ Hypersexuality and sexual aggression
Tosto et al., 2008 (197)	$N = 1$ AD	Citalopram 40 mg	Open	→ Pursuit of sexual acts and frustration when refused
Stewart et al., 1997 (198)	$N = 1$ dementia	Paroxetine 20 mg/day	Open	→ Hypersexuality by 95% (estimate)
Wiseman et al., 2000 (201)	$N = 20$ dementia	Cimetidine 600–1600 mg/day	Open	→ Hypersexual behaviors, libido
Leo et al., 1995 (202)	$N = 2$ dementia	Clomipramine	Open	→ Paraphilias
Miller 2001 (168)	$N = 1$ vascular dementia	Gabapentin	Open	→ Sexual inappropriateness, lability, agitation
Alkhalil et al., 2003 (203)	$N = 1$ AD	Gabapentin	Open	→ Public masturbation, fondling others
Alkhalil et al., 2004 (204)	$N = 3$ dementia	Gabapentin	Open	→ Sexual disinhibition
Freymann et al., 2005 (205)	$N = 1$ AD	Carbamazepine 200 mg	Open	→ Hypersexual behavior
MacKnight et al., 2000 (206)	$N = 1$ dementia	Quetiapine	Open	→ Excessive masturbation
Prakash et al., 2009 (207)	$N = 1$ Lewy body dementia	Quetiapine	Open	→ Sexual inappropriate behaviors
Rosenthal et al., 2003 (208)	$N = 1$ AD	Haloperidol	Open	→ Urethral masturbation and sexual disinhibition
Alagiakrishnan et al., 2003 (209)	$N = 1$ mixed dementia	Rivastigmine	Open	→ Sexual aggression
Cooper, 1987 (210)	$N = 4$ dementia	Medroxyprogesterone	Open	→ Sexual acting out
Britton, 1998 (211)	$N = 1$ traumatic brain injury	Medroxyprogesterone	Open	→ Hypersexuality
Amadeo, 1996 (212)	$N = 3$ dementia	Medroxyprogesterone plus leuprolide acetate	Open	→ Disruptive sexual behavior, ↓ agitation
Rich et al., 1994 (213)	$N = 1$ Huntington's disease	Leuprolide	Open	→ Exhibitionism
Ott, 1995 (214)	$N = 1$ dementia	Leuprolide	Open	→ Sexual aggressiveness
Shelton et al., 1999 (215)	$N = 2$ dementia (1 AD, 1 vascular)	Estrogen	Open	→ Physical and sexual aggressiveness

AD, Alzheimer's disease; ALS-FTD, amyotrophic lateral sclerosis with frontotemporal dementia.

are well known to cause sexual dysfunction (199). More studies are clearly needed (200). Cimetidine is an H_2 antagonist and a nonhormonal antiandrogen. There was one study showing that it may be useful in reducing libido and hypersexual behaviors in demented patients (201). Cimetidine has been known to cause mental confusion in the elderly but in general is very well tolerated.

If an SSRI is not effective, there are several other medication choices that can be used. Clomipramine has been reported to reduce sexually inappropriate conduct seen in dementia patients and its effect was thought to be unrelated to any decreased ability to sustain an erection or orgasm (202). Although, clomipramine has anticholinergic properties that can cause memory loss, it is very effective in my experience. Sexual inappropriateness declined with gabapentin in one patient with vascular dementia (168), one with AD (203), and three with dementia (204). Carbamazepine was reported to reduce hypersexual behavior in an AD patient (205). Quetiapine and haloperidol in separate case reports reduced masturbation and hypersexuality in demented patients and sexually inappropriate behaviors in a patient with Lewy body disease (206–208). A woman with mixed dementia (AD and vascular dementia) had reduced sexual aggressiveness while using rivastigmine (209). Two antiandrogen agents, medroxyprogesterone acetate and leuprolide acetate, in several studies, were reported to reduce aggression, sexual aggression, exhibitionism, and public masturbation symptoms in demented men (210–214). For men, estrogen preparations also may reduce physical and sexual aggression (215). However, the antiandrogen treatments should be used cautiously in men due to their potential side effects.

Aberrant Motor Behaviors (Psychomotor Activity Disturbances)

Disturbances of psychomotor activity are frequent in AD patients. Wandering is seen in 3% to 26% of AD patients (216). Some patients feel that they have to go or keep moving. They want to leave or want to "go home" even if they are already at their home. They may be thinking about the home where they grew up or may be looking for their parents or children. They may have a physical need such as needing to urinate. Pacing is often seen. Motor restlessness or hyperkinesia is seen in about 46% of AD patients (1,4,216). They display purposeless activity including opening and closing pocketbooks, packing and unpacking clothing, putting on and taking off clothes, opening and closing drawers, and pacing. Storing, hoarding, or hiding objects in inappropriately places (throwing clothes in a wastebasket or putting clean plates in an oven) occur. Insistent repeating of demands or questions becomes tiresome to caregivers. Intrusiveness with touching, petting, and getting to close to others is commonly associated with increased restless activities. Patients may tap, fidget, or pound on walls. Hyperverbalness or singing can be another manifestation. Some of these behaviors may be due to akathisias seen with antipsychotic use. Environmental changes, sundowning, and anxiety may also contribute to these behaviors.

Treatment of Aberrant Motor Behaviors in Dementia

There is very little data on the treatments for aberrant motor behaviors in dementia. Suggested preferred pharmacotherapies for aberrant motor behaviors in dementia are listed in Table 21 and specific studies are listed in Table 22. In virtually the only study designed specifically to measure drug efficacy for reducing aberrant motor behaviors in dementia, citalopram was reported to significantly

Table 21   Suggested Preferred Treatments for Aberrant Motor Behaviors in Dementia

---
Aberrant motor behaviors: First-line suggested preferred treatments
1. Citalopram
2. Valproate[a]
3. Galantamine[a] and rivastigmine

Aberrant motor behaviors: Second-line suggested preferred treatments
1. Sertraline, paroxetine, and trazodone
2. Risperidone[a], quetiapine
3. Gabapentin

---
[a]Positive double-blind studies.

reduce nonaggressive restless activity (217). Other SSRIs have helped hyperverbalness and disruptive vocalizations, which can be a manifestation of motor restlessness (218–220). Sertraline showed a trend in improving aggression and aberrant motor behaviors versus placebo (221). I have experienced that citalopram and sertraline are helpful in decreasing general restlessness, purposeless activities, and repetitive compulsive-like behaviors. Trazodone has been reported to reduce restlessness as well (123). Valproate has been shown to help with impulsivity, restless behaviors, and nonaggressive physical agitation in demented patients (149,222,223). I have found that valproate is very helpful in reducing symptoms of pacing, intrusiveness, hyperverbalness, and hyperkinesis (cannot stay still or sit for any length of time). Some of the cholinesterase inhibitors have shown significant reductions in aberrant motor behaviors in AD patients (65,87,141,153–155). Clinically I have seen a reduction in the wanting to go home symptoms with those agents. In double-blind or placebo-controlled trials (24,26,224–226) and in open-label studies (136,160,227), antipsychotic agents have demonstrated improvement in psychomotor restlessness, diurnal rhythm disturbances, persistent vocalizations, wandering, and/or activity disturbances. Another anticonvulsant, gabapentin reduced restlessness and incessant vocalizations in a single AD patient (228). However, reports of using gabapentin in dementia with Lewy body patients caused increased confusion and hypersomnolence (229). Light therapy for 30 minutes a day for two weeks was also reported to reduce restlessness in dementia subjects (16).

Obsessive–Compulsive Traits

Obsessive-compulsive–like behaviors are seen commonly in those with the frontal variant of FTD while only approximately 2% of AD patients may exhibit these symptoms (1). These obsessive–compulsive behaviors may not meet the *DSM-IV* diagnostic criteria for obsessive–compulsive disorder (OCD). These types of behaviors may include ritualistic behaviors, significantly repetitive behaviors, pacing or walking in a very set path, excessive ritualistic touching, excessive picking of the skin, or counting behaviors. Some of these behaviors overlap with aberrant motor activities. However, these behaviors feature an obsessive thought and not just the motor action. Individuals with excessive motor restlessness who pace will avoid obstacles along the way, whereas those with obsessive–compulsive pacing must walk in a very set pathway, perhaps touching a railing

Table 22 Studies for the Treatment of Aberrant Motor Behaviors in Dementia

Study	Subjects	Agents	Design	Results
Scharre et al., 2003 (217)	$N = 19$ AD	Citalopram 20–40 mg/day	Open	↓ Aberrant motor behaviors, restless activity
Pollock et al., 1997 (218)	$N = 16$ dementia	Citalopram	Open	↓ Mean disruptive vocalizations
Kim et al., 2000 (219)	$N = 2$ dementia	Citalopram	Open	↓ Verbal agitation
Ramadan et al., 2000 (220)	$N = 15$ dementia	Paroxetine 10–40 mg/day	Open	↓ Verbal agitation
Lanctot et al., 2002 (221)	$N = 22$ AD	Sertraline	DBPC	NS; 38% ↓ aberrant motor behaviors, aggression
Sival et al., 2002 (149)	$N = 42$ dementia	Valproate	DBPC	↓ Restless behaviors, no help in aggression
Kunik et al., 1998 (222)	$N = 13$ dementia	Valproate	Chart review	↓ Nonaggressive physical agitation
Buchalter et al., 2001 (223)	$N = 1$ vascular dementia	Valproate	Open	↓ Impulsivity
Kaufer et al., 1998 (141)	$N = 40$ AD	Tacrine 80–160 mg	Open	↓ Apathy, aberrant motor behaviors, disinhibition, anxiety
Cummings et al., 2005 (65)	$N = 173$ Nursing home AD	Rivastigmine 3–12 mg	Open	↓ Delusions, hallucinations, agitation, apathy, lability, aberrant motor behaviors, sleep disturbance, eating changes
Tariot et al., 2000 (153); Cummings et al., 2004 (154)	$N = 978$ AD	Galantamine 8–24 mg	DBPC	↓ Aberrant motor behaviors, anxiety, disinhibition, hallucinations
Herrmann et al., 2005 (155)	$N = 2033$ AD	Galantamine 16–32 mg ($N = 1347$) or placebo ($N = 686$)	Post hoc analysis of 3 DBPC trials	↓ Anxiety, disinhibition, aberrant motor behaviors, and agitation
Monsch et al., 2004 (87)	$N = 124$ AD	Galantamine 8–24 mg	Open	30% improvement in anxiety, aberrant motor behaviors, delusions, euphoria, sleep disturbance
Gutzmann et al., 1997 (224)	$N = 156$ dementia	Tiapride 100 mg/morning, 100 mg/noon, 200 mg/evening and melperone	DB	Global improvement in psychomotor restlessness

(Continued)

Table 22 Studies for the Treatment of Aberrant Motor Behaviors in Dementia (*Continued*)

Study	Subjects	Agents	Design	Results
Chan et al., 2001 (24)	N = 58 AD or vascular dementia	Risperidone 0.5–2 mg (mean 0.85 mg) or Haloperidol 0.5–2 mg	DB 12-wk	Improved diurnal rhythm, ↓ activity disturbances, and ↓ agitation in both groups
Gareri et al., 2004 (225)	N = 60 Vascular dementia and AD	Risperidone 1–2 mg, olanzapine 5–10 mg, promazine 50–100 mg	DB	↓ Wandering behaviors with risperidone
Suh et al., 2006 (26)	N = 114 dementia nursing home with behaviors	Risperidone 0.5–1.5 mg or haloperidol 0.5–1.5 mg	DB	↓ Agitation, wandering, and anxiety with risperidone
Meguro et al., 2004 (226)	N = 34 AD	Risperidone	PC	↓ Wandering behaviors with risperidone
Kopala et al., 1997 (227)	N = 2 mixed AD or vascular	Risperidone	Open	↓ By 80% persistent vocalizations
Yoon et al., 2003 (136)	N = 48 AD	Risperidone 1 mg average dose/day	Open 8-wk study	↓ Restlessness, sleep disturbances, & depression
Fujikawa et al., 2004 (160)	N = 16 AD	Quetiapine 77 mg average dose/day	Open 8-wk study	↓ Restlessness, sleep disturbances, and anxiety
Goldenberg et al., 1998 (228)	N = 1 AD	Gabapentin 200 mg tid	Open	↓ Incessant vocalizations and restlessness
Haffmans et al., 2001 (16)	N = 10 dementia	Melatonin with and without light therapy	DBPC crossover	↓ Restlessness with light therapy alone; melatonin no help

AD, Alzheimer's disease; DB, double blind; ns, nonsignificant; PC, placebo control.

Table 23 Suggested Preferred Treatments for Obsessive–Compulsive Traits in Dementia

---

Obsessive–compulsive traits: First-line suggested preferred treatments
1. Fluvoxamine
2. Other SSRIs

Obsessive–compulsive traits: Second-line suggested preferred treatments
1. Clomipramine
2. Risperidone and other atypical antipsychotics

---

along the way, and will run into objects or knock others over who block their path. Restless behaviors, as opposed to obsessive–compulsive behaviors, can be redirected fairly easily. Yelling or moaning behaviors may in some cases be obsessive–compulsive if the yelling becomes repetitive and does not seem to be related to pain, discomfort, or other obvious reason. Other examples of obsessive–compulsive behaviors include craving and eating the same type of food, prepared in the same way day after day with variation only infrequently. Compulsions may include eating at one sitting, an entire bag of chips, a box of candy, or a package of cookies until all food in sight is gone. Other patients might demand and watch the same TV shows or videos over and over without boredom. These behaviors can cause additional health issues. Excessive eating may result in obesity and secondary infections might occur when there is excessive picking of the skin causing excoriations.

Treatment of Obsessive–Compulsive Traits in Dementia

Fluvoxamine and other SSRIs have been approved for the treatment of OCD. However, there are no double-blind or placebo-controlled studies for the treatment of obsessive–compulsive traits in dementia subjects. The few open-label studies that exist have very small numbers of subjects. Suggested preferred pharmacotherapies for obsessive–compulsive traits in dementia are listed in Table 23, and specific studies are listed in Table 24. Fluvoxamine, in dementia and FTD subjects, was found to be helpful for control of stereotypic behaviors (230,231) compulsive pain complaints (231). Fluvoxamine also has been shown to reduce psychogenic excoriation independent of mood (232). I have found excellent results with fluvoxamine for these behaviors but it needs to be titrated up to high doses, usually 200 to 300 mg total dose per day to be effective. Citalopram eliminated trichotillomania in one FTD patient (233) and fluoxetine dramatically reduced recitations and excessive crying out of people's names in one AD patient (234). Paroxetine and other serotonergic agents may help vocally disruptive behaviors (235,236). All the SSRIs in high doses seem to be effective for OCD (119,237).

If high doses of an SSRI are not helpful, use of clomipramine should be considered. It works well for obsessive–compulsive traits but has more side effects than fluvoxamine and the other SSRIs (238). There was a case report of an AD patient responding better to clomipramine than to fluvoxamine for obsessive–compulsive traits (239). However, clomipramine should still be used second line due to its anticholinergic and sedative properties. Risperidone is not typically

Table 24 Studies for the Treatment of Obsessive–Compulsive Traits in Dementia

Study	Subjects	Agents	Design	Results
Trappler et al., 1997 (230)	$N = 3$ dementia	Fluvoxamine up to 150 mg/day	Open	↓ Stereotypic behaviors
Ishikawa et al., 2006 (231)	$N = 2$ FTD	Fluvoxamine	Open	↓ Stereotypic behaviors and compulsive pain complaint
Mittal et al., 2001 (233)	$N = 1$ FTD	Citalopram 60 mg/day	Open	↓ Trichotillomania
Marksteiner et al., 2003 (234)	$N = 1$ AD	Fluoxetine 60 mg/day	Open	↓ Obsessive–compulsive traits
Meares et al., 1999 (235)	$N = 1$ AD	Paroxetine	Open	↓ Vocally disruptive behaviors
Swartz et al., 1997 (119)	$N = 11$ FTD	Fluoxetine, sertraline, or paroxetine	Open	↓ Compulsions, carbohydrate craving, disinhibition, and depression in at least half
Trappler 1999 (239)	$N = 1$ AD	Clomipramine	Open	↓ Obsessive–compulsive traits
Kopala et al., 1997 (227)	$N = 2$ dementia	Risperidone	Open	↓ Persistent vocalizations

AD, Alzheimer's disease; FTD, frontotemporal dementia.

used for these obsessive–compulsive traits, but it lessened persistent vocalizations in two demented women (227).

SUMMARY

Behavioral disturbances are protean in dementia conditions. The key to the management of these difficult symptoms is to correctly identify the specific underlying behaviors. To do this, health care providers should seek the details of what may have precipitated the behavior disturbance. They should try to perceive the circumstances through the eyes of the patient. They should first look for environmental triggers and correct those that they can. Next, checking for any medical causes of behaviors is prudent. Laboratory evaluations may be indicated. Then, ensure that the patient's basic needs are met (comfort, food, drink, sleep, toileting, activity). Educating caregivers on techniques to reduce behaviors are very useful. Once the specific underlying behaviors are discovered, treatment can be directed right to the core symptoms. Polypharmacy is typical as there may be several underlying behaviors that are best treated with different agents. It is not always wise to continue to go higher and higher on the dose of one specific medication and expect it to effectively treat every difficult behavior that the patient is exhibiting. This typically leads to increased adverse effects with little to show for it in regards to behavior reduction. More often, the effective strategy is to use low doses of medications with each drug targeting a specific underlying behavior, which improves tolerability by reducing dose-dependent side effects and usually provides improved behavior control. Finally, by eliminating or rarely using benzodiazepines and anticholinergics the health care provider can reduce sedation, improve balance, and maximize cognition.

REFERENCES

1. Mega MS, Cummings JL, Fiorello T, et al. The spectrum of behavioral changes in Alzheimer's disease. Neurology 1996; 46:130–135.
2. Brun A, Gustafson L. Clinical and pathological aspects of frontotemporal dementia. In: Miller BL, Cummings JL, eds. The Human Frontal Lobes: Functions and Disorders. New York, NY: The Guilford Press, 1999:349–369.
3. Mega MS, Masterman DL, Benson DF, et al. Dementia with Lewy bodies: Reliability and validity of clinical and pathologic criteria. Neurology 1996; 47:1403–1409.
4. Teri L, Larson EB, Reifler BV. Behavioral disturbances in dementia of the Alzheimer's type. J Am Geriatr Soc 1988; 36:1–6.
5. Steele C, Rovner B, Chase GA, Folstein M. Psychiatric symptoms and nursing home placement of patients with Alzheimer's disease. Am J Psychiatry 1990; 147:1049–1051.
6. Scharre DW, Cummings JL. Dementia. In: Yoshikama TT, Cobbs EL, Brummel-Smith K, eds. Practical Ambulatory Geriatrics. 2nd ed. St. Louis, MO: Mosby Year Book, 1998:290–301.
7. Jackson GR, Lang AE. Hyperkinetic movement disorders. In: Coffey CE, Cummings JL, eds. Textbook of Geriatric Neuropsychiatry. 2nd ed. Washington, DC: American Psychiatric Press, 2000:531–557.
8. Cummings JL, Arciniegas DB, Brooks BR, et al. Defining and diagnosing involuntary emotional expression disorder (IEED). CNS Spectr 2006; 11(suppl 6):1–7.
9. Scharre DW. Infectious, inflammatory, and demyelinating disorders of the frontal lobes. In: Miller BL, Cummings JL, eds. The Human Frontal Lobes: Functions and Disorders. 2nd ed. New York: The Guilford Press, 2006:518–539.
10. Alexopoulos GS, Meyers BS, Young RC, et al. The course of geriatric depression with 'reversible dementia': A controlled study. Am J Psychiatry 1993; 150:1693–1699.
11. Carlson DL, Fleming KC, Smith GE, et al. Management of dementia-related behavioral disturbances: A nonpharmacologic approach. Mayo Clin Proc 1995; 70:1108–1115.
12. Beck CK. Psychosocial and behavioral interventions for Alzheimer's disease patients and their families. Am J Geriatr Psychiatry 1998; 6:S41–S48.
13. Namazi K, Gwinnup P, Zadorozny C. A low intensity exercise/movement program for patients with Alzheimer's disease: The TEMP-AD Protocol. J Aging Phys Activity 1994; 2:80–92.
14. Gerdner L. Effects of individualized versus classical "relaxation" music on the frequency of agitation in elderly persons with Alzheimer's disease and related disorders. Int Psychogeriatr 2000; 12:49–65.
15. Churchill M, Safaoui J, McCabe B, et al. Using a therapy dog to alleviate the agitation and desocialization of people with Alzheimer's disease. J Psychosoc Nurs 1999; 37:16–22.
16. Haffmans PM, Sival RC, Lucius SAP, et al. Bright light therapy and melatonin in motor restless behaviour in dementia: A placebo-controlled study. Int J Geriatr Psychiatry 2001; 16:106–110.
17. Ballard CG, O'Brien JT, Reichelt K, et al. Aromatherapy as a safe and effective treatment for the management of agitation in severe dementia: The results of a double-blind, placebo-controlled trial with Melissa. J Clin Psychiatry 2002; 63:553–558.
18. Knopman DS, Berg JD, Thomas R, et al. Nursing home placement is related to dementia progression: Experience from a clinical trial. Neurology 1999; 52:714–718.
19. Pollock BG, Mulsant BH, Rosen J, et al. Comparison of citalopram, perphenazine, and placebo for the acute treatment of psychosis and behavioral disturbances in hospitalized, demented patients. Am J Psychiatry 2002; 159:460–465.
20. Pollock BG, Mulsant BH, Rosen J, et al. A double-blind comparison of citalopram and risperidone for the treatment of behavioral and psychotic symptoms associated with dementia. Am J Geriatr Psychiatry 2007; 15:942–952.
21. Sultzer DL, Gray KF, Gunay I, et al. A double-blind comparison of trazodone and haloperidol for treatment of agitation in patients with dementia. Am J Geriatr Psychiatry 1997; 5:60–69.

22. Devanand DP, Marder K, Michaels KS, et al. A randomized, placebo-controlled dose-comparison trial of haloperidol for psychosis and disruptive behaviors in Alzheimer's disease. Am J Psychiatry 1998; 155:1512–1520.

23. De Deyn PP, Rabheru K, Rasmussen A, et al. A randomized trial of risperidone, placebo, and haloperidol for behavioral symptoms of dementia. Neurology 1999; 53:946–955.

24. Chan W, Lam LC, Choy CN, et al. A double-blind randomized comparison of risperidone and haloperidol in the treatment of behavioural and psychological symptoms in Chinese dementia patients. Int J Geriatr Psychiatry 2001; 16:1156–1162.

25. Verhey FR, Verkaaik M, Lousberg R, Olanzapine-Haloperidol in Dementia Study Group. Olanzapine versus haloperidol in the treatment of agitation in elderly patients with dementia: Results of a randomized controlled double-blind trial. Dement Geriatr Cogn Disord 2006; 21:1–8.

26. Suh G-H, Greenspan AJ, Choi S-K. Comparative efficacy of risperidone versus haloperidol on behavioural and psychological symptoms of dementia. Int J Geriatr Psychiatry 2006; 21;654–660.

27. Katz IR, Jeste DV, Mintzer JE, et al. Comparison of risperidone and placebo for psychosis and behavioral disturbances associated with dementia: A randomized, double-blind trial. J Clin Psychiatry 1999; 60:107–115.

28. Brodaty H, Ames D, Snowdon J, et al. A randomized, placebo-controlled trial of risperidone for the treatment of aggression, agitation, and psychosis of dementia. J Clin Psychiatry 2003; 64:134–143.

29. Holmes C, Wilkinson D, Dean C, et al. Risperidone and rivastigmine and agitated behaviour in severe Alzheimer's disease: A randomized double blind placebo con-trolled study. Int J Geriatr Psychiatry 2007; 22:380–381.

30. Schneider LS, Tariot PN, Dagerman KS, et al. Effectiveness of atypical antipsychotic drugs in patients with Alzheimer's disease. N Engl J Med 2006; 355:1525–1538.

31. Rainer M, Haushofer M, Pfolz H, et al. Quetiapine versus risperidone in elderly patients with behavioural and psychological symptoms of dementia: Efficacy, safety and cognitive function. Eur Psychiatry 2007; 22:395–403.

32. Zhong KX, Tariot PN, Mintzer J, et al. Quetiapine to treat agitation in dementia: A randomized, double-blind, placebo-controlled study. Curr Alzheimer Res 2007; 4:81–93.

33. Tariot PN, Schneider L, Katz IR, et al. Quetiapine treatment of psychosis associated with dementia: A double-blind, randomized, placebo-controlled clinical trial. Am J Geriatr Psychiatry 2006; 14:767–776.

34. Street JS, Clark WS, Gannon KS, et al. Olanzapine treatment of psychotic and behav-ioral symptoms in patients with Alzheimer's disease in nursing care facilities. Arch Gen Psychiatry 2000; 57:968–976.

35. De Deyn PP, Carrasco MM, Deberdt W, et al. Olanzapine versus placebo in the treatment of psychosis with or without associated behavioral disturbances in patients with Alzheimer's disease. Int J Geriatr Psychiatry 2004; 19:115–126.

36. Meehan KM, Wang H, David SR, et al. Comparison of rapidly acting intramuscular olanzapine, lorazepam and placebo: A double-blind randomized study in acutely agitated patients with dementia. Neuropsychopharmacology 2002; 26:494–504.

37. Mintzer JE, Tune LE, Breder CD, et al. Aripiprazole for the treatment of psychoses in institutionalized patients with Alzheimer's dementia: A multicenter, randomized, double-blind, placebo-controlled assessment of three fixed doses. Am J Geriatr Psy-chiatry 2007; 15:918–931.

38. Streim JE, Porsteinsson AP, Breder CD et al. A randomized, double-blind, placebo-controlled study of aripiprazole for the treatment of psychosis in nursing home patients with Alzheimer's disease. Am J Geriatr Psychiatry 2008; 16:537–550.

39. Porsteinsson AP, Tariot PN, Erb R, et al. Placebo-controlled study of divalproex sodium for agitation in dementia. Am J Geriatr Psychiatry 2001; 9:58–66.

40. Tariot PN, Erb R, Leibovici A, et al. Carbamazepine treatment of agitation in nursing patients with dementia: A preliminary study. J Am Geritr Soc 1994; 42:1160–1166.

41. Tariot PN, Erb R, Podgorski CA, et al. Efficacy and tolerability of carbamazepine for agitation and aggression in dementia. Am J Psychiatry 1998; 155:54–61.
42. Olin JT, Fox LS, Pawluczyk S, et al. Pilot randomized trial of carbamazepine for behavioral symptoms in treatment-resistant outpatients with Alzheimer's disease. Am J Geriatr Psychiatry 2001; 9:400–405.
43. Gauthier S, Wirth Y, Mobius HJ. Effects of memantine on behavioural symptoms in Alzheimer's disease patients: An analysis of the Neuropsychiatric Inventory (NPI) data of two randomized, double-blind, placebo-controlled 6-month study. Int J Geriatr Psychiatry 2005; 20:459–464.
44. Cummings JL, Schneider E, Tariot PN, et al.; Memantine MEM-MD-02 Study Group. Behavioral effects of memantine in Alzheimer disease patients receiving donepezil treatment. Neurology 2006; 67:57–63.
45. Huertas D, Lopez-Ibor Alino JJ, Molina JD, et al. Antiaggressive effect of cyproterone versus haloperidol in Alzheimer's disease: A randomized double-blind pilot study. J Clin Psychiatry 2007; 68:439–444.
46. Hawkins JW, Tinklenberg JR, Sheikh JI, et al. A retrospective chart review of gabapentin for the treatment of aggressive and agitated behavior in patients with dementia. Am J Geriatr Psychiatry 2000; 8:221–225.
47. Kitamura Y, Kudo Y, Imamura T. Trazodone for the treatment of behavioral and psychological symptoms of dementia (BPSD) in Alzheimer's disease: A retrospective study focused on the aggression and negativism in caregiving situations. No To Shinkei 2006; 58:483–488.
48. Lopez-Pousa S, Garre-Olmo J, Vilalta-Franch J, et al. Trazodone for Alzheimer's disease: A naturalistic follow-up study. Arch Gerontol Geriatr 2008; 47:207–215.
49. Lavretsky H, Sultzer DL. An open-label trial of risperidone for the treatment of agitation in dementia. Am J Geriatr Psychiatry 1998; 6:127–135.
50. Onor ML, Saina M, Trevisiol M, et al. Clinical experience with risperidone in the treatment of behavioral and psychological symptoms of dementia. Prog Neuropsychopharmacol Psychiatry 2007; 31:205–209.
51. Scharre DW, Chang S-I. Cognitive and behavioral effects of quetiapine in Alzheimer disease patients. Alzheimer Dis Assoc Disord 2002; 16:128–130.
52. Onor ML, Saina M, Aguglia E. Efficacy and tolerability of quetiapine in the treatment of behavioral and psychological symptoms of dementia. Am J Alzheimers Dis Other Demen 2006; 21:448–453.
53. Lee HB, Hanner JA, Yokley JL, et al. Clozapine for treatment-resistant agitation in dementia. J Geriatr Psychiatry Neurol 2007; 20;178–182.
54. Cole SA, Saleem R, Shea WP, et al. Ziprasidone for agitation or psychosis in dementia: Four cases. Int J Psychiatry Med 2005; 35:91–98.
55. Rocha FL, Hara C, Ramos MG, et al. An exploratory open-label trial of ziprasidone for the treatment of behavioral and psychological symptoms of dementia. Dement Geriatr Cogn Disord 2006; 22:445–448.
56. Rais AR, Wiliams K, Rais T, et al. Use of intramuscular ziprasidone for the control of acute psychosis or agitation in an inpatient geriatric population: An open-label study. Psychiatry (Edgmont) 2010; 7:17–24.
57. Lott AD, McElroy SL, Keys MA. Valproate in the treatment of behavioral agitation in elderly patients with dementia. J Neuropsychiatry Clin Neurosci 1995; 7:314–319.
58. Porsteinsson AP, Tariot PN, Jakimovich LJ, et al. Valproate therapy for agitation in dementia: Open-label extension of a double-blond trial. Am J Geriatr Psychiatry 2003; 11:434–440.
59. Forester B, Vanelli M, Hyde J, et al. Report on an open-label prospective study of divalproex sodium for the behavioral and psychological symptoms of dementia as monotherapy and in combination with second-generation antipsychotic medication. Am J Geriatr Pharmacother 2007; 5:209–217.
60. Gleason RP, Schneider LS. Carbamazepine treatment of agitation in Alzheimer's outpatients refractory to neuroleptics. J Clin Psychiatry 1990; 51:115–118.

61. Lemke M. Effect of carbamazepine on agitation and emotional lability associated with severe dementia. Eur Psychiatry 1995; 10:259–262.
62. Fhager B, Meiri IM, Sjogren M, et al. Treatment of aggressive behavior in dementia with the anticonvulsant topiramate: A retrospective pilot study. Int Psychogeriatr 2003; 15:307–309.
63. Calkin PA, Kunik ME, Orengo CA, et al. Tolerability of clonazepam in demented and non-demented geropsychiatric patients. Int J Geriatr Psychiatry 1997; 12:745–749.
64. Holzer JC, Gitelman DR, Price BH. Efficacy of buspirone in the treatment of dementia with aggression. Am J Psychiatry 1995; 152:812.
65. Cummings JL, Koumaras B, Chen M, et al.; Rivastigmine Nursing Home Study Team. Effects of rivastigmine treatment on the neuropsychiatric and behavioral disturbances of nursing home residents with moderate to severe probable Alzheimer's disease: A 26-week, multicenter, open-label study. Am J Geriatr Pharmacother 2005; 3:137–148.
66. Gauthier S, Juby A, Rehel B, et al. EXACT: Rivastigmine improves the high prevalence of attention deficits and mood and behaviour symptoms in Alzheimer's disease. Int J Clin Pract 2007; 61:886–895.
67. Weiler PG, Mungas D, Bernick C. Propranolol for the control of disruptive behavior in senile dementia. J Geriatr Psychiatry Neurol 1988; 1:226–230.
68. Shankle WR, Nielson KA, Cotman CW. Low-dose propranolol reduces aggression and agitation resembling that associated with orbitofrontal dysfunction in elderly demented patients. Alzheimer Dis Assoc Disord 1995; 9:233–237.
69. Tariot PN, Raman R, Jakimovich, et al. Divalproex sodium in nursing home residents with possible of probable Alzheimer's disease complicated by agitation: A randomized, controlled trial. Am J Geriatr Psychiatry 2005; 13:942–949.
70. Herrmann N, Lanctot KL, Rothenburg LS, et al. A placebo-controlled trial of valproate for agitation and aggression in Alzheimer's disease. Dement Geriatr Cogn Disord 2007; 23:116–119.
71. Auchus AP, Bissey-Black C. Pilot study of haloperidol, fluoxetine, and placebo for agitation in Alzheimer's disease. J Neuropsychiatry Clin Neurosci 1997; 9:591–593.
72. Ballard C, Margallo-Lana M, Juszczak E, et al. Quetiapine and rivastigmine and cognitive decline in Alzheimer's disease: Randomised double blind placebo controlled trial. BMJ 2005; 330:874–876.
73. Teri L, Logsdon RG, Peskind E, et al. Treatment of agitation in AD: A randomized, placebo-controlled clinical trial. Neurology 2000; 55:1271–1278.
74. Sultzer DL, Gray KF, Gunay I, et al. Does behavioral improvement with haloperidol or trazodone treatment depend on psychosis or mood symptoms in patients with dementia? J Am Geriatr Soc 2001; 49:1294–1300.
75. Wragg RE, Jeste DV. Overview of depression and psychosis in Alzheimer's disease. Am J Psychiatry 1989; 146:577–587.
76. Alexopoulos GS, Streim J, Carpenter D, et al. Using antipsychotic agents in older patients. Expert Consensus Guideline Series. J Clin Psychiatry 2004; 65(suppl 2):1–102.
77. Clark WS, Street JS, Feldman, et al. The effects of olanzapine in reducing the emergence of psychosis among nursing home patients with Alzheimer's disease. J Clin Psychiatry 2001; 62:34–40.
78. Cummings JL, Street J, Masterman D, et al. Efficacy of olanzapine in the treatment of psychosis in dementia with Lewy bodies. Dem Geriatr Cogn Disord 2002; 13:67–73.
79. De Deyn P, Jeste DV, Swanink R, et al. Aripiprazole for the treatment of psychosis in patients with Alzheimer's disease: A randomized, placebo-controlled study. J Clin Psychopharmacol 2005; 25:463–467.
80. Hamuro A. Aripiprazole for treatment of behavioural psychological symptoms of dementia. Aust N Z J Psychiatry 2007; 41:556.
81. Kurlan R, Cummings J, Raman R, et al; Alzheimer's Disease Cooperative Study Group. Quetiapine for agitation or psychosis in patients with dementia and parkinsonism. Neurology 2007; 68:1356–1363.

82. Paleacu D, Barak Y, Mirecky I, et al. Quetiapine treatment for behavioural and psychological symptoms of dementia Alzheimer's disease patients: A 6-week, double-blind, placebo-controlled study. Int J Geriatr Psychiatry 2008; 23:393–400.
83. Mintzer JE, Greenspan A, Caers I, et al. Risperidone in the treatment of psychosis of Alzheimer's disease: Results from a prospective clinical trial. Am J Geriatr Psychiatry 2006; 14;280–291.
84. Fernandez HH, Trieschmann ME, Burke MA, et al. Quetiapine for psychosis in Parkinson's disease versus dementia with Lewy bodies. J Clin Psychiatry 2002; 63:513–515.
85. Tanaka M, Kita T. Paroxetine and improvement of visual hallucinations in patients with dementia with Lewy bodies. J Am Geriatr Soc 2005; 53:732–733.
86. Cummings JL, McRae T, Zhang R. Effects of donepezil on neuropsychiatric symptoms in patients with dementia and severe behavioral disorders. Am J Geriatr Psychiatry 2006; 14:605–612.
87. Monsch AU, Giannakopoulos P; GAL-SUI Study Group. Effects of galantamine on behavioural and psychological disturbances and caregiver burden in patients with Alzheimer's disease. Curr Med Res Opin 2004; 20:931–938.
88. Tangwongchai S, Thavichachart N, Senanarong V, et al. Galantamine for the treatment of BPSD in Thai patients with possible Alzheimer's disease with or without cerebrovascular disease. Am J Alzheimers Dis Other Demen 2008; 23:593–601.
89. Erkinjuntti T, Kurz A, Gauthier S, et al. Efficacy of galantamine in probable vascular dementia and Alzheimer's disease combined with cerebrovascular disease: A randomised trial. Lancet 2002; 359:1283–1290.
90. Litvinenko IV, Odinak MM, Mogil'naia VI, et al. Efficacy and safety of galantamine (reminyl) for dementia in patients with Parkinson's disease (an open controlled trial). Neurosci Behav Physiol 2008; 38:937–945.
91. Edwards K, Royall D, Hershey L, et al. Efficacy and safety of galantamine in patients with dementia with Lewy bodies: 24-week open-label study. Dement Geriatr Cogn Disord 2007; 23:401–405.
92. Caligiuri MR, Jeste DV, Lacro JP. Antipsychotic-induced movement disorders in the elderly: Epidemiology and treatment recommendations. Drugs Aging 2000; 17:363–384.
93. Kryzhanovskaya LA, Jeste DV, Young CA, et al. A review of treatment-emergent adverse events during olanzapine clinical trials in elderly patients with dementia. J Clin Psychiatry 2006; 67:933–945.
94. Schneider LS, Dagerman KS, Insel P. Risk of death with atypical antipsychotic drug treatment for dementia: Meta-analysis of randomized placebo-controlled trials. JAMA 2005; 294:1934–1943.
95. Ray WA, Chung CP, Murray KT, et al. Atypical antipsychotic drugs and the risk of sudden cardiac death. N Engl J Med 2009; 360:225–235.
96. Al-Khatib SM, LaPointe NMA, Kramer JM, et al. What clinicians should know about the QT interval. JAMA 2003; 289:2120–2127.
97. Consensus development conference on antipsychotic drugs and obesity and diabetes. J Clin Psychiatry 2004; 65:267–272.
98. Frenchman B, Prince T. Clinical experience with risperidone, haloperidol, and thioridazine for dementia-associated behavioral disturbances. Int Psychogeriatr 1997; 9:431–435.
99. Diagnostic and Statistical Manual of Mental Disorders. 4th ed. Text Revision (DSM-IV-TR). Washington, DC: American Psychiatric Association, 2000.
100. Zubenko GS, Moossy J. Major depression in primary dementia: Clinical and neuropathologic correlates. Arch Neurol 1988; 45:1182–1186.
101. Reding M, Haycox J, Blass J. Depression in patients referred to a dementia clinic: A three-year prospective study. Arch Neurol 1985; 42:894–896.
102. Cummings JL, Victoroff JI. Noncognitive neuropsychiatric syndromes in Alzheimer's disease. Neuropsychiatry Neuropsychol Behav Neurol 1990; 3:140–158.

103. Kaufer DI, Cummings JL, Christine D, et al. Assessing the impact of behavioral disturbances in Alzheimer's disease: The Neuropsychiatric Inventory Caregiver Distress Scale. J Am Geriatr Soc 1998; 46:210–215.
104. Nyth AL, Gottfries G. The clinical efficacy of citalopram in treatment of emotional disturbances in dementia disorders: A Nordic multicenter study. Br J Psychiatry 1990; 157:894–901.
105. Nyth A, Gottfries C, Lyby K, et al. A controlled multicenter clinical study of citalopram and placebo in elderly depressed patients with and without concomitant dementia. Acta Psychiatr Scand 1992; 86:138–145.
106. Karlsson I, Godderis J, Augusto De Mendonca, et al. A randomized, double-blind comparison of the efficacy and safety of citalopram compared to mianserin in elderly, depressed patients with or without mild to moderate dementia. Int J Geriatr Psychiatry 2000; 15:295–305.
107. Rao V, Spiro JR, Rosenberg PB, et al. An open-label study of escitalopram (Lexapro) for the treatment of 'depression of Alzheimer's disease' (dAD). Int J Geriatr Psychiatry 2006; 21:273–274.
108. Lyketsos CG, Sheppard JM, Steele CD, et al. Randomized, placebo-controlled, double-blind clinical trial of sertraline in the treatment of depression complicating Alzheimer's disease: Initial results from the Depression in Alzheimer's Disease Study. Am J Psychiatry 2000; 157:1686–1689.
109. Lyketsos CG, Lourdes D, Steinberg M, et al. Treating depression in Alzheimer's disease. Efficacy and safety of sertraline therapy, and the benefits of depression reduction: The DIADS. Arch Gen Psychiatry 2003; 60:737–746.
110. Munro CA, Brandt J, Sheppard JM, et al. Cognitive response to pharmacological treatment for depression in Alzheimer's disease: Secondary outcomes from the Depression in Alzheimer's Disease Study (DIADS). Am J Geriatr Psychiatry 2004; 12:491–498.
111. Finkel SI, Mintzer JE, Dysken M, et al. A randomized, placebo-controlled study of the efficacy and safety of sertraline in the treatment of the behavioral manifestations of Alzheimer's disease in outpatients treated with donepezil. Int J Geriatr Psychiatry 2004; 19:9–18.
112. Oslin DW, Ten Have TR, Streim JE, et al. Probing the safety of medications in the frail elderly: Evidence from a randomized clinical trial of sertraline and venlafaxine in depressed nursing home residents. J Clin Psychiatry 2003; 64:875–882.
113. Volicer L, Rheaume Y, Cyr D. Treatment of depression in advanced Alzheimer's disease using sertraline. J Geriatr Psychiatry Neurol 1994; 7:227–229.
114. Burke WJ, Dewan V, Wengel SP, et al. The use of selective serotonin reuptake inhibitors for depression and psychosis complicating dementia. Int J Geriatr Psychiatry 1997; 12:519–525.
115. Katona CL, Hunter BN, Bray J. A double-blind comparison of the efficacy and safety of paroxetine and imipramine in the treatment of depression with dementia. Int J Geriatr Psychiatry 1998; 13:100–108.
116. Moretti R, Torre P, Antonello RM, et al. Frontotemporal dementia: Paroxetine as a possible treatment of behavior symptoms. A randomized, controlled, open 14-month study. Eur Neurol 2003;49;13–19.
117. Taragano FE, Lyketosos CG, Mangone CA, et al. A double-blind, randomized, fixed-dose trial of fluoxetine vs. amitriptyline in the treatment of major depression complicating Alzheimer's disease. Psychosomatics 1997; 38:246–252.
118. Sobow TM, Maczkiewicz M, Kloszewska I. Tianeptine versus fluoxetine in the treatment of depression complicating Alzheimer's disease. Int J Geriatr Psychiatry 2001; 16:1108–1109.
119. Swartz JR, Miller BL, Lesser IM, et al. Frontotemporal dementia: Treatment response to serotonin selective reuptake inhibitors. J Clin Psychiatry 1997; 58:212–216.
120. Olassfon K, Jorgensen S, Jensen HV, et al. Fluvoxamine in the treatment of demented elderly patients: A double-blind, placebo-controlled study. Acta Psychiatry Scand 1992; 85:453–456.

121. Raji MA, Brady SR. Mirtazapine for treatment of depression and comorbidities in Alzheimer's disease. Ann Pharmacother 2001; 35:1024–1027.
122. Lebert F, Stekke W, Hasenbroekx C, et al. Frontotemporal dementia: A randomized, controlled trial with trazodone. Dem Geriatr Cogn Dis 2004; 17:355–359.
123. Lebert F, Pasquier F, Petit H. Behavioral effects of trazodone in Alzheimer's disease. J Clin Psychiatry 1994; 55:536–538.
124. Magai C, Kennedy G, Cohen CI, et al. A controlled clinical trial of sertraline in the treatment of depression in nursing home patients with late-stage Alzheimer's disease. Am J Geriatr Psychiatry 2000; 8:66–74.
125. Petracca GM, Chemerinski E, Starkstein SE. A double-blind, placebo-controlled study of fluoxetine in depressed patients with Alzheimer's disease. Int Psychogeriatr 2001; 13:233–240.
126. de Vasconcelos Cunha UG, Lopes Rocha F, Avila de Melo R, et al. A placebo-controlled double-blind randomized study of venlafaxine in the treatment of depression in dementia. Dement Geriatr Cogn Disord 2007; 24:36–41.
127. Caballero J, Hitchcock M, Beversdorf D, et al. Long-term effects of antidepressants on cognition in patients with Alzheimer's disease. J Clin Pharm Ther 2006; 31:593–598.
128. Deakin JB, Rahman S, Nestor PJ, et al. Paroxetine does not improve symptoms and impairs cognition in frontotemporal dementia: A double-blind randomized controlled trial. Psychopharmacology (Berl) 2004; 172:400–408.
129. Petracca G, Teson A, Chemerinski E, et al. A double-blind placebo-controlled study of clomipramine in depressed patients with Alzheimer's disease. J Neuropsychiatry Clin Neurosci 1996; 8:270–275.
130. Roth M, Mountjoy C, Amrein R; International Collaborative Study Group. Moclobemide in elderly patients with cognitive decline and depression. Br J Psychiatry 1996; 168:149–157.
131. Fuchs A, Hehnke U, Erhart Ch, et al. Video rating analysis of effect of maprotiline in patients with dementia and depression. Pharmacopsychiatry 1993; 26:37–41.
132. Reifler B, Teri L, Raskind M, et al. Double-blind trial of imipramine in Alzheimer's disease patients with and without depression. Am J Psychiatry 1989; 146:45–49.
133. Bartlome P, King KS, Matsuo F, et al. Cognitive decline with nortriptyline use in a patient with dementia of the Alzheimer's type. Western J Med 1992; 156:75–77.
134. Tekin S, Aykut-Bingöl C, Tarnridag T, et al. Antiglutamatergic therapy in Alzheimer's disease—Effects of lamotrigine. J Neural Transm 1998; 105:295–303.
135. Belzie LR. Risperidone for AIDS-associated dementia: A case series. AIDS Patient Care and STDS 1996; 10:246–249.
136. Yoon JS, Kim JM, Lee H, et al. Risperidone use in Korean patients with Alzheimer's disease: Optimal dosage and effect on behavioural and psychological symptoms, cognitive function and activities of daily living. Hum Psychopharmacol Clin Exp 2003; 18:627–633.
137. Fontaine CS, Hynan LS, Koch K, et al. A double-blind comparison of olanzapine versus risperidone in the acute treatment of dementia-related behavioral disturbances in extended care facilities. J Clin Psychiatry 2003; 64:726–730.
138. Catsman-Berrevoets CE, von Harskamp F. Compulsive pre-sleep behavior and apathy due to bilateral thalamic stroke: Response to bromocriptine. Neurology 1988; 38:647–649.
139. Scharre DW, Johnson RH, Wu X, et al. SPECT imaging in fronto-temporal degeneration: Anatomical correlations with apathy and disinhibition. Neurology 1996; 46:A178.
140. Landes AM, Sperry SD, Strauss ME. Apathy in Alzheimer's disease. J Am Geriatr Soc 2001; 49:1700–1707.
141. Kaufer D, Cummings JL, Christine D. Differential neuropsychiatric symptom responses to tacrine in Alzheimer's disease: Relationship to dementia severity. J Neuropsychiatry Clin Neurosci 1998; 10:55–63.

142. Gauthier S, Feldman H, Hecker J, et al. Efficacy of donepezil on behavioral symptoms in patients with moderate to severe Alzheimer's disease. Int Psychogeriatr 2002; 14:389–404.
143. Marin R, Fogel B, Hawkins J, et al. Apathy: A treatable syndrome. J Neuropsychiatry Clin Neurosci 1995; 7:23–30.
144. Padala PR, Burke WJ, Bhatia SC. Modafinil therapy for apathy in an elderly patient. Ann Pharmacother 2007; 41:346–349.
145. Negron AE, Reichman WE. Risperidone in the treatment of patients with Alzheimer's disease with negative symptoms. Int Psychogeriatr 2000; 12:527–536.
146. Rankin ED, Layne RD. The use of olanzapine in the treatment of negative symptoms in Alzheimer's disease. J Neuropsychiatry Clin Neurosci 2005; 17:423–424.
147. Sival RC, Duivenoorden HJ, Jansen PA, et al. Sodium valproate in aggressive behaviour in dementia: A twelve-week open label follow-up study. Int J Geriatr Psychiatry 2004; 19:305–312.
148. Keck PE, McElroy SL, Friedman LM. Valproate and carbamazepine in the treatment of panic and posttraumatic stress disorders, withdrawal states, and behavioral dyscontrol syndromes. J Clin Psychopharmacol 1992; 12:35S–41S.
149. Sival RC, Haffmans PMJ, Jansen PAF, et al. Sodium valproate in the treatment of aggressive behavior in patients with dementia—a randomized placebo controlled clinical trial. Int J Geriatr Psychiatry 2002; 17:579–585.
150. Moretti R, Torre P, Antonello RM, et al. Gabapentin for the treatment of behavioural alterations in dementia: Preliminary 15-month investigation. Drugs Aging 2003; 20:1035–1040.
151. Kunik ME, Yudofsky SC, Silver JM, et al. Pharmacologic approach to management of agitation associated with dementia. J Clin Psychiatry 1994; 55(suppl 2):13–17.
152. Colenda CC. Buspirone in treatment of agitated demented patient. Lancet 1988; 1(8595):1169.
153. Tariot PN, Solomon PR, Morris JC, et al. A 5-month, randomized, placebo-controlled trial of galantamine in AD. Neurology 2000; 54:2269–2276.
154. Cummings JK, Schneider L, Tariot PN, et al. Reduction of behavioral disturbances and caregiver distress by galantamine in patients with Alzheimer's disease. Am J Psychiatry 2004; 161:532–538.
155. Herrmann N, Rabheru K, Wang J, et al. Galantamine treatment of problematic behavior in Alzheimer disease: Post-hoc analysis of pooled data from three large trials. Am J Geriatr Psychiatry 2005; 13:527–534.
156. Petrie WM, Ban TA. Propranolol in organic agitation. Lancet 1981; 1(8215):324.
157. Mintzer J, Faison W, Street JS, et al. Olanzapine in the treatment of anxiety symptoms due to Alzheimer's disease: A post hoc analysis. Int J Geriatr Psychiatry 2001; 16:S71–S77.
158. Street JS, Clark WS, Kadam DL, et al. Long-term efficacy of olanzapine in the control of psychotic and behavioral symptoms in nursing home patients with Alzheimer's dementia. Int J Geriatr Psychiatry 2001; 16:S62–S70.
159. Moretti R, Torre P, Antonello RM, et al. Olanzapine as a possible treatment for anxiety due to vascular dementia: An open study. Am J Alzheimers Dis Other Demen 2004; 19:81–88.
160. Fujikawa T, Takahashi T, Kinoshita A, et al. Quetiapine treatment for behavioral and psychological symptoms in patients with senile dementia of Alzheimer type. Neuropsychobiology 2004; 49:201–204.
161. Hogan DB, Maxwell CJ, Fung TS, et al. Prevalence and potential consequences of benzodiazepine use in senior citizens: Results from the Canadian Study of Health and Aging. Can J Clin Pharmacol 2003; 10:72–77.
162. Stonnington CM, Snyder PJ, Hentz JG, et al. Double-blind crossover study of the cognitive effects of lorazepam in healthy apolipoprotein E (APOE)-epsilon4 carriers. J Clin Psychiatry 2009; 70:1379–1384.
163. Salzman C. Treatment of agitation, anxiety, and depression in dementia. Psychopharmacol Bull 1988; 24:39–42.

164. Scharre DW. Neoplastic, demyelinating, infectious, and inflammatory brain disorders. In: Coffey CE, Cummings JL, eds. Textbook of Geriatric Neuropsychiatry. 2nd ed. Washington, DC: American Psychiatric Press, Inc., 2000:669–697.
165. De Leon OA. Antiepileptic drugs for the acute and maintenance treatment of bipolar disorder. Harv Rev Psychiatry 2001; 9:209–222.
166. Haas S, Vincent K, Holt J, et al. Divalproex: A possible treatment alternative for demented, elderly, aggressive patients. Ann Clin Psychiatry 1997; 9:145–147.
167. Essa M. Carbamazepine in dementia. J Clin Psychopharmacol 1986:6:234–236.
168. Miller LJ. Gabapentin for treatment of behavioral and psychological symptoms of dementia. Ann Pharmacother 2001; 35:427–431.
169. Devarajan S, Dursun SM. Aggression in dementia with lamotrigine treatment. Am J Psychiatry 2000; 157:1178.
170. Ng B, Camacho A, Bardwell W, et al. Lamotrigine for agitation in older patients with dementia. Int Psychogeriatr 2009; 21:207–208.
171. Tiller JW, Dakis JA, Shaw JM. Short-term buspirone treatment in disinhibition with dementia. Lancet 1988; 2(8609):510.
172. Vitiello MV, Prinz PN, Williams DE, et al. Sleep disturbances in patients with mild-stage Alzheimer's disease. J Gerontol Med Sci 1990; 45:131–138.
173. Bliwise DL. Sleep disorders in Alzheimer's disease and other dementias. Clin Cornerstone 2004; 6(suppl 1A):S16–S28.
174. McGaffigan S, Bliwise DL. The treatment of sundowning. A selective review of pharmacological and nonparmacological studies. Drugs Aging 1997; 10:10–17.
175. Saletu-Zyhlarz GM, Abu-Bakr MH, Anderer P, et al. Insomnia related to dysthymia: Polysomnographic and psychometric comparison with normal controls and acute therapeutic trials with trazodone. Neuropsychobiology 2002; 44:139–149.
176. Haffmans PM, Vos MS. The effects of trazodone on sleep disturbances induced by brofaromine. Eur Psychiatry 1999; 14:167–171.
177. Mashiko H, Niwa S, Kumashiro H, et al. Effect of trazodone in a single dose before bedtime for sleep disorders accompanied by a depressive state: Dose-finding study with no concomitant use of hypnotic agent. Psychiatry Clin Neurosci 1999; 53:193–194.
178. Shelton PS, Hocking LB. Zolpidem for dementia-related insomnia and nighttime wandering. Ann Pharmacother 1997; 31:319–322.
179. Wirz-Justice A, Werth E, Savaskan E, et al. Haloperidol disrupts, clozapine reinstates the circadian rest-activity cycle in a patient with early-onset Alzheimer disease. Alzheimer Dis Assoc Dis 2000; 14:212–215.
180. Garfinkel LD, Laudon M, Nof D, et al. Improvement of sleep quality in elderly people by controlled-release melatonin. Lancet 1995:346:541–544.
181. Haimov IP, Lavie P, Laudon M, et al. Melatonin replacement therapy of elderly insomniacs. Sleep 1995; 18:589–603.
182. Mishima K, Tozawa T, Satoh K, et al. Melatonin secretion rhythm disorders in patients with senile dementia of Alzheimer's type with disturbed sleep-walking. Biol Psychiatry 1999; 45:417–421.
183. Asayama K, Yamadera H, Ito T, et al. Double blind study of melatonin effects on the sleep-wake rhythm, cognitive and non-cognitive functions in Alzheimer type dementia. J Nippon Med School 2003; 70:334–341.
184. Jean-Louis G, Zizi F, von Gizycki H, et al. Effects of melatonin in two individuals with Alzheimer's disease. Percept Mot Skills 1998; 87:331–339.
185. Brusco LI, Marquez M, Cardinali DP. Monozygotic twins with Alzheimer's disease treated with melatonin: Case report. J Pinneal Res 1998; 25:260–263.
186. Brusco LI, Fainstein I, Marquez M, et al. Effect of melatonin in selected populations of sleep-disturbed patients. Biol Signals Recept 1999; 8:126–131.
187. Cardinali DP, Brusco LI, Liberczuk C, et al. The use of melatonin in Alzheimer's disease. Neuroendocrinol Lett 2002; 23(suppl 1):20–23.
188. Serfaty M, Kennell-Webb S, Warner J, et al. Double blind randomized placebo controlled trial of low dose melatonin for sleep disorders in dementia. Int J Geriatr Psychiatry 2002; 17:1120–1127.

189. Singer C, Tractenberg RE, Kaye J, et al. A multicenter, placebo-controlled trial of melatonin for sleep disturbance in Alzheimer's disease. Sleep 2003; 26:893–901.
190. Gehrman PR, Connor DJ, Martin JL, et al. Melatonin fails to improve sleep or agitation in a double-blind randomized placebo-controlled trial of institutionalized patients with Alzheimer's disease. Am J Geriatr Psychiatry 2009; 17:166–169.
191. McCarten JR, Kovera C, Maddox MK, et al. Triazolam in Alzheimer's disease: Pilot study on sleep and memory effects. Pharmacol Biochem Behav 1995; 52:447–452.
192. Power DA, Noel J, Collins R, et al. Circulating leptin levels and weight loss in Alzheimer's disease patients. Dement Geriatr Cogn Disord 2001; 12:167–170.
193. Gillette-Guyonnet S, Nourhashemi F, Andrieu S, et al. Weight loss in Alzheimer disease. Am J Clin Nutr 2000; 71:637S–642S.
194. Knittweis J. Weight loss in cancer and Alzheimer's disease is mediated by a similar pathway. Med Hypotheses 1999; 53:172–174.
195. Levitsky AM, Owens NJ. Pharmacologic treatment of hypersexuality and paraphilias in nursing home residents. J Am Geriatr Soc 1999; 47:231–234.
196. Anneser JM, Jox RJ, Borasio GD. Inappropriate sexual behaviour in a case of ALS and FTD: Successful treatment with sertraline. Amyotroph Lateral Scler 2007; 8:189–190.
197. Tosto G, Talarico G, Lenzi GL, et al. Effect of citalopram in treating hypersexuality in an Alzheimer's disease case. Neurol Sci 2008; 29:269–270.
198. Stewart JT, Shin KJ. Paroxetine treatment of sexual disinhibition in dementia. Am J Psychiatry 1997; 154:1474.
199. Gitlin MJ. Psychotropic medications and their effects on sexual function: Diagnosis, biology, and treatment approaches. J Clin Psychiatry 1994; 55:406–413.
200. Kafka MP. Sertraline pharmacotherapy for paraphilias and paraphilia-related disorders: An open trial. Ann Clin Psychiatry 1994; 6:189–195.
201. Wiseman SV, McAuley JW, Freidenberg GW, et al. Hypersexuality in patients with dementia: Possible response to cimetidine. Neurology 2000; 54:2024.
202. Leo RJ, Kim KY. Clomipramine treatment of paraphilias in elderly demented patients. J Geriatr Psychiatry Neurol 1995; 8:123–124.
203. Alkhalil C, Hahar N, Alkhalil B, et al. Can gabapentin be a safe alternative to hormonal therapy in the treatment of inappropriate sexual behavior in demented patients? Clin Pharmacol Physiol Conf 2003; 35:299–302.
204. Alkhalil C, Tanvir F, Alkhalil B, et al. Treatment of sexual disinhibition in dementia: Case reports and review of the literature. Am J Ther 2004; 11:231–235.
205. Freymann N, Michael R, Dodel R, et al. Successful treatment of sexual disinhibition in dementia with carbamazepine—as case report. Pharmacopsychiatry 2005; 38:144–145.
206. MacKnight C, Rojas-Fernandez C. Quetiapine for sexually inappropriate behavior in dementia. J Am Geriatr Soc 2000; 48:707.
207. Prakash R, Pathak A, Munda S, et al. Quetiapine effective in treatment of inappropriate sexual behavior of Lewy body disease with predominant frontal lobe signs. Am J Alzheimers Dis Other Demen 2009; 24:136–140.
208. Rosenthal M, Berkman P, Shapira A, et al. Urethral masturbation and sexual disinhibition in dementia: A case report. Israel J Psychiatry Rel Sci 2003; 40:67–72.
209. Alagiakrishnan K, Sclater A, Robertson D. Role of cholinesterase inhibitor in the management of sexual aggression in an elderly demented woman. J Am Geriatr Soc 2003; 51:1326.
210. Cooper AJ. Medroxyprogesterone acetate (MPA) treatment of sexual acting out in men suffering from dementia. J Clin Psychiatry 1987; 48:368–370.
211. Britton KR. Medroxyprogesterone in the treatment of aggressive hypersexual behavior in traumatic brain injury. Brain Inj 1998; 12:703–707.
212. Amadeo M. Antiandrogen treatment of aggressivity in men suffering from dementia. J Geriatr Psychiatry Neurol 1996; 9:142–145.
213. Rich SS, Ovsiew F. Leuprolide acetate for exhibitionism in Huntington's disease. Mov Disord 1994; 9:353–357.

214. Ott BR. Leuprolide treatment of sexual aggression in a patient with dementia and the Kluver-Bucy syndrome. Clin Neuropharmacol 1995; 18:443–447.
215. Shelton PS, Brooks VG. Estrogen for dementia-related aggression in elderly men. Ann Pharmacother 1999; 33:808–812.
216. Merriam AE, Aronson MK, Gaston P, et al. The psychiatric symptoms of Alzheimer's disease. J Am Geriatr Soc 1988; 36:7–12.
217. Scharre DW, Davis RA, Warner JL, et al. A pilot open-label trial of citalopram for restless activity and aberrant motor behaviors in Alzheimer's disease. Am J Geriatr Psychiatry 2003; 11:687–691.
218. Pollock BG, Mulsant BH, Sweet R, et al. An open pilot study of citalopram for behavioral disturbances of dementia. Plasma levels and real-time observations. Am J Geriatr Psychiatry 1997; 5:70–78.
219. Kim KY, Bader GM, Jones E. Citalopram for verbal agitation in patients with dementia. J Geriatr Psychiatry Neurol 2000; 13:53–55.
220. Ramadan FH, Naughton BJ, Bassanelli AG. Treatment of verbal agitation with a selective serotonin reuptake inhibitor. J Geriatr Psychiatry Neurol 2000; 13:56–59.
221. Lanctot KL, Herrmann N, van Reekum R, et al. Gender, aggression and serotonergic function are associated with response to sertraline for behavioral disturbances in Alzheimer's disease. Int J Geriatr Psychiatry 2002; 17:531–541.
222. Kunik ME, Puryear L, Orengo CA, et al. The efficacy and tolerability of divalproex sodium in elderly demented patients with behavioral disturbances. Int J Geriatr Psychiatry 1998; 13:29–34.
223. Buchalter EN, Lantz MS. Treatment of impulsivity and aggression in a patient with vascular dementia. Geriatrics 2001; 56:53–54.
224. Gutzmann H, Kuhl K, Kanowski S, et al. Measuring the efficacy of psychopharmacological treatment of psychomotoric restlessness in dementia: Clinical evaluation of tiapride. Pharmacopsychiatry 1997; 30:6–11.
225. Gareri P, Cotroneo A, Lacava R, et al. Comparison of the efficacy of new and conventional antipsychotic drugs in the treatment of behavioral and psychological symptoms of dementia (BPSD). Arch Gerontol Geriatr Suppl 2004; 9:207–215.
226. Meguro K, Meguro M, Tanaka Y, et al. Risperidone is effective for wandering and disturbed sleep/wake patterns in Alzheimer's disease. J Geriatr Psychiatry Neurol 2004; 17:61–67.
227. Kopala LC, Honer WG. The use of risperidone in severely demented patients with persistent vocalizations. Int J Geriatr Psychiatry 1997; 12:73–77.
228. Goldenberg G, Kahaner K, Basavaraju N, et al. Gabapentin for disruptive behaviour in an elderly demented patient. Drugs Aging 1998; 13:183–184.
229. Rossi P, Serrao M, Pozzessere G. Gabapentin-induced worsening of neuropsychiatric symptoms in dementia with Lewy bodies: Case reports. Eur Neurol 2002; 47:56–57.
230. Trappler B, Vinuela LM. Fluvoxamine for stereotypic behavior in patients with dementia. Ann Pharmacother 1997; 31:578–581.
231. Ishikawa H, Shimomura T, Shimizu T. Stereotyped behaviors and compulsive complaints of pain improved by fluvoxamine in two cases of frontotemporal dementia. Seishin Shinkeigaku Zasshi 2006; 108:1029–1035.
232. Arnold LM, Mutasim DF, Dwight MM, et al. An open clinical trial of fluvoxamine treatment of psychogenic excoriation. J Clin Psychopharmacol 1999; 19:15–18.
233. Mittal D, O'Jile J, Kennedy R, et al. Trichotillomania associated with dementia: A case report. Gen Hosp Psychiatry 2001; 23:163–165.
234. Marksteiner J, Walch T, Bodner T, et al. Fluoxetine in Alzheimer's disease with severe obsessive compulsive symptoms and a low density of serotonin transporter sites. Pharmacopsychiatry 2003; 36:207–209.
235. Meares S, Draper B. Treatment of vocally disruptive behaviour of multifactorial aetiology. Int J Geriat Psychiatry 1999; 14:285–290.
236. Greenwald BS, Marin DB, Silverman SM. Serotonergic treatment of screaming and banging in dementia. Lancet 1986; 2(8521–8522):1464–1465.

237. Mundo E, Bianchi E, Bellodi L. Efficacy of fluvoxamine, paroxetine, and citalopram in the treatment of obsessive-compulsive disorder: A single-blind study. J Clin Psychopharmacol 1997; 17:267–271.
238. Milanfranchi A, Ravagli S, Lensi P, et al. A double-blind study of fluvoxamine and clomipramine in the treatment of obsessive-compulsive disorder. Int Clin Psychopharmacol 1997; 12:131–136.
239. Trappler B. Treatment of obsessive-compulsive disorder using clomipramine in a very old patient. Ann Pharmacother 1999; 33:686–690.

5 Management of function: instrumental activities of daily living

Catherine Anne Bare and Martha S. Cameron

INTRODUCTION

Instrumental activities of daily living (IADLs) are those activities that require a higher level of cognitive functioning than activities of daily living (ADLs). They are multistep activities that are critical to successful independent living within a community and include such areas as occupation, driving, financial management, medication administration, household management, and computer technology (1,2). Deficits in these areas may be among the first indicators that an individual is having challenges with reasoning skills, intellectual abilities, and memory. IADLs may also become the first "battleground" for the caregiver and the person with dementia in terms of what are appropriate independent activities for the person with dementia. It becomes a fine balance between an individual's autonomy and the safety of the person, family, and/or the community. As the disease progresses, the individual has increased memory and visuospatial deficits, declines in problem-solving abilities, impaired decision-making skills and logical sequential reasoning skills, and consequently exhibits increased anxiety. Therefore, they become less able to accomplish these multistep activities. Because their insight into their abilities is diminished, what appears abundantly clear and logical to a caregiver or a doctor will have little relevance or meaning to the individual with dementia.

Individuals with dementia have the same needs as those without dementia: the need to feel productive and to participate in purposeful activity. Throughout the course of the disease, the abilities and therefore the needs of the individual will change and consequently the IADLs must be adapted accordingly.

The caregiver must assume considerable responsibility and serve as the gatekeeper as well as the advocate. When no caregiver is available, the community may need to assume the responsibility through adult protective services or a court-appointed guardian.

A question that must be asked in every situation is, "How much risk are we willing to take?"

The physician should play a key role in assessing and managing the client's functional abilities as well as providing support to the caregiver (3). Several assessment scales are available such as the Instrumental Activities of Daily Living Scale by Lawton and Brody.

(4) Results from these assessments may provide important data regarding the individual's ability to live safely on their own. For results to be valid, it is important to interview the caregiver separately and, when possible,

conduct an in-home functional and safety assessment. Observation of the family in their own home provides data that are helpful in developing a realistic plan. Some local Alzheimer's Association chapters can be helpful in providing this service (5). As the physician shares the results of the testing with the individual and family, it is important to provide some resources for the family to take home, such as an information packet from the Alzheimer's Association (5). They have a number of services to help the family as well as up-to-date knowledge regarding many community resources. This approach equips the family with a "next step" to follow rather than leaving them with only a physician's diagnosis and/or report.

OCCUPATION/LIFE ROLE

Occupations or life roles are an important part of an individual's identity and must be considered. Roles include one's profession, volunteering, homemaking, and leisure activities. The complexity of these roles will determine if and how long they can be sustained during the course of the disease. Indicators suggesting the need for adaptation include missing appointments, increased anxiety, getting lost, lack of initiative, and if working, calls from the workplace. The caregiver is typically in the best position to determine when adjustments must be made in these activities. There may be a need to simplify or modify an activity and ultimately find new activities as the disease progresses.

One of the hallmarks of dementia is apathy or loss of initiative. Caregivers may perceive this inactivity as laziness. Specific skills may still be present, but without cueing or encouragement by the caregiver, participation in the activity will not occur.

A person with dementia, who is still employed, presents additional challenges to the family as well as to the work place. As the person's cognitive skills, ability to reason, and problem solving continue to decline, there are increased errors and lapses in performance of the tasks for which they were hired and for which they are responsible. As coordination and physical abilities also deteriorate, job safety must be assessed particularly if the person is using power tools or driving vehicles. The complexity of the job needs to be considered to prevent unrealistic expectations that can cause anxiety. Job responsibilities or positions must be re-evaluated. If the person is responsible for employee supervision and welfare and/or finances, a trusted assistant may need to be hired. When the disease has been identified, it is important for the family to work with the employer to increase their understanding of what is happening and why. Hopefully, the employer will be cooperative. Coworkers may begin to see a change in work output. Some employers are more helpful and may be willing to adapt or redesign job responsibilities as the person's disease progresses. Cooperation with the workplace is important in order to establish qualifications for disability, rather than being fired for incompetence. It is critical for the physician to become involved and serve as an advocate for the individual and the family.

While it may be desirable for the person to retain their job for immediate financial remuneration, future financial implications must also be considered. Disability cannot be accessed as long as the person is employed fulltime. Ongoing health insurance is vital. When there is no health insurance with the job or after retirement, it is advantageous for the person to take Social Security Disability since the person will not become eligible for Medicare until the 25th month after the date of disability is established. Families should check with the Social Security Administration as qualifications for benefits may change (6). Initial application can be made online, by calling 1(800)772–1212, or through their local Social Security Office.

Many individuals with dementia have retired and have retained a set of skills or interests from their former jobs. They may also have leisure activities that fill their days and have become a part of their identity. When possible, caregivers should build on these learned skills and interests, simplifying the activities as the disease progresses, rather than introducing an activity that requires learning new skills.

Examples:

- A person who was involved in sales and still demonstrates strong social skills: Working 4 to 8 hours per week at a large warehouse type store may be appropriate and create a sense of fulfillment.
- A person who used to enjoy knitting or crocheting in the past but can no longer follow complex patterns: Try to interest the person in rolling balls of yarn.
- A person who has previously worked with children but can no longer be responsible for their care: The person may enjoy going to parks to watch children play.
- A person who had worked in the church kitchen: Enlist their help in setting the tables for church functions.
- A person who has a welcoming spirit: Enroll them in adult day services and ask the program if they can wear a "greeter" badge, and welcome people as they arrive.

While it may seem easier to allow the individual with dementia to sit and do nothing, building on their former skills and interests will ultimately lead to a more contented individual and consequently a less stressed caregiver.

DRIVING

Driving is one of the most difficult issues to deal with for the caregiver/family and the person with dementia. Driving is a means of independence in most areas of the United States. It is the way for the person to stay connected to family and activities. Many consider driving a right versus a privilege. Caregivers frequently hear the argument,

"I've been driving for more than 50 years without an accident or with one accident etc."

This is a difficult argument to counter as the person often overestimates his abilities and minimizes the complexities of driving. Another argument occurs when the state readily renews the person's driver's license without significant examination or evaluation.

Although a diagnosis of dementia does not mean that driving must stop immediately, there does need to be monitoring and ongoing informal assessment.

Hints for assessing driving skills

- Monitor mileage on the car on a weekly basis if possible. Usually the person is only driving short distances. Mileage increases that are out of character may indicate that the person is getting lost.
- Monitor the car for new dents and scrapes.
- If possible, follow the person on an errand and observe driving skills and compliance with traffic laws.
- Study options for dealing with driving issues. The Hartford has developed a guide, "At the Crossroads, Family conversations about Alzheimer's Disease, Dementia & Driving." (7) This free manual provides a list of warning signs to observe in persons with dementia, as well helpful suggestions for families.

Driving requires good vision, hearing, judgment, reaction time, memory, visuospatial skills, and the ability to make instant decisions. Impairment in any of these areas is a cause for concern. Many hospitals and universities offer geriatric driving evaluation programs. Medicare and private insurance may or may not cover some of the cost. These programs are typically managed by an occupational therapist and consist of an evaluation of knowledge of current traffic laws, a simulated driving skill test using a computer and on-the-road supervised driving. These evaluations can take 4 to 8 hours and are frequently administered in two sessions. A neutral third party then makes the decision that a person can drive safely.

A brief assessment tool used in the office setting, the 4-Turn Test, has been designed to assist in the determination of driving abilities of dementia patients (8). This simple test consists of having the patient follow the examiner along a short course in the clinic that arrives at four separate intersections where the individual turns to the right on two occasions and to the left on two occasions. The patient is provided visual clues at each intersection to remind them where to make a turn. They are then brought back to the starting point and asked to walk the same path again, but this time they must lead the way. One study (8) using the 4-Turn Test shows that if the mild Alzheimer's disease individual makes any nonself correcting error and ends up going in the wrong direction, 88% failed a behind the wheel driver's assessment by a professional driving instructor. If the person made all four turns correct and ended successfully at the end of the course, 92% of them passed the behind the wheel driver's evaluation.

If the person is willing to stop driving, it is important to remove the car from the home or hide the keys as they may forget and try to drive at a later date. It is helpful to have alternative driving options in place such as prearranging for friends to drive. Such plans can help to lessen potentially explosive situations.

What to do if there is resistance to assistance

- Tell the person that an adult child or grandchild needs to borrow the car because of a needed repair to his car that is going to take a couple weeks. Some are easily persuaded with this technique. Frequently after a couple

> weeks, the person stops asking to drive or wants the family member to keep the car.
> - Make the car inoperable. Early in the disease, the person may call a dealer or mechanic to fix it. If one suspects that this may happen, place a note under the hood requesting that the repairs not be made.
> - Sometimes getting to the car first and getting in the driver's seat will work and eventually this becomes a habit.

It is advisable that the caregiver not be the one to actually stop the person's driving if the person is resistant. Though there are short-term memory deficits, frequently the person with dementia will remember who was responsible for taking away their driving privilege and will constantly "blame" this person of this disservice.

The physician plays a key role with driving safety. Physician expertise in this decision is crucial. Techniques that the physician may find useful include:

- Write a prescription stating that the person should not drive or that the person needs a driver. Suggesting that this ban is "temporary" often is more palatable than telling them it may be permanent. This works for some and, if so, copies of the prescription should be made since the initial prescriptions may get lost.
- Tell the person with dementia that the doctor has no problem with the person continuing to drive as long as the person is willing to take the Older Adult Driver's Evaluation. The doctor needs to write a prescription for this to remind the person with dementia about the need to take the test. The doctor's office should try to assist with possible reimbursement for this evaluation through the patient's insurance company or Medicare.
- Request that the person stop driving until the next appointment because of starting a new medication.
- Ask the person's ophthalmologist to advise no driving due to vision losses, if appropriate. This can be a more acceptable recommendation when it is blamed on vision rather than memory problems.
- Use a direct approach. Tell the person that they cannot drive any longer. This may be traumatic and some people will refuse to return to the physician. Others may feel relieved that they do not have to drive and are willing to accept this directive from the physician.
- The American Medical Association, in conjunction with the National Traffic Safety Administration has developed the "Physician's Guide to Assessing and Counseling Older Drivers." (9) It is an excellent guide and includes such topics as counseling the patient who is no longer safe to drive, the legal and ethical responsibilities of physicians, and medical conditions and medications that may impair driving.

In some states the physician is required to notify the Bureau of Motor Vehicles if he deems it unsafe for the person to drive. Physicians should check their specific state law.

HINT—SAMPLE LETTER THE PHYSICIAN CAN WRITE TO THE CAREGIVER

Dear Mrs. Smith:

Unfortunately, because of Harold's difficulties with memory and concentration, and because of the medications that he is taking, he may no longer drive. As you are well aware, driving is a very complex task that involves the ability to focus and concentrate not only on where you are going, but where the other vehicles are around you. Because of his medical condition, he may not drive at this time.

I hope this is helpful to you in clarifying his driving and insurance status.

Sincerely,
Jane Jones, MD

TRAVELING

Traveling can be done successfully with a person with dementia, but will require additional planning to ensure their safety and comfort. Changes in routine and environment can increase their confusion and distress (10). It may be beneficial not to discuss a trip ahead of time with a person who has dementia due to anticipatory anxiety. Anticipatory anxiety, a common symptom in dementia, is worrying about an upcoming event, whether it is a pleasurable event or not. If there is known anticipatory anxiety, wait until it is time to leave before discussing the trip with the individual. Avoid vacation areas where there is overstimulation such as Las Vegas, noisy restaurants or places with crowds. Sightseeing trips can cause added confusion and may not be enjoyed by the person with dementia. Events such as weddings, family reunions, and other celebrations may need to be abbreviated. It is helpful to talk with the extended family about the possible need to shorten stays at events and the need for flexibility. Have the person with dementia seated in a quiet place where they are able to greet guests one or two at a time to reduce overstimulation and confusion. Fatigue can increase behavioral symptoms; try to schedule rest periods to avoid this. Environmental changes, such as new and unfamiliar surroundings, have the potential to increase confusion and cause wandering in someone who has not attempted to wander in the past.

The Alzheimer's Association has cards that are called "Pardon My Companion" cards. These usually state that the person with me has memory loss and thank you for understanding. The cards can be helpful in restaurants or stores where the person with dementia has difficulty making decisions or responding in an appropriate manner. They are also beneficial when traveling particularly with security checks at the airport. The cards can be given to the sales or security person, without embarrassing the person with dementia.

Traveling Tips

- Enroll the person in Medic Alert Safe Return through the local Alzheimer's Association or go to www.alz.org.
- Notify the doctor about the planned trip to see if a prescription can be obtained for a fast acting medication in the event that a behavioral problem occurs.

- Consider taking a motion detector to use in the bedroom or hotel room in the event that the person attempts to wander at night. (These can be bought at electronic stores relatively inexpensively.)
- Take at least an extra 24-hour supply of medications. Have a current list of medications with you.
- Create an itinerary to have with you at all times. Give a copy to family members and emergency contacts.
- Have an emergency bag that is easily accessible with medications, an extra change of clothing, snacks, drinks, and disposable underwear, if needed.
- Take "Pardon My Companion" cards.

Driving Tips

To lessen anxiety, it is advised to decrease daily miles traveled so that the person is not in the car longer than six to eight hours. Plan for more frequent stops. Safety locks on the car are helpful if the person with dementia has attempted to open the door unexpectedly and is an exit risk. Avoid traveling in the late afternoon if there is a history of sundowning symptoms such as increased agitation or aggressive behavior. Be observant for signs of agitation. If these symptoms begin to escalate while driving, pull over to the side of the road and have a snack or take a walk. If possible, having a third person available in the car will make it easier for the caregiver and the person with dementia. If staying at a hotel, inform the staff of any special needs.

Toileting can be a challenge if one is traveling with a spouse or a person of the opposite sex. Most restaurants and roadside stops do not have unisex bathrooms. However, department stores and malls may have family bathrooms. Plan stops around malls so that toileting can be done without difficulty. If the person is independent with toileting, it is important to keep an eye on the restroom as the person with dementia may be confused when coming out of the restroom and turn the wrong way, especially when there are separate entrance and exit doors.

Air Travel Tips

Airports can be very busy and confusing for someone with dementia. Security checks can cause fear and resulting agitation. Planning ahead is, again, key to a successful flight.

Planning Hints

- Avoid flights that require tight connections. Nonstop flights, if available, may be worth any additional expense.
- Notify the airlines at least 48 hours ahead of time of any special needs. If there is potential for a long walk between gates, request shuttle services to and from gates.
- "Pardon My Companion" cards need to be accessible to assist with any challenges that may occur at the airport or on the plane. Security personnel may perceive anxious behavior as an indication of a security risk.
- Travel insurance may be a wise purchase in the event of the need to change plans unexpectedly.

Allow for extra time for traveling and activities. Attempt to keep as close as possible to a normal schedule. Try to avoid placing unrealistic expectations on the person with dementia to keep frustration to a minimum. Weigh the benefits and challenges that travel may produce. If it appears that the challenges will outweigh the benefits, consider arranging either a respite stay at a facility or home care for the person with dementia, rather than taking the person with you (11).

MANAGEMENT OF FINANCES

Management of finances and bill paying are often compromised early in individuals with cognitive loss. This could potentially cause long-term financial problems that may affect the entire family. Problems may include difficulty making change, overdrawn accounts, bills lift unpaid or paid more than once, and falling for financial scams. These situations cause embarrassment for the cognitively impaired person and occasionally are completely denied. Statements such as, "My son has been stealing from me" or "The bank lost my money" are frequent justifications used by the individual.

One of the most important actions a caregiver can do is to locate the person's health insurance cards, social security card, credit cards, and military discharge papers. These documents should be secured in a safe place as they frequently become misplaced. Military discharge papers are valuable because of the myriad of services that the VA offers a person with dementia.

When the person with dementia has always paid the bills, it can be difficult to take that responsibility away from them. Offering assistance with these tasks may be effective though some will refuse this help, particularly when there is no recognition of deficiencies. It may help to offer the assistance in conjunction with a lunch or dinner out on a monthly basis so that there is a pleasurable activity associated with the task.

If offering assistance fails, the Internet may be useful for checking bank and credit card balances. It may be beneficial to have just the bills or occasionally all mail redirected to the power of attorney or to a post office box. Direct deposit of social security checks and pension checks is a protection against theft. When there is a financial power of attorney in place, that person can go to the bank and obtain information concerning the bank account(s). Some banks will allow a financial power of attorney to establish an amount of money that the person with dementia can spend on a monthly basis. If more money is withdrawn or spent, the bank then notifies the power of attorney.

Insurance payments also need to be monitored closely. Some insurance companies will discontinue a policy if the payments are not paid in a timely manner. This can affect not only Medicare and supplements but long-term care insurance policies as well.

Safety concerns go beyond the failure to pay bills and poor management of funds. Vulnerability to financial exploitation through telephone marketers, mail or computer solicitations, or someone on the street who recognizes that a person has some memory loss is an ongoing concern. Impaired judgment frequently leads to financial scams. Protective measures should be taken although scam artists continually devise new ways to operate. Place the person on the "Do Not Call List" to decrease telemarketing calls that may entice the person to spend funds unwisely (12). When there are telemarketers calling frequently, forwarding the calls to another number may help. Later, as the disease progresses, an answering machine may be an effective way to screen calls.

Contests can be very attractive to an older adult. These contest offers usually come through the mail or by telephone. Watch for new magazine subscriptions and an increased number of boxes being delivered to their home.

An overlooked means of protection is keeping the landscaping around the home in good condition. Overgrown shrubs may identify an older adult living alone. Someone who may be offering to repair a roof or cement walk that may or may not need repair looks for these signals and offers to make repairs for "cash." Frequently, the work is not completed or the person pays more than a fair amount for the work completed. Landscape assistance can be a wonderful birthday or Mothers/Fathers Day gift for an older adult.

Investments can be a challenge if controlled by the person with dementia. When there is a financial planner involved, this person needs to be notified of the memory loss. A financial power of attorney can ask to be notified of any changes to the portfolio. Debt load needs to be monitored as well. Often people who have paid off their mortgages obtain loans and incur a new mortgage and sometimes secondary mortgages as well. Many times, the cost of in-home care and services is income-based. A sliding scale may be used to set the fees. The provider's sliding scale may consider income only and not recognize debts in setting the cost of the service. If all the funds are being used to pay debts and these debts are not considered in the sliding scale, there will be nothing available to pay for needed care.

Financial management is one of the most challenging tasks for the person with dementia; yet taking away this function can be devastating. Until the person with dementia is completely unable to assist with financial decision making, allowing them to continue to have some input and having them participate in the process is the kindest way to gain their trust and for them to feel that they have some control of their finances.

MEDICATION ADMINISTRATION

Medication administration is a challenge for individuals with dementia, particularly if the person lives alone. Common problems that may occur are: denying that medication is necessary, forgetting to take medications, inadvertently dropping the pills, taking the wrong dose, or taking the pills at the wrong time of day.

The first thing to do is enlist the family physician's help. Ask the doctor to reassess medications to make certain that they all are needed. Attempt to get medication schedules adjusted to daily or, at most, twice daily. Blood thinning medications such as Coumadin can present an added challenge if the doses are varied on different days of the week. More intense monitoring is required while using this medication. Discuss this problem with the physician to see if there is a way that the same dose can be given daily.

Hints for medication safety

- After confirming the current medication schedule, make a list of all medications, preferably on a computer, using bold letters at a font of 12 or higher including the name of the person taking the medications and the date. It

is much easier for the older adult to read on light yellow paper with black print.
- List allergies and the name and phone number of the pharmacy. Include the name of the medication, dose, and timing of doses.
- Make several copies, retaining one for the caregiver. Place one on the refrigerator door and one with the medication bottles. If paramedics are called, they frequently check the refrigerator for information particularly if the person lives alone.
- Keep the list updated and be certain to date each update.

Medication bottles may need to be hidden or kept in one of the caregiver's homes so the person cannot inadvertently overdose. It may be helpful for the caregiver to set up medications in a weekly container or pill box, as this allows for monitoring and mistakes can be minimized or identified much earlier.

There are many types of containers; some have one compartment per day for seven days, others have two to four compartments per day. Keep it as simple as possible. Try to use only one type of container as using different ones may cause confusion. Due to the shift to more generic medications, many of the tablets are white. When there is a visual problem, it may help to use a dark colored container so the pills will be seen. If two containers are used, one for morning and one for night, using a yellow one for mornings denoting the sun and a dark blue one for night denoting the darker sky may help. Round containers can be confusing and should be avoided. Sliding door containers are also difficult to use, as it is easy to slide the door too far and pour out the entire day's medications at once. Open and close the container before purchase to make sure it is easily opened. For those who live alone, it is usually better to set up medications one week at a time.

If the person has never used medication containers and appears to be taking the medications correctly, it may be better not to introduce a weekly container. For someone with dementia, learning new things presents a challenge, and this can cause increased anxiety and possibly even more medication errors. For those individuals who are taking their medication directly from the pill bottles themselves, one of the best ways to assure that medications are being taken correctly is to check the date on the pill bottle and then count the remaining pills. When using sample cards of medications, date them as soon as they are received so a count can be used to make sure they are being taken as ordered by the physician.

Electronic medication dispensers are available that emit a sound when doses are scheduled to be taken. Some dispensers will notify a remote caregiver if the dose was not taken. These can be effective, but sometimes the person will take the medication from the container, become distracted, lay the pills down, and subsequently forget to take the medication. These dispensers can be expensive but, if effective, may be worthwhile. Call your local Alzheimer's Association for further information (5).

A person with memory loss may need a daily call as a reminder when medications are due to be taken. Caregivers who live close by may be able to stop in daily to give the medications. Continuing the daily newspaper can be a help for some who are very compliant with medications but become confused about the day of the week. Reminding the person to look at the newspaper just before taking medications may help identify the correct day in the medication container.

Ethical challenges can come into play concerning medications. Everyone has the right to refuse medications. However, when someone refuses medications and is not competent to make the decision, the family or health care power of attorney may decide to give the medications by disguising them. If swallowing problems occur, an alternative to whole pills may also need to be used. Some medications come in sprinkles or concentrated liquids that need only one or two drops to be effective. Some medications may be available in a patch. Others may need to be crushed. It is wise to purchase a pill crusher so that it can be made into a fine powder. The medications can then be mixed in applesauce, ice cream, yogurt, puddings, etc. When mixing the crushed medications in food, try using a consistency of mashed potatoes as it may be easier than liquids for the person to swallow. Mixing medications in liquids can be tricky if the person does not drink the full glass right away or just drinks a portion because powders may settle on the bottom of the glass. There are some pills that cannot be crushed so it is wise to check with the pharmacist prior to crushing medications.

Sometimes a person will refuse medications. However, when given later, the person may take them without difficulty. Directing, rather than asking, may ease the burden for someone with dementia. Decision making can cause anxiety in a person with dementia. It also may help to tell the person that the medications are like vitamins since this is a more understandable term for a person with memory loss.

HOUSEHOLD MANAGEMENT

Household management incorporates a myriad of activities and skills, such as shopping, meal planning and preparation, cleaning, laundry, and yard maintenance. The complexity of an activity as well as its implicit danger will determine the length of time the individual can continue to participate independently and without adjustments by the caregiver. It is desirable to maintain as much independence as possible without jeopardizing the safety of the individual or the family. In many instances, the individual will lose initiative to begin an activity. This may be perceived as lack of interest, but they will happily participate when someone gets them started.

Activities that require multiple steps and proper sequencing will be more difficult to accomplish than repetitive activities. The concept of task breakdown or simplification becomes a useful technique to use when working toward the goal of keeping the individual involved. Each activity can be broken down into a subset of activities. The role of the caregiver is to analyze the activity and simplify it to the point that the individual with dementia can safely and successfully complete the activity.

Meal Preparation

Though a wife has been an outstanding cook for many years, it may become apparent to her husband, through burned meals and complete chaos in the kitchen, that she can no longer accomplish this task independently. She is unable to get a meal on the table correctly and has increased anxiety when preparing a meal. In the early stages of the disease, the caregiver may need to simplify meal preparation by helping to plan menus, buying prepared food, or being available to assist. By mid-stage in the disease, the caregiver may need to take the lead, handle the stove, and transform the impaired individual into an assistant, giving them one task to accomplish at a time. Sharp knives should be secured. With the progression of the disease, the person with dementia will be able to do less and less without supervision. Finding the stove left on with burned pans or being used to heat the room would be indicators to the caregiver that judgment is impaired to the extent that the stove needs to be disabled for fire prevention. This can be done by removing the knobs on the stove, flipping the circuit breaker when not in use, or adding a shut-off valve.

When the person with dementia lives alone, challenges in the kitchen are magnified because there is no in-home caregiver to observe changes in the individual's skills. Disabling the stove may need to occur earlier in the disease. A simplified microwave and an electric teakettle with an automatic turn off may be a satisfactory solution early in the disease process. Community resources such as meals on wheels may be useful.

Cleaning
Cleaning includes multiple activities, such as sweeping, dusting, cleaning toilets, and removing clutter. The individual components can be successfully accomplished throughout much of the course of the dementing illness. Many of these activities do not require problem-solving and higher level cognitive skills, but rather are repetitive no-fail activities—the perfect activity for an individual with dementia. Cleaning supplies that are a health hazard should be removed as judgment becomes increasingly impaired.

Laundry care
In the early stages of the disease, this activity can be accomplished independently with few problems. As the disease progresses, the caregiver will need to break the task down into easier steps. In some instances, posting the steps for laundry care may be adequate direction for the individual. The caregiver may need to sort the laundry, buy premeasured tablets, and/or start the washer. It is wise to remove bleaches or other additives that could ruin the clothing or constitute a health hazard. In later stages, the individual may participate by folding the laundry.

Yard Maintenance
In the early stages of the disease, an individual can continue to mow the yard, plant flowers, and rake leaves. For safety reasons, mowing must be supervised carefully as a serious accident could occur with sharp blades. Judgment becomes an ongoing issue as the disease progresses. Planting and tending flowers can be a pleasurable activity throughout much of the disease. Raised flower beds are a worthwhile accommodation if balance becomes an issue. Raking leaves is a no fail activity that can provide hours of enjoyment and the feelings of being productive.

In each instance, the caregiver observes the activity, determines the specific point of challenge, and simplifies the activity to meet the needs and abilities of the individual, always with an eye towards safety. Praise and encouragement for the successful accomplishment of a task are critical for an individual who is confronting failure or an inability to perform in many IADLs.

The physician can serve as a sounding board as well as a support for the caregiver. The caregiver may erroneously consider one failure in completing an activity as an indication that no more participation should take place in this area. It would be valuable for the physician to give recommendations for increased supervision, while encouraging ongoing participation in household activities.

TECHNOLOGY

The use of technology to support an individual with dementia is beginning to play an important role in improving their quality of life (13). Technology has been used for some time to provide surveillance through the use of alarm systems. Bed alarms are used to alert caregivers that the individual with dementia is out of bed. Baby monitors can alert family members when activity is taking place behind closed doors. Door alarms with motion detectors alert caregivers when the individual moves towards an exit. Automatic shut-off devices may keep individuals from leaving burners on the stove, water temperature guards may keep water from scalding an individual who has become less sensitive to water temperature, water shut-off valves may keep the tub from overflowing, and light sensors can be installed to light pathways when there is movement at night. These safety items are available at local security stores, hardware stores, specialty home adaptation stores, or can be located online.

Global positioning systems in automobiles are helpful for individual in the early stages of dementia, who are still driving. These systems have been adapted for individuals to wear and can be used to track individuals who may wander.

Medication reminders are available that sound a buzzer as a reminder to take medicine. Some machines dispense medications at the appropriate time. These can be effective in the early stages of the disease, however as the disease progresses they become less effective; while they do alert the client, there is no guarantee that the medicines will actually be taken.

Emergency response systems can be effective if the client remembers to push the alert button when help is needed. However, as the disease progresses and confusion increases, the individual may in fact go looking for the voice that is offering to help, not realizing it is coming from a phone line.

Computer technology can be used successfully by individuals in the early stages of the disease, especially if the individual was computer savvy prior to having memory impairment. Some individuals with dementia have organized their computers with lists that serve as reminders of important tasks or activities. Others use the computer to develop a support system with other individuals through e-mails, blogs, and chat rooms. This allows for communication around the world and provides tremendous support for individuals with dementia. In a similar manner, caregivers have found the Internet to be a useful tool to research the disease and find assistance and support. For some, it is their only link to the outside world and one that they can access at any time, day or night. Organizations such as the Alzheimer's Association (5) and the Alzheimer's Foundation of America (14) maintain websites that provide connection to individuals in similar circumstances.

Physicians may find e-mail a useful way to communicate with families. All family members can be included in communications at one time, decreasing the opportunity for miscommunication among family members. Families should also be encouraged to e-mail concerns to the physician prior to office visits so that the physician is aware of behaviors occurring at home, without the family member having to describe them in front of the patient. In such e-mails, note the time/date of the scheduled visit so that the staff can alert the physician to these communications prior to the visit.

As technologies advance, undoubtedly more systems will be put into place, which can assist both individuals with dementia and caregivers.

CONCLUSION

IADLs have been examined in this chapter. It is clear that with the support of the caregiver, the physician, and the community, the individual with dementia can live a life that continues to have value and purpose as well as extend the time they are able to remain in their home or familiar surroundings. Flexibility and creativity become key with adjusting care to compensate as additional functional loses occur.

REFERENCES

1. http://www.cdc.gov/nchs/datawh/nchsdefs/iadl.htm. Accessed April, 2007.
2. http://en.wikipedia.org/wiki/Daily_living_skills. Accessed April, 2007.
3. Cummins JL, Cherry D, Kohatsu ND, et al. Guidelines for managing Alzheimer's disease: Part I. Assessment. AAFP 2002; 65:2263–2272.
4. Lawton MP, Brody EM. Assessment of older people: Self-maintaining and instrumental activities of daily living. Gerontologist 1969; 9:179–186.
5. http://www.alz.org. Accessed January, 2008.
6. http://www.socialsecurity.gov/disability. Accessed January, 2008.
7. http://www.thehartford.com/alzheimers. Accessed January, 2008.
8. http://neurology.osu.edu/cognitive/4turn.html. Accessed January, 2008).
9. http://www.ama-assn.org/ama/pub/category/print/10791.html. Accessed January, 2008.
10. http://www.alzfdn.org/education-care/traveling_shtml. Accessed January, 2008.
11. http://www.alz.org/national/documents/topicssheet_travelsaafety.pdf. Accessed January, 2008.
12. http://www.donotcall.gov. Accessed January, 2008.
13. Sixsmith A. New technologies to support independent living and quality of life for people with dementia. Alzheimers Care Q 2006; 7(3):194–202.
14. http://www.alzfdn.org/connect/careconnection. Accessed January, 2008.

6   Management of function: basic activities of daily living

Gail A. Greenley

INTRODUCTION

Basic activities of daily living (ADLs) can be defined as those tasks that we perform everyday, with little thought, often times with little effort, such as dressing, bathing, eating, walking, and toileting. ADLs were taught to us at a very young age, they have become our daily rituals, important to our overall well-being and general health.

If we have done these basic ADLs for so long, then why is it so challenging for someone with dementia to manage these basic ADLs that they have learned so long ago and perform daily? Why does the caregiver have such a difficult time in assisting the individual with dementia to complete the ADLs?

In this chapter, we explore the ways to increase independence with these activities, address some safety concerns that may arise, when to increase supervision, when to restrict the activity, how to restrict the activity, and the role of both the physician and the caregivers.

Routine is the key. When possible, stay as close to the patient's nature or customary routines. We are creatures of habit. As the dementia progresses this becomes more and more important. There is comfort, a sense of safety, and most importantly familiarity in routines. Choose the same time every day or as close as possible, including Saturday and Sunday to perform the activity. Allow plenty of time and do not rush a task. If necessary, or when possible, break the tasks down into simple, visual steps. The caregiver must maintain a sense of calm even during episodes of verbal and/or physical aggression. Always keep your emotions in check, using warm, calm voice tones. De-escalation of such situations can also be helped by the use of open body language and offering reassurances. Keep a sense of humor. Be creative. Be flexible. What works today might not work next week, and what did not work before might work now.

As a caregiver it is necessary to distinguish your reality from their reality. In the early stages of dementia, reality orientation may be appropriate, or even a necessary exchange between the caregiver and the patient to provide acknowledgement and a feeling of trust. In the middle stages of dementia it is much more difficult to continue to provide reality orientation. The caregiver will need to decide when to use reality and when not to. This is where the no harm no foul rule applies. If someone is looking for their mom or dad, is telling them that their parents are deceased going to cause mental anguish? If they believe someone is stealing their money and they want you to help, is telling them that it is only their imagination and that no one has stolen any money going to make them angry and untrusting of you? If so, what is the harm in telling them that you are going to help them find mom and dad, or in telling them that you will help them get their money back? They perceive reality differently then you. Sometimes nothing you say is going to be acceptable. Keep trying. Redirect their attention to a different place and time or a more distant pleasant memory. Remain calm and in control of your emotions. If necessary, take a 5-minute personal time out to regain control of your emotions and then reapproach—refreshed.

DRESSING

Dressing is a very complex task, especially for the cognitively impaired. It requires object identity. Is that a shirt or pants and where does it go? Gross and fine motor skills, zipping zippers, buttoning buttons, tying our shoes, and the balance to stand up and pull one's pants on are all complex skills we often take for granted. Patience and time are what are needed the most when assisting others to dress.

Early stage dementia clients may only require minimal assistance with dressing. Keep a routine. Limit the amount of clothing choices. Lay the clothing out. Allow plenty of time for them to complete the task. Provide them the opportunity to be independent and provide as much privacy as possible.

As one progresses through the middle stages of dementia they will require more and more assistance with the tasks associated with dressing. Keeping a routine is more important now than ever. Choose the clothing for them. Lay the clothing out in the order in which they should go on. Assist by prompting, using simple instructions, and visual cues when possible. As you are handing them clothing items give instruction and ample time to complete the task. For example: Stand up, pull down your pants, step out of your pants, sit down, put your foot in your sock, now the other foot, take your pants and put your feet in your pants legs, stand up, pull your pants up, now pull up the zipper. Addressing each item of clothing in this manner will provide independence and a sense of self worth. Allow plenty of time to complete the task. If frustration sets in, you need to be the cheerleader; simple praises go a long way. Do not reprimand or correct—assist with the task. Do not disagree—acknowledge. Limit questions—allow time for a response. During care it is also important to look for visual signs of pain or discomfort.

The later stages of dementia require the caregiver to perform the task of dressing for the individual. Stay with the routine you established in the earlier stages. While performing the task of dressing allow the individual to help as much as possible, even if it is only holding an item for you such as a sock. When possible the use of button front shirts and elastic wasted pants/slacks are easier to put on. The clothing should be comfortable with proper fitting. Keep in mind that this population tends to get cold easier. Undressing and redressing one item at a time will provide greater warmth and provide a sense of dignity. Do not be in a rush. This only leads to frustration for yourself as well as the dementia patient. They do not understand your emotions. But your emotion will soon become theirs. The more positive your emotions the greater the experience is for the dementia patient. It is important that you tell them everything you are doing before as well as during the task. This helps in eliminating the fear of harm. Remember to give praise frequently during the task. Even if you are the recipient of cursing, yelling, and hitting, use low, calm, warm, reassuring tones.

GROOMING

Bathing

With bathing, comes a new set of obstacles. The thought of having someone watch you bathe, someone helping you with your bath, or being bathed is embarrassing. Now imagine someone who requires help but believes they can do it themselves, or the one who is already confused and does not understand what it is that you are about to do to them. Either way it is a very personal, embarrassing, and even an emotional experience. Bathing does not need to be a challenge or a negative experience for either the patient or the caregiver. It is helpful to find out what their bathing routines have been. For instance: How often did they bath; what time of day; did they prefer a bath or a shower; and how often did they shampoo their hair? Knowing this in advance will allow you to continue with the routine that they are most familiar with. Make the bathroom user-friendly. Remove clutter and unnecessary items and objects. Colors should be warm and inviting. When possible use the décor that they are familiar with. When it becomes necessary to use shower chairs or benches make sure the seat is padded for comfort and adjust the height of the chair so that their feet are comfortably on the ground or use a stool. This provides an increased sense of security and lessens the fear of falling.

For individuals with recent onset of dementia, the bathing experience should remain fairly independent. Reminders may be all that is required for some time. Eventually you may need to lay out bathing products, such as towel, washcloth, soap, and shampoo when needed. Provide for their privacy as much as possible. Stay close by to monitor compliance as well as safety. Do not allow yourself to become distracted. Shaving is a precision skill and when possible change to an electric razor. This will provide greater independence for a greater length of time.

Many dementia conditions are progressive. As the dementia progresses the caregiver will be performing more and more of the bathing tasks. Continue to encourage the person to do as much as possible. This provides them with a sense of control, independence, and a feeling of respect. This allows for a more positive bathing experience. Do not rush the patient as this only leads to frustration, which increases negative behaviors. It may be true that not rushing the individual requires a great deal more time than providing the care yourself. However, the alternative could mean increased verbal or physical aggression. There are going to be times when you as the caregiver will need to provide bathing instructions. Give instructions in short simple terms using visual cues when possible. For instance, hand them the washcloth and ask them to get the washcloth wet and then with a wet washcloth place the soap on or in the washcloth. Continue giving simple one-statement instruction until the desired task is complete. Allow them to do as much as possible giving praise even if you must redo the area.

In the later stages of dementia it is important to maintain the routine established earlier. The dementia client finds comfort in routines. At this time in the dementia process the caregiver is most likely the one performing the bathing task. Involve them in the bath as much as possible; ask them to hold a washcloth or some other item for you. Talk to them during the entire bathing process. Tell them what you are doing before, as well as during the bath to help decrease their fears, both real and perceived. Speak in low calming tones. Involve them in stories/memories of long ago; this helps to distract the attention away from the task to a more enjoyable time. Be patient. Trying to rush tends to increase the amount of time needed to complete the bath. It is not necessary to expose the entire body at one time. This is especially important when giving a shower. Cover the parts of the body that are not being washed. Leaving a t-shirt on or draping a large bath towel or sheet around the shoulders helps in keeping the client warm and alleviate feelings of being completely exposed and vulnerable. This also provides them with a sense of dignity and comfort and makes the bathing experience a more pleasant experience for both the individual as well as the caregiver. Start with the least invasive body part, the feet, and work upward toward their head, face, and hair.

When it becomes necessary to give bed baths, the same techniques can work for you. Maintain a conversation throughout the bed bath. Talk about things that are familiar to the person, even if it is a one-way conversation—keep it going. Keep as much of the body covered as possible. Work on one part at a time. As you are bathing look for visuals signs of pain or discomfort. Report changes to their physician.

Oral Hygiene

Oral hygiene can be one of the most difficult tasks. Patients with mild dementia may require assistance with set up, reminders to brush, or prompting to brush. Maintaining a sense of independence is the key. Their oral hygiene routines should be established for a long time. It is important to find out and maintain as much of their routine as possible.

As one advances through the middle stages of dementia setting up the toothbrush becomes difficult for the patient; reminders and prompting work some of the time. It often becomes more and more difficult to convince them to brush their teeth or even for them to allow you to brush their teeth. If they get upset or frustrated, approach them later.

For those who wear dentures, often times they refuse to take the dentures out or may not allow you to remove them. Sometimes the opposite occurs. There are times when they take their dentures out, refusing to put them in, and misplacing the dentures becomes increasingly common. If they do not want their dentures in—that is OK. Diets and food textures can easily be altered to accommodate the lack of teeth. Talk to the physician or dietician for correct food consistency. Keeping the dentures out rarely bothers the individual. Often times it is the family members who want the dentures to be worn. This can be problematic at times. For the individual it can be stressful and frightening and may result in verbal exchange of words or physical aggression. At a certain point, it may not be worth the safety risk to wear the dentures. It is important to remember that the individual person is changing, as well as their needs. What was once important to them may be of little or of no importance now. Choose your battles, if they are getting upset or frustrated—stop. Reproach later. You are not always going to be successful. Be patient. Be creative. Do not take it personally. It is not about you. It is about the individual. What works today might not work tomorrow. Do not be afraid to try things that had not previously worked. You will not know until you try. Following each meal or snack with an 8 ounce glass of water will help his or her overall oral hygiene especially when usual oral hygiene has been unsuccessful.

Generally the caregiver provides the oral care in late stage dementia. Dentures are by now usually ill fitting due to weight changes and decreased facial tone. Whether using a toothbrush, toothette (a small sponge tip on a stick) or water pick, oral care is equally important with or without teeth. If one easily accepts the toothbrush—use it. If you are attempting to force the toothbrush in, use a toothette. The sponge tip will not cause injury to the lips or gums. Use toothettes with caution. If the toothette is in their mouth and they bite down, do not attempt to pull it out. The sponge tip could become dislodged and become a chocking hazard. Gently place your thumb across their chin and push in and down, this should open the jaw. Safety must always be the first priority.

NUTRITIONAL ISSUES

Weight Loss
The only thing that can be counted on with dementia is that things change as the disease progresses. Patient's food choices, appetite, and weight are no different. In the early stages of dementia it seems that they are eating constantly, not remembering that they have just eaten. As the caregiver it is important to monitor their eating and make available nutritional foods. Early weight gains are usually seen. Limit caffeine intake where possible. Talk with their physician for suggestions regarding vitamin supplements and much needed calcium to promote bone health.

As one moves into the middles stages of dementia, convincing them to eat sometimes presents new challenges. Foods that used to be considered their favorites—they may not eat. The foods they disliked are foods they may now prefer. While eating utensils become confusing, limit the needs for utensils to a spoon or a fork. As the dementia advances, the appetite will start to dwindle. Maintaining their weight is increasingly difficult. Taste buds keep changing; they tend to be overwhelmed by the amount of food placed before them. Presenting the food, one item at a time and preparing the food items so that they can be eaten with one utensil, helps to eliminate the confusion. Eventually preparing foods that can be eaten with one's fingers will work better; further eliminating the utensil confusion and maintaining some independence. Sometimes adding honey, syrup, or even yogurt to the food items helps to stimulate the taste buds and the hunger mechanism in the brain. Sometimes the sweeter the taste they find it more apt to eat. The thought of mixing honey, syrup, or even yogurt in scrambled eggs is probably not very appetizing to you. The good news is twofold. Firstly, it is not for you. Secondly, as the taste buds decline in ability, the sweetened food is more appetizing and palatable to them so that they eat more and maintain their weight longer. When the weight starts to decrease, the addition of a high calorie, high protein supplement may be recommended. Checking with their physician and perhaps a referral to a Speech Therapist for additional interventions will be necessary.

Communication between the caregiver and physician is essential. Diets may change depending on the underlying medical conditions such as diabetes, hypertension, and renal failure, just to name a few. The ability to tolerate different food consistencies can change with the progression of dementia. If the consistency of food becomes problematic, the caregiver might see the patient keep chewing and chewing, rarely swallowing, or holding large amounts of chewed food in their cheeks. When this begins to happen, call the physician immediately and avoid stringy foods such as pork, ham, and beef (nonground). If they are still independently feeding themselves cut the food into smaller pieces. To control the portion size the patient is attempting to put into their mouth, using a plastic spoon or toddler spoon is helpful. If they tend to cough after swallowing food or liquid, a referral for a swallowing study is usually needed to evaluate their risk for aspiration pneumonia. A change in food texture from regular to chopped or even puree consistency may be recommended. Changing the consistency of liquids from thin to a nectar, honey, or pudding consistency may also be recommended.

With the progression of dementia, the risk of aspiration continues to increase. In the event that the individual advances to the final stages of dementia, the likelihood that the brain cannot control the complex task of swallowing increases.

The subject of placing a feeding tube (a surgical procedure in which a latex or silicone tube is inserted into the stomach) as a means to administer liquid nutrition and necessary medication(s) is a very personal decision. A decision to place a feeding tube needs to be discussed with their physician. Providing liquid nutrition through a feeding tube represents its own set of complications and risks of infection and aspiration. Issues of quality of life versus quantity of life are inevitable. Sometimes the most difficult position to be in is the decision maker position. The ability to act on behalf of someone who can no longer independently make their own health decisions is the most challenging of tasks. The mental anguish one tends to place on oneself as the caregiver, trying to separate his/her personal beliefs/choices from the belief/choices of the one he/she is acting on behalf of, is extremely difficult. Their physician can discuss the pros and cons of tube feeding. Just remember, there is no right or wrong decision when you act in their best interest. The only person judging you is you.

TOILETING/SPINCTER ISSUES

Toileting is the most personal and private activity of daily living. Emotions of embarrassment, helplessness, and shame just to name a few complicate this task. Helping another adult in toileting is unnatural for both the recipient and the caregiver.

Allow the individual to do as much as possible. At first, oversight might be all that is necessary. Provide privacy. Be patient. Try to stick to a routine. Giving reminders upon waking, an hour after a meal and before bed helps. Toileting in advance of need can be very helpful to reduce accidents. Limit fluids and caffeine an hour before bedtime. Leave a light on in the restroom with the door open when unused, if possible. As more assistance is needed, it is important that you allow them to do as much as possible even if it requires additional time. Do not rush the individual. When caregiver assistance is needed, be sure to let them know what you are doing before and as you are proceeding with the personal care.

Prompting and cueing, ensuring a clear path to the restroom, leaving a light on in the restroom after dark and possibly hanging a picture on the restroom door will help the cognitively impaired individual. At times they may realize the need to do something but do not understand what it is they need to do. Relieving oneself in inappropriate places may occur. Watch for nonverbal cues such as wondering aimlessly or fidgeting around in one's seat and then direct them to the toilet. When hands-on care to toilet is required, good peri-care and strict hand washing are important to decrease the risk of infection. Always monitor for signs of skin breakdown and notify their physician immediately if this occurs. Assisting one with peri-care after toileting is a task that needs a great deal of patience and creativity. Engaging them in conversations of interest, which may require going back to a memory from long ago which is still familiar to them, can help change the focus from the task at hand to a more pleasant one.

As the dementia progresses, sphincter control becomes more impaired because inhibitory control is lost. The brain is no longer telling the individual to hold their urine. Inhibitory control is lost in end stage dementia. This is the main cause of urinary incontinence. Knowing when it is time to wear incontinence products such as pads, pull-ups or adult diapers (which I like to refer to as adult briefs) is challenging. In the early stages, the cognitively impaired person may only require a pad for minimal leakage. Those who become frequently to totally incontinent require an adult brief. Proper fitting adult briefs are necessary to prevent accidental leakage. Good hygiene and skin care are essential.

Urinary tract infections (UTIs) not only can affect the health of patients but they can also affect their gait and may lead to increased aggression and confusion. Signs and symptoms of a UTI may include but are not limited to: strong or offensive odor; increase frequency of urination; fatigue; fever; increasing confusing; increasing aggression; pain upon urination; gait disturbances. If you suspect a UTI call their physician immediately. Individuals in advanced stages of dementia requiring extensive or total care, who are nonambulatory, are at an increased risk for UTIs.

It is equally as important to continue taking the individual to the toilet every two hours for as long as one can transfer safely. Maintaining a toileting routine will assist them with a more effective bowel movement. Not everyone has a bowel movement daily. Diet, fluids, and exercise play a big role in bowel motility. It is necessary, however, to track bowel movements to potentially prevent fecal impactions or even a bowel obstruction. If you as the caregiver notice that one is straining, having loose stools, or ribbon-like stools, contact their physician immediately for medical interventions.

APRAXIA

Apraxia is the impairment in the ability to perform purposeful acts. Dressing apraxia is the inability to perform the complex sequence of dressing including the inability to manipulate buttons, zippers, or shoe laces. Those with early onset dementia may initially be able to dress by themselves. Later on, some may physically be able to perform the task but have difficulty with properly identifying the articles of clothing or the sequence in which they are to be performed. Others may be able to tell you in words but cannot physically perform the steps to complete the task. A referral to occupation therapy can assist you with techniques and suggest modifications for dressing routines.

Walking or gait apraxia is the inability to properly use the legs or lower limbs to walk. This diagnosis is given in the absence of other potential causes such as muscle weakness, bone and joint degeneration, and medication side effects. When noticing gait or walking disturbances contact their physician to rule other potential causes. Physical therapy may be beneficial.

Eating and swallowing apraxia is the impairment in the ability to perform the complex sequence of events necessary to swallow and swallow safely. Facial muscles, the coordination of the tongue, the ability to move saliva or food to the back of the mouth, and the brain's ability to identify air from food or saliva, all play a role in swallowing. With swallowing apraxia the impairment in the ability to swallow can come with significant consequences. Medical intervention is necessary to decrease the risk of choking as well as aspiration pneumonia. A referral to speech therapy for eating and swallowing techniques will be beneficial. Speech therapy can be beneficial in assisting you as the caregiver in feeding techniques, cueing techniques, as well as food textures to encourage and promote a safer eating experience. Speech therapists can assess for risks of aspiration or other swallowing impairments that can go on unnoticed. This can be done at the bedside or in an outpatient hospital setting. If facial muscle weakness is identified, they may recommend exercises to improve facial tone. If thin liquids are identified to be a risk they may recommend that liquids be given at a nectar, honey, or pudding consistency.

AMBULATION AND FALLS

Safety is the first goal. Open, uncluttered hallways, unrestricted rooms, a clear pathway to the restroom, and good lighting are needed to promote safe ambulation. Eliminating the number of steps and reducing or eliminating when possible the use of throw or area rugs will reduce the risk of one tripping or falling. Keeping one ambulatory for as long as possible is essential. Gait or walking disturbances increase with the progression of dementia, thus, increasing the risk of falls. Decreased coordination in ambulation presents a new set of challenges. When is it time to use a cane, a walker, or a wheelchair? Each device has its own risks; one's physical and mental ability to use the device safely is a major concern. Physical therapy will evaluate walking and trunk movement, rising from a chair, rate and width of steps, direction of the steps, as well as the coordination of the arms, truck, and legs. Coordination and the ability to safely support one's own weight is required to use a cane or a walker. A quad (a three or four prong) cane provides greater stability. Initially, a wheelchair may be necessary for distance. As the dementia progresses a wheelchair may be necessary due to one's inability to ambulate safely or at all. When or if this should occur, exercising the lower extremities is important to decrease the risk of blood clots forming in the legs and to maintain range of motion of the joints. A referral to physical therapy will aid in increasing one's understanding and knowledge of maintaining good joint and muscle tone through the use of home exercises.

HOME SAFETY

When someone is diagnosed with and progresses through the stages of dementia, home safety takes on a new meaning. With each stage, dementia brings with it new safety concerns. The need is to adult proof your home, not childproof. Adults are smarter, taller, and more creative. Do not underestimate them. A referral to occupational therapy can help safeguard everyone in the household as well as the dwelling. Occupational therapists will help identify potential hazards initially and throughout the course of the illness. They can make recommendations related to furniture placement, lighting, as well as special equipment designed to assist with care. For example, handrails to assist with ambulation, tub rails or shower seats for safety, perhaps an electric bed or special lifts for ease of transfers. Occupational therapists will educate and work with all caregivers on the use of equipment in your home. A review of safety issues can also be addressed. Early in the disease process it is important to think ahead and start safeguarding your home. This is especially important in regards to gas stoves, microwaves, and all medications, both prescribed and over-the-counter medications.

All health care providers are there for you. They are not there to judge, they are there to help you. Only you know what it is like to care for someone with dementia day and night. The patient's physician can and will help, but the physician can only help if you let them know. It is equally important to ask for help. We sometimes fool ourselves into believing that our family and friends know what we are going through and either do not care or do not want to be bothered. In most cases this is only our perception and not reality. Even those close to us cannot read our mind. Ask for help before you think you need it. Networking with others in similar situations through support groups or other organizations can prove to be very beneficial for everyone's well-being.

I have often heard from the caregivers, "Unless you have walked in my shoes there is no way you can understand what I'm going through." It is important to note that I do understand. I have walked in their shoes. For nine years I walked daily in their shoes with my mother. I was my mothers' caregiver, first personally, then professionally. This was the worst of times and the best of times. I was the lucky one; my mom not so lucky. Caregivers are not in this alone. Many professionals and support groups are there to help just for the asking. I admire caregivers for the love and the dedication they show every day. Being a caregiver can be the most challenging of times, as well as the most rewarding of times.

7

Health economics and financial decision making

Christopher Leibman and Trent McLaughlin

INTRODUCTION

Dementia—including its most common form, Alzheimer's disease (AD)—is characterized by progressive memory impairment, confusion, loss of independence, and a variety of other cognitive and functional deficits. AD affects predominantly the elderly and is usually insidious in onset. A patient with AD generally undergoes a relatively rapid progression from being a healthy, independent person to being a completely dependent, uncomprehending person who lacks insight and self-awareness. This progression makes AD one of the most feared disorders in the elderly (1).

Although AD is primarily regarded as a disease that results in cognitive impairment and disability, it is increasingly recognized as an underlying cause of death (2,3). Research reveals that AD accounts for about 7% of all deaths in the United States and is one of the leading causes of mortality in older people (4). The life expectancy of patients with AD is markedly lower than the life expectancy of the general population (Fig. 1) (5). For example, a woman diagnosed with AD at the age of 70 years will likely survive only half as long as a 70-year-old woman without AD. However, some patients with AD survive for many years, often requiring long-term care and supervision (5).

The relationship between age and the prevalence of AD (Fig. 2) (6) is especially pertinent when considered from a societal perspective. The percentage of the U.S. population that is elderly (≥65 years of age) is projected to grow over in the coming decades (Fig. 3) (7), mirroring trends in many other regions of the world (8). This aging of the population translates to an increasing number of people at the highest level of risk of developing AD. In fact, it has been predicted that the prevalence of AD worldwide will grow from an estimated 26.6 million cases in 2006 to 106 million cases by 2050 (6).

As the prevalence of AD increases, so will its economic burden. Currently, the annual estimated cost of caring for patients with AD in the United States is more than $100 billion (9). These costs are borne not only by society, but also by extended care networks and—more importantly—by patients and families. Although family members and caregivers may often find themselves overwhelmed by the physical, emotional, and mental demands of the disease, there are steps they can take, particularly in the early stages of the disease, to ease some of the financial uncertainties they are facing, especially when it comes to providing for the care of their loved ones.

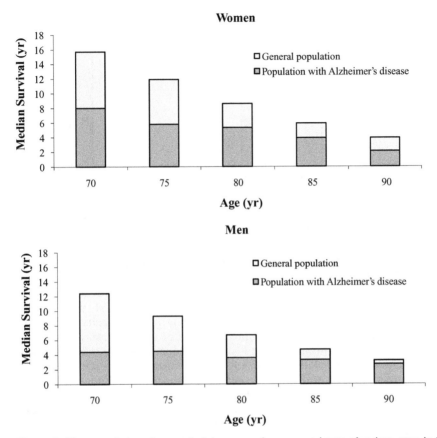

Figure 1 The expected median survival, in years, of women and men of various ages in the general population and in the population with Alzheimer's disease (5).

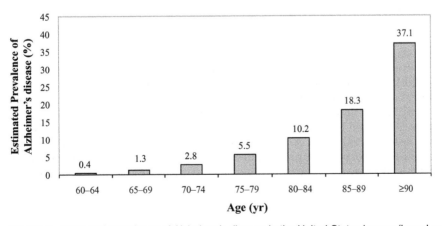

Figure 2 Estimated prevalence of Alzheimer's disease in the United States by age (based on the methodology of Ref. 6).

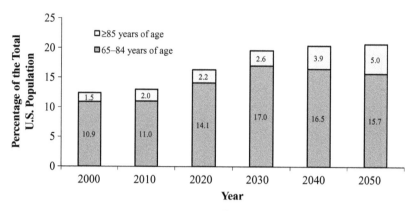

Figure 3 Past and projected percentages of total U.S. population between 65 and 84 years of age and ≥85 years of age for the decades 2000 to 2050 (7).

STAGES OF DEMENTIA AND LEVEL OF CARE REQUIRED AT EACH STAGE

Although no two people will experience dementia in exactly the same way, the progression of the disease is fairly predictable. Typically, the first symptoms are subtle short-term memory problems. Patients may have difficulty finding the right words, planning meals, managing finances or medications, using a telephone, and driving without getting lost. Many capacities may initially remain intact, including social skills and the ability to perform self-care activities. However, changes in mood and behavior, such as personality alterations, irritability, anxiety, or depression, may occur at an early stage of the disease (10). In the middle and late stages of AD, delusions, hallucinations, aggression, and wandering often occur (10). The late stages of dementia are also characterized by an inability to recall information acquired early in life (e.g., names of relatives) and the deterioration of other cognitive functions (e.g., language, orientation, judgment) (10).

To determine where a patient falls on the AD continuum (and thus the level of care and services he or she might require), one of several classification systems can be used. The most commonly used system divides dementia (and AD) into three stages: mild, moderate, and severe (Table 1) (11,12). These classifications are often based on patient scores from the Folstein Mini-Mental State Examination (MMSE), which measures memory, attention, orientation, and other cognitive abilities (13). The maximum score on the MMSE is 30; patients who score between 20 and 25 are considered to have mild dementia, those with scores between 10 and 20 are considered to have moderate dementia, and those with scores less than 10 are considered to have severe dementia (14). However, these classifications may underestimate or not transparently describe the level of care a patient requires. For example, because of impairments associated with the disease, a patient classified with *mild* dementia on the basis of an MMSE score may still require a home health aide or informal caregiver for help in choosing clothing and performing household chores.

The degree of independence that a patient has lost as a result of cognitive, functional, and behavioral problems is another means of classifying disease

Table 1   Patient Capabilities and Needs at Each Stage of Dementia (11,12)

	Disease stage		
	Mild	Moderate	Severe
What patients are generally able to do	• Remember many important facts about themselves and others • Remember their own name • Remember the names of their spouse and children	• Almost always remember their own name • Can generally distinguish between familiar and unfamiliar people they meet	• Sporadically remember their own name or the names of immediate family members
What patients are sometimes unable to do or may require assistance to do	• Always remember a familiar address or telephone number • Always remember the names of grandchildren • Always remember the high school or college that they attended • Always remember the day of the week and the year • Perform simple household chores	• Always remember the name of their spouse • Remember recent events and experiences • Remember the year and the season • Perform everyday activities without help	• Recognize or remember people • Eat without assistance
Additional assistance that may be required by patients	• May need to be reminded to eat or use the toilet • May need help choosing clothing	• May have bladder or bowel control problems requiring assistance • May have irregular sleep patterns, necessitating additional supervision	• Generally unable to control their body requiring much assistance

severity. This system may be a more relevant measure of dementia progression than is the use of broad descriptors such as mild, moderate, and severe (Table 2). Characterization of the stages by level of dependence on others for service or care (15) permits estimates of the costs and resources necessary to care for patients at each stage of dementia. This information, in turn, allows the patient, the family, and health care professionals to begin to investigate agencies that can provide the needed services and to identify ways of paying for them. For example, a patient in Stage 3 dementia dependence will need assistance with most daily activities and may require the services of a home health aide or the use of an adult day care facility (Table 2). Anticipating this, family members can begin discussing options or even touring day care facilities and comparing costs. Even if a spouse or caregiver decides to continue caring for a patient at home full-time, this information can be used to coordinate help from other family members and friends or to ask more informed questions about patient care.

Although it is often in the best interest of patients (and their families, insurance payers, and society) that they remain at home as long as possible (14); at some point, more supervision and protection will likely be required than some families may be able to provide at home. In fact, loss of independence by a patient with AD is often associated with nursing home placement (16). This is not a decision that most families make lightly; in fact, moving a loved one into a long-term care facility is often one of the most difficult and painful decisions a family will make during the course of the disease. Family members may wrestle with feelings of failure or guilt over "giving up," experience a deep sense of loss and sadness, or worry about the financial implications of long-term care. In many cases, however, family members will look back on nursing home placement as the right decision, not only from the patient's perspective, but also from their own perspective.

COSTS OF CARE

Because dementia is a complex, long-term illness, the costs of caring for patients can be considerable (Table 3). In general, as the severity of the disease increases, so do the associated expenditures and required services (Fig. 4) (18,19). However, other factors can also influence the costs of care. One is the setting in which the care is given, typically either community based (e.g., the patient's home, a residential community) or a nursing home. Disease severity most markedly affects the costs of caring for patients in community-based settings (Fig. 4), where the majority of patients with dementia (approximately 59%) live (20). The costs associated with community-based settings are partially the result of the lost income of caregivers (i.e., as patients lose independence and require more supervision, caregivers are apt to work less) and an increase in their out-of-pocket expenditures (18).

Entry into a nursing home or skilled nursing facility is often associated with large increases in resource use and cost. This is partly due to the expanded range of services that assisted living and nursing home providers offer for patients with dementia. Although the majority of the increased costs are easily measured direct costs (e.g., the cost of caring for a patient in a nursing home), it should be noted that less easily measured costs (e.g., informal care costs) are also incurred while the patient is still in the community, and entry into a nursing home only shifts these costs (21). Despite the large costs seen on entry to a nursing facility, dementia care costs appear to continue to increase after patients have been placed

Table 2 Patient Capabilities and Needs Associated with Loss of Independence

	Stage 1 (reminders)	Stage 2 (increased assistance needs)	Stage 3 (supervision required)	Stage 4 (functional assistance required)	Stage 5 (complete dependence)
Level of assistance required by patients	• Occasional need for advice about how to cook, handle money, and do chores • Occasional need to be reminded about appointments, recent events, and names of family members and friends • May be unable to continue working	• More frequent need to be reminded about appointments, recent events, and names of family members and friends • Unable to do most household chores	• Almost constant supervision required • Need to be escorted when outside • May require a home health aide, day care, or respite care	• Need to be supervised while bathing and eating • Need to be dressed, washed, and groomed	• Require full-time care
Functional, behavioral, and psychological symptoms	• May experience depression or anxiety	• Limited ability to perform instrumental activities of daily living	• Wandering behavior or other psychological symptoms may be present	• Possible incontinence	• Unable to perform most, if not all, activities of daily living without assistance

Table 3   Costs[a] Associated with Care of Patients with Dementia

Fixed costs: Fixed costs do not vary with the volume of output; however, they can vary over time, independently of the volume of output. Fixed costs may include rent, equipment lease payments, and some wages and salaries. An example is the cost of maintaining the physical structure of an outpatient clinic once it is built; this cost is the same regardless of the number of patients who use the facility.

Variable costs: Variable costs vary with the volume of output. Examples include drugs, devices, supplies, and medical procedures. For example, if an increasing number of patients are treated with a drug at a hospital, the hospital's cost for that drug will increase because more of the drug is being used.

Direct medical costs: Direct medical costs are directly associated with a medical condition or health care intervention; they may be fixed or variable. Direct medical costs include services and products used for the care of patients, such as hospital stays, physician visits, emergency department visits, home health care visits, dental visits, drugs, and medical equipment and supplies. The direct medical costs for drugs include acquisition, storage, administration, and monitoring costs. For example, the direct cost of an outpatient intravenous drug therapy session includes the cost of the drug, the cost of the syringe and needle, the wages of the health care professionals who administer the treatment, and a portion of the cost to run the outpatient clinic. As a general rule, direct costs can be reimbursed through an insurance payer.

Direct nonmedical costs: Direct nonmedical costs are the costs of providing the patient with nonmedical assistance such as food, lodging, and transportation. For example, commercial or volunteer home-delivered meals programs (e.g., Meals on Wheels) provided to homebound patients with Alzheimer's disease (AD) would be considered a direct nonmedical cost. Care provided by professional home health aides or caregivers, paid for by either the patient's family or insurers, is also considered a direct nonmedical cost.

Indirect costs: Indirect costs (also known as productivity costs) are the costs of lost productivity that may result from morbidity, premature mortality, or informal care costs. Morbidity costs include goods and services not produced by the patient because of illness. Mortality costs include goods or services not produced by the patient because of premature death. Informal care costs are described below. As a general rule, insurance payers do not reimburse indirect costs.

Informal care costs: Family members or friends provide informal care to a patient. Informal care costs are generally calculated in one of two ways. When the input method is used, the total number of informal care hours is multiplied by the price per hour, which may be calculated using market replacement cost. For example, if a family member cares for a patient with AD 40 hr per week, and it would cost $20 per hour to hire someone to perform the same job, the informal care cost is $800 per week. When the output method is used, the value of the caregiver's labor on the open market is considered. For example, if a family member quits his or her job to take care of a patient with AD, and that family member earned $650 per week, the informal care cost is $650 per week.

Perspective: The costs of AD care are considered from one of three perspectives: institutional (i.e., government or private insurer), societal (i.e., all of society), or individual (i.e., the patient and his or her family). From an institutional perspective, informal care costs are not important because they are not reimbursed. From a societal perspective, informal care accounts for the majority of the costs associated with AD. From an individual perspective, informal care costs may be associated with the decision to place a patient in a nursing home.

Long-term care: Long-term care is generally defined as continuing health and social care provided to individuals with chronic impairments and/or a reduced degree of independence. Long-term care is thought of as primarily low-tech, although it is becoming more high-tech as the prevalence of patients with severe illnesses in long-term care has increased (17).

[a]The total value of all resources used in the production of a good or service: fixed costs, variable costs, direct medical costs, direct nonmedical costs, indirect costs, and informal care costs are included.

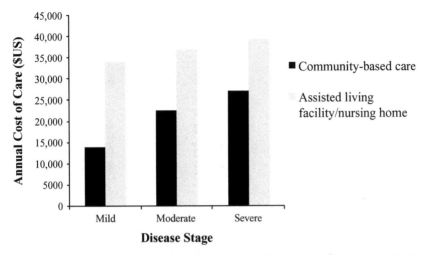

Figure 4 Estimated annual costs (including formal and informal costs) associated with the care of patients with dementia, based on disease stage and care setting; data are from 1996 (19).

in institutionalized care, regardless of the stage of the disease (22,23). Table 4 details some common direct medical and nonmedical costs associated with caring for patients with dementia in either setting (24–34).

Another factor that can increase the costs of dementia care is the presence of comorbid disease (e.g., congestive heart failure, arthritis), which is often more common as a patient ages (22,23,35). Addressing comorbid diseases in a patient with dementia can be particularly challenging because treatment often requires adherence to lifestyle changes (e.g., diet) or drug regimens (14).

Dementia care costs can be overwhelming for patients and their families. Information on how to anticipate and finance the costs of care is presented in the next section.

FINANCING THE COSTS OF CARE

In 2006, the average annual cost of nursing home care was $75,190, more than three times the median income of households headed by an older person ($24,509) (9). Not surprisingly, it has been estimated that 57% of the elderly population in the United States and 75% of the elderly population at high risk of needing nursing home care do not have adequate assets to cover even one month of nursing home care (9). Planning for long-term care is one way that families and caregivers can help to ensure the well-being of the patient with dementia, while also ensuring their own welfare throughout all stages of the disease.

Anticipating and Planning for Long-Term Care Expenses

Long-term planning for any event, especially when it involves anticipating expenses, is challenging. Long-term planning for the care of a patient with dementia can be particularly difficult because the nature of the care is so complex (e.g., drug treatments, arranging for transportation to physicians, individual variability in disease progression, nursing home placement). In addition, available services

Table 4   Direct Medical and Nonmedical Costs Associated with Caring for Patients with Dementia

Element	Purpose	Unit	Cost per unit
Office visit: primary care physician	Routine office visit	Visit	$59.80 (24)[a]
Initial visit: neurologist	Evaluation/management of new patient	Visit	$91.03 (24)[a]
Initial visit: psychiatrist	Evaluation/management of new patient	Visit	$174.06 (24)[a]
Office consultation: neurologist	Cognitive assessment	Visit	$122.26 (24)[a]
Office consultation: psychiatrist	Behavioral and psychological assessment	Visit	$89.12 (24)[a]
Computerized tomography (CT) scan	Imaging scan that shows the internal structure of the brain; when dementia is diagnosed, CT scans can also reveal tumors and small strokes in the brain	Scan	$203.77 (24)[a]
Electroencephalography (EEG)	Recording of natural electrical activity of the brain that involves placement of small recording electrodes on the scalp	Assessment	$231.95 (24)[a]
Magnetic resonance imaging (MRI)	Scanning technique that generates cross sectional images of the brain by detecting small molecular changes; reveals the contrast between normal and abnormal tissue	Scan	$572.45 (24)[a]
Positron emission tomography (PET) scan	Imaging scan that gauges the activity or functional level of the brain by measuring the use of glucose	Scan	$1229.79 (24)[a]
Donepezil (Aricept)	Acetylcholinesterase inhibitor, indicated for treatment of mild to severe AD	One day supply	$9.83
Galantamine (Razadyne)	Acetylcholinesterase inhibitor, indicated for treatment of mild to moderate AD	One day supply	$6.10
Rivastigmine (Exelon) oral capsules	Acetylcholinesterase inhibitor, indicated for treatment of mild to moderate AD and mild to moderate Parkinson's disease	One day supply	$9.73
Rivastigmine (Exelon) transdermal patches	Acetylcholinesterase inhibitor, indicated for treatment of mild to moderate AD and mild to moderate Parkinson's disease	One day supply	$7.48
Memantine (Namenda)	N-methyl-D-aspartate (NMDA) receptor antagonist indicated for the treatment of moderate to severe AD	One day supply	$6.64
Hospital stay	Average stay in a hospital	8.6 days (26)[b]	$6709.00
Emergency department visit	Single visit to an emergency department	Visit	$561.00 (27)[c]
Hired transportation	Often provided by county or municipal programs to transport patients to physician appointments or to perform errands	Hour	$18.00 (28)[d]
Walker	Nonadjustable walker	Each	$66.85 (29)
Rails	Full-length side rails for bed	Pair	$185.18 (29)

Service	Description	Unit	Cost
Home health aide (noncertified but licensed provider)	Licensed individual who provides assistance with nonmedical care such as assisting with activities of daily living and providing supervision and companionship	Hour	$18.57 (30)
Home health aide (certified home care provider)	Licensed and certified individual who provides assistance with nonmedical care such as assisting with activities of daily living and providing supervision and companionship	Hour	$32.37 (30)
Registered Nurse home visit	Registered nurse who assists with medical care of patient in the home	Per visit	$121.00 (30)
Adult day care	Programs that provide care and companionship during the day	Day	$60.00–150.00 (31)[d]
Volunteer respite care (noncertified but licensed homemaker services)	Patient care usually provided by local church groups or local agencies	Hour	$17.46 (30)
In-home respite care	Assistance/companionship provided to the patient and the caregiver; possible assistance with housekeeping chores or personal care	Hour	$14.24 (32)[d]
Residential respite care	Respite care provided by nursing homes and hospitals, allowing for overnight and/or extended services	Day	$75.00–250.00 (33)[d]
Assisted living facility	Care provided for seniors who need some help with activities of daily living but who wish to remain as independent as possible; facilities are typically residential in nature and offer help with personal or custodial care but limited or no medical care	Day	$89.24 (30)
Assisted living facility entrance fee	One-time fee, commonly referred to as a *community* or *entrance* fee	One-time fee	$1621.08 (30)
Private room in a nursing home	Private room	Day	$204.95 (30)[e]
Semiprivate room in a nursing home	Typically shared with one other patient	Day	$180.78 (30)[e]
Hospice care	End-of-life care provided in a patient's home, a nursing home, an assisted living facility, or wherever the patient resides	Total stay	$24034.00–29309.00 (34)[f]

Aricept is a registered trademark of Eisai Co., Ltd.
Razadyne is a registered trademark of Ortho-McNeil Neurologics Division of Ortho-McNeil-Janssen Pharmaceuticals, Inc.
Exelon is a registered trademark of Novartis Pharmaceuticals Corporation.
Namenda is a registered trademark of Forest Pharmaceuticals.
[a] Nonfacility price.
[b] Average length of hospital stay for patients with delirium, dementia, and/or amnestic and cognitive disorders.
[c] Visit for a patient ≥65 years of age.
[d] Will vary, depending on the patient's location and needs.
[e] Among those assisted living facilities that provide dementia care services, 54% charge additional fees for dementia-related care, at an additional average monthly cost of $1110.
[f] Median cost per patient with Alzheimer's disease; costs depend on whether the patient chooses to be in a facility or nursing home or chooses to stay at home.

may vary from region to region. Determining how to pay for care can also be a complicated process, given the wide variety of assets and insurance sources that may have to be investigated and coordinated and the significant variability in costs from patient to patient. Furthermore, because the patient's judgment may be impaired and because family members and caregivers may be stressed by the day-to-day demands of care, others may need to be involved in financial decisions. Families are encouraged to seek professional advice on legal and financial matters involving the patient and his or her care. However, family members can also begin laying the groundwork for future decisions. One useful financial planning tool, the PLAN process, is introduced and described below.

The **PLAN** process is a set of guidelines for making arrangements for the eventual care of a patient with dementia. It can be summarized in four steps.

1. Prepare health insurance and asset information.
2. Look for dementia resources in your area.
3. Ask about availability and costs of services that may be required at each stage of the disease.
4. Note potential resources that can be used in addition to asset and insurance sources to cover costs.

Prepare Health Insurance and Asset Information

The first step in the PLAN process is to identify and collect all the patient's health insurance and asset information to determine how his or her future care might be financed. Some combination of the following programs may apply.

Medicare

Americans aged 65 years and older are eligible for Medicare (9). Many individuals are older than 65 years when they are diagnosed with dementia, and Medicare is often their primary source of health coverage. Medicare covers acute medical costs such as inpatient hospitalizations and physician visits, but the program does not pay for long-term care. Medicare pays out nearly three times as much annually on patients with AD and other dementias than it pays out on patients without dementias ($13207 vs. $4454 per patient, respectively) (36). Many of these expenditures are for hospital stays, which are more frequent among Medicare patients with dementia than among those without dementia (36).

Medigap insurance

Medicare does not cover all medical services, and it does not pay the entire cost of many of the services and supplies that are covered, which leaves the patient responsible for these costs. Medigap insurance (also known as Medicare supplemental insurance) can be purchased to close the coverage gap left by Medicare. However, long-term care in a nursing home is generally not covered by Medigap insurance (31).

Medicaid

Medicaid provides medical coverage to low-income individuals or families, regardless of age (31). Although there are national guidelines for Medicaid, coverage varies from state to state. Medicaid does cover long-term care; however, some providers of long-term care either limit the number of Medicaid beneficiaries they accept or do not accept Medicaid beneficiaries at all. Consequently, a Medicaid recipient in need of long-term care may have limited options. Despite this, an estimated 51% of nursing home residents with AD use Medicaid to help pay for their care (9). Under Medicaid rules, a married person with a spouse in a long-term care facility is allowed to keep his or her primary residence, as well as a portion of the couple's assets. The dollar amount of the assets allowed varies by state.

Private insurance
Private insurance, supplemental insurance, and managed care organizations generally pay for acute medical costs but rarely cover the costs of long-term care.

Long-term care insurance
Long-term care insurance is designed to help pay for nursing home care required by patients with disabilities or chronic illnesses. However, few people have this type of insurance. If people wait until they are elderly to purchase a long-term care policy, insurance carriers may consider insuring them to be too great a risk; in fact, many long-term care policies have restrictions on age and health status. If an older person does qualify for coverage, the premiums are likely to be very high.

Veterans' benefits
The Department of Veterans Affairs (VA) has nursing care facilities available for veterans. The VA also has contracts with state and private nursing homes to care for veterans. However, priority goes to those veterans with service-related disabilities. In addition, unless a veteran requires long-term care because of a service-related illness or injury, the VA has income and asset criteria that must be met for long-term care coverage eligibility.

State-specific programs
Many state-funded programs subsidize various services, including home health care. Services and eligibility standards vary from state to state. Generally, these services are reserved for people with limited incomes and few assets and provide a means of preventing or postponing placement of patients into expensive nursing home environments. The Eldercare Locator service (1–800–677–1116 or http://www.eldercare.gov), a program of the U.S. Department of Health and Human Services, may be of assistance in finding state-specific agencies by region (37).

Health care tax benefits
Taxpayers who itemize their federal income taxes may deduct all unreimbursed medical expenses and insurance premiums once those expenses exceed a certain percentage of the taxpayer's adjusted gross income (currently, 7.5%) (38). This deduction may benefit people with catastrophic medical costs.

After insurance information has been gathered, all of the patient's and family's financial records should be collected. Since nursing home care is sometimes paid for by patients and their families, care should be taken to examine each type of income and asset. Only then can informed decisions be made regarding the allocation of resources for the long-term care of the patient. If assets are overestimated, caregivers and family members may overspend on the patient, or if all expenses of the spouse and family are not taken into account when resources are allocated, a financial crisis may develop down the road. Some common retirement benefits and assets are detailed below.

Pensions
Pensions are steady sources of income paid to retirees. The company or institution that employed the retiree generally pays benefits.

Individual retirement accounts
These are investment tools used to save money for retirement. Individual retirement accounts have certain tax benefits that regular savings accounts lack. Contributions to these accounts are generally made while an individual is still working.

Social Security benefits
Most persons older than 65 years (or older than 62 years, in some cases) are already receiving or are entitled to receive Social Security benefits from the U.S. government. These benefits are paid on a monthly basis and increase at the rate of inflation. Persons with dementia who are younger than 65 years may be eligible for Social Security Disability Insurance.

Stocks
Stocks are shares of ownership in corporations. Some stocks pay dividends (payments made by companies to shareholders).

Bonds.   Bonds are debt securities; the issuer owes the holder of the bond a debt and is obliged to repay both the principal and interest at the time of its maturity.

Savings accounts
Savings accounts may be in banks or credit unions.

Home equity/real estate
Many older people own their primary residence and have equity in it. Home equity is the difference between the market value of a home and the unpaid balance of the mortgage(s) and any outstanding debts on the home. Some people also have other real estate assets such as income property, second homes, and vacant land.

Personal property
Personal property includes cars, jewelry, and other items of value.

Look for Dementia Resources in Your Area
The next step in the PLAN process is to identify and locate providers of services that may be needed by the patient in the future. Sources of information about

area services include health care providers, hospital social workers and discharge planners, religious organizations, and local offices of the Alzheimer's Association. The Eldercare Locator service can provide information about state programs and community resources and can direct families to local agencies (37). Some of these services, such as meals delivered to the home, respite care, transportation, and support groups for both patients and caregivers, may be available either at no cost or at minimal cost.

Ask About Availability and Costs of Services That May Be Required at Each Stage of the Disease

After resources have been identified, patients and their families and caregivers can contact the appropriate agencies to find out whether help (e.g., home health aides) will be available when needed and how much these services will cost. It is important to anticipate and plan for all the costs that may be incurred over the entire course of a patient's dementia. Because of the progressive nature of the disease, these costs may range from modifications to the patient's current home (e.g., handrails in the shower) to placement of the patient into a new care setting. A contingency plan should also be considered. For example, if a spouse or family member is no longer able to care for the patient because of deteriorating health, additional caregivers may have to be recruited. To help in estimating the services that may be needed at each stage of dementia, a table with examples has been provided (Table 5), along with a blank table for family members to complete (Table 6).

Note Potential Resources That Can Be Used in Addition to Asset and Insurance Sources to Cover Costs

Table 7 can be used to plot the estimated needs of the patient at each stage of dementia, the estimated costs of the services, and the various assets or insurance policies that will be used to pay for those services. Table 8 provides an example of a completed plot based on the following case study of a hypothetical patient.

In this example, the patient is a 72-year-old man with AD and Stage 2 loss of independence. His cognitive abilities have steadily declined since he received a diagnosis of AD 2 years ago. He has a history of type 2 diabetes and hyperlipidemia. His current medications include donepezil 10 mg/day, atorvastatin 20 mg/day, metformin extended release 1000 mg/day, and glyburide 1.2 mg/day. Every three months, he visits his primary care physician, who monitors his diabetes and hyperlipidemia. Recently, the patient began using a walker, and rails were installed on his bed to prevent falls during the night. The patient's wife lives with him in their home; however, because she has osteoporosis and arthritis, her ability to care for him is limited. The patient's son lives nearby and visits several times each week. The patient's daughter works full-time and lives an hour's drive away, but she would consider moving closer if her father needed additional assistance. Despite the family's efforts, a home health aide is also required four times each week to perform household chores and help the patient with daily activities. The patient has Medicare coverage and receives Social Security benefits and a modest pension.

Table 5 Potential Care and Service Needs Determined by Loss of Independence

	Stage 1 (reminders)	Stage 2 (increased assistance needs)	Stage 3 (supervision required)	Stage 4 (functional assistance required)	Stage 5 (complete dependence)
Direct medical costs	• Ongoing medical treatments including treatment for conditions other than dementia (e.g., prescription drugs, laboratory tests, physician office visits, hospitalizations); these costs will be present across all stages and likely will increase as the patient ages				
Direct nonmedical costs	• Adult day care • In-home respite care • Home health aide • Transportation costs • Home-delivered meals			• Adult day care • In-home or residential respite care • Home-delivered meals • Home health aide	• In-home or residential respite care
Indirect/informal care resources	• Assistance needed from spouse or family member to perform some daily activities	• Assistance needed to perform many daily activities	• Assistance needed to perform most daily activities • Some supervision required	• Assistance needed to perform almost all daily activities • Almost constant supervision required	• Assistance needed to perform virtually all daily activities • 24-hr supervision required
Living situation/long-term care	• Rails in shower or bathtub • Walker		• Assisted living facility or nursing home care (private or semiprivate room)		• Assisted living facility or nursing home care (private or semiprivate room) • Hospice care

Table 6 Plot for Estimating Care and Service Needs at Each Stage of Dementia

	Stage 1 (reminders)	Stage 2 (increased assistance needs)	Stage 3 (supervision required)	Stage 4 (functional assistance required)	Stage 5 (complete dependence)
Direct medical costs					
Direct nonmedical costs					
Indirect/informal care resources					
Living situation/long-term care					

Table 7 Plot of Anticipated Services and Costs[a]

Anticipated cost or service	Anticipated provider	Insurance or asset covering the cost or service
Direct medical costs		
Direct nonmedical costs		
Indirect/informal care resources[b]		
Living situation/long-term care		

[a]Use a blank page for each of the following stages:
Stage 1 (Reminders)
Stage 2 (increased assistance needs)
Stage 3 (supervision required)
Stage 4 (functional assistance required)
Stage 5 (complete dependence)
[b]Specify who will provide the care, and specify a backup provider, in case the first provider is unavailable.

Table 8 Sample Plot of Anticipated Services and Costs for the Case Study (Stage 2 Loss of Independence)

Anticipated cost or service	Anticipated provider	Insurance or asset covering the cost or service
Direct medical costs		
• Donepezil 10 mg/day ($20.00 monthly co-pay)	• Pharmacy	• Social Security and Medicare
• Atorvastatin 20 mg/day ($20.00 monthly co-pay)	• Pharmacy • Pharmacy	• Social Security and Medicare
• Metformin extended release 1000 mg/day ($10.00 monthly co-pay)	• Pharmacy • Primary care physician	• Social Security and Medicare
• Glyburide 1.2 mg/day ($10.00 monthly co-pay)		• Social Security and Medicare
• Physician visit ($40.00 co-pay per visit)		• Social Security and Medicare
Direct nonmedical costs		
• Home health aide for 20 hr per week (about $1500 per month)	• Local agency	• Pension
Indirect/informal care resources		
• 5–10 hr per day of support and supervision	• Spouse and son; daughter as a backup	• None required
Living situation/long-term care		
• Walker ($66.85)	• Local medical equipment provider	• Pension
• Rails for bed ($185.18)	• Local medical equipment provider	• Pension

CONCLUSION

The financial costs associated with caring for a patient with AD or another form of dementia can be overwhelming. Unfortunately, decisions about care and how to pay for it often must be made at a time when patients and their families are struggling with grief and trying to cope with the day-to-day demands of a very debilitating disease. If families avoid making decisions or planning for future costs, they may ultimately limit their options down the road. However, careful planning for services that will be needed and an understanding of how to pay for them can help to maximize the well-being of the patient and family throughout the course of the disease.

REFERENCES

1. MetLife Foundation Alzheimer's survey: What America thinks. Conducted by Harris Interactive. Metropolitan Life Insurance Company Web site. Published May 11, 2006. Accessed January 19, 2008.
2. Dodge HH, Shen C, Pandav R, et al. Functional transitions and active life expectancy associated with Alzheimer disease. Arch Neurol 2003; 60(2):253–259.
3. Agüero-Torres H, Fratiglioni L, Guo Z, et al. Mortality from dementia in advanced age: A 5-year follow-up study of incident dementia cases. J Clin Epidemiol 1999; 52(8):737–743.
4. Rosenberg H, Ventura S, Maurer J, et al. Births, marriages, divorces, and deaths for March 1996. Month Vital Stat Rep 1996; 45(3):1–20.
5. Larson EB, Shadlen MF, Wang L, et al. Survival after initial diagnosis of Alzheimer disease. Ann Intern Med 2004; 140(7):501–509.
6. Brookmeyer R, Johnson E, Ziegler-Graham K, et al. Forecasting the global burden of Alzheimer's disease. Alzheimers Dement 2007; 3(3):186–191.
7. Projected population of the United States, by age and sex: 2000 to 2050. US Census Bureau Web site. http://www.census.gov/ipc/www/usinterimproj/natprojtab02a.pdf. Published March 18, 2004. Accessed January 21, 2008.
8. Lloyd-Sherlock P. Population ageing in developed and developing regions: implications for health policy. Soc Sci Med 2000; 51(6):887–895.
9. Alzheimer's disease facts and figures: 2007. Alzheimer's Association Web site. http://www.alz.org/national/documents/Report_2007FactsAndFigures.pdf. Published March 20, 2007. Accessed March 20, 2007.
10. Small GW, Rabins PV, Barry PP, et al. Diagnosis and treatment of Alzheimer disease and related disorders. Consensus statement of the American Association for Geriatric Psychiatry, the Alzheimer's Association, and the American Geriatrics Society. JAMA 1997; 278(16):1363–1371.
11. Morris JC. The Clinical Dementia Rating (CDR): Current version and scoring rules. Neurology 1993; 43(11):2412–2414.
12. Hughes CP, Berg L, Danziger WL, et al. A new clinical scale for the staging of dementia. Br J Psychiatry 1982; 140:566–572.
13. Folstein MF, Folstein SE, McHugh PR. "Mini-mental state". A practical method for grading the cognitive state of patients for the clinician. J Psychiatr Res 1975; 12(3):189–198.
14. Stander P. Management of Alzheimer's disease in the managed care setting. J Manag Care Med 2007; 10(4):8–13.
15. Stern Y, Albert SM, Sano M, et al. Assessing patient dependence in Alzheimer's disease. J Gerontol 1994; 49(5):M216–M222.
16. Yaffe K, Fox P, Newcomer R, et al. Patient and caregiver characteristics and nursing home placement in patients with dementia. JAMA 2002; 287(16):2090–2097.
17. Stone RI. Long-term care for the elderly with disabilities: Current policy, emerging trends, and implications for the twenty-first century. The Milbank Memorial Fund Web site. http://milbank.org/reports/0008stone/index.html. Published August 2000. Accessed January 21, 2008.

18. Moore MJ, Zhu CW, Clipp EC. Informal costs of dementia care: Estimates from the National Longitudinal Caregiver Study. J Gerontol B Psychol Sci Soc Sci 2001; 56(4):S219–S228.

19. Leon J, Chen CK, Neumann PJ. Alzheimer's disease care: Costs and potential savings. Health Aff (Millwood) 1998; 17(6):206–216.

20. Gruber-Baldini AL, Stuart B, Zuckerman IH, et al. Treatment of dementia in community-dwelling and institutionalized Medicare beneficiaries. J Am Geriatr Soc 2007; 55(10):1508–1516.

21. Rice DP, Fox PJ, Max W, et al. The economic burden of Alzheimer's disease care. Health Aff (Millwood) 1993; 12(2):164–176.

22. Zhu CW, Scarmeas N, Torgan R, et al. Longitudinal study of effects of patient characteristics on direct costs in Alzheimer disease. Neurology 2006; 67(6):998–1005.

23. Leon J, Moyer D. Potential cost savings in residential care for Alzheimer's disease patients. Gerontologist 1999; 39(4):440–449.

24. Physician fee schedule search. Centers for Medicare and Medicaid Services Web site. http://www.cms.hhs.gov/PFSlookup/02_PFSSearch.asp#TopOfPage. Published January 2008. Accessed January 22, 2008.

25. VitaminLife, Inc. VitaminLife.com Web site search function. http://www.vitaminlife.com/. Accessed February 1, 2008.

26. Owens P, Myers M, Elixhauser A, et al. Care of Adults with Mental Health and Substance Abuse Disorders in U.S. Community Hospitals, 2004—HCUP Fact Book No. 10. AHRQ Publication No. 07–0008. Agency for Healthcare Research and Quality Web site. http://www.ahrq.gov/data/hcup/factbk10/. Published January 2007. Accessed February 4, 2008.

27. Machlin SR. Expenses for a hospital emergency room visit, 2003. Medical expenditure panel survey, Statistical Brief No. 111. Agency for Healthcare Research and Quality Web site. http://www.meps.ahrq.gov/mepsweb/data_files/publications/st111/stat111.pdf. Published January 2006. Accessed January 22, 2008.

28. St. Leonard senior living community housing rates. St. Leonard Web site. Accessed January 31, 2008.

29. Fee schedule for durable medical equipment & prosthetic devices. State of New Jersey Web site. http://www.nj.gov/dobi/ad062201b.pdf. Accessed January 22, 2008.

30. Genworth Financial 2007 cost of care survey: Home care providers, assisted living facilities and nursing homes. Genworth Financial Web site. http://www.genworth.com/content/etc/medialib/genworth/us/en/pdfs/ltc_pdfs.Par.34346.File.dat/Cost_Of_Care_Survey.pdf. Published March 31, 2007. Accessed January 22, 2008.

31. Alzheimer's disease continuing care information. Fisher Center for Alzheimer's Research Foundation Web site. Accessed January 22, 2008.

32. Frequently asked questions. Serve Link Home Care Web site. http://www.servelinkhomecare.com/faq.html. Accessed February 1, 2008.

33. The RCCCWA respite resource guide: Description of respite services. The Arc of King County Web site. Accessed January 22, 2008.

34. Pyenson B, Connor S, Fitch K, et al. Medicare cost in matched hospice and non-hospice cohorts. J Pain Symptom Manage 2004; 28(3):200–210.

35. Murman DL, Von Eye A, Sherwood PR, et al. Evaluated need, costs of care, and payer perspective in degenerative dementia patients cared for in the United States. Alzheimer Dis Assoc Disord 2007; 21(1):39–48.

36. Alzheimer's disease and chronic health conditions: The real challenge for 21st century Medicare. Alzheimer's Association Web site. http://www.alz.org/national/documents/report_chroniccare.pdf. Published 2003. Accessed January 22, 2008.

37. Eldercare search. Department of Health and Human Services Eldercare Locator Web site. Accessed January 31, 2008.

38. Lyke B, Whittaker JM. Tax benefits for health insurance and expenses: Overview of current law and legislation. Order Code RL 33505. Congressional Reports for the People Web site. Updated July 20, 2007. Accessed January 23, 2008.

8 The primary care physician's role in the recognition, diagnosis, and management of dementia

Larry W. Lawhorne

INTRODUCTION

Managing the chronic health care needs of the elderly, including those with Alzheimer's disease, will place an enormous burden on the health care system in the United States (1–4). The number of people aged 65 years and older will essentially double between now and 2030 (from approximately 36 million to 72 million), representing an increase from 12% to 20% of the U.S. population (5). The increase in the over-85 age group is noteworthy as well, reaching over 10 million by 2030 (5). Both the relative and absolute increase in the number of elderly people will affect the health care delivery system, including the relationship that exists between the primary care provider and the elderly consumer of health services (1,2). Family physicians, internists, nurse practitioners, and physician assistants will see more and more elderly patients as each wave of aging baby boomers becomes Medicare-eligible. The challenge of their increasing numbers will be matched by the heterogeneity of their health care expectations and needs, ranging from requests for anti-aging therapies and health maintenance on one end of the spectrum to management of frail elders with multiple medical and neuropsychiatric conditions on the other. In particular, the primary care clinician's ability to diagnose and manage Alzheimer's disease will become increasingly important for at least two reasons. First, it is prevalent and the number of people with Alzheimer's disease is expected to increase dramatically. There are now 4.5 million Americans with Alzheimer's disease, with an expected increase to 13.2 million by 2050 (4). Second, Alzheimer's disease has a devastating effect on the people suffering from it, on those around them, especially their caregivers, and on society as a whole (1–5).

Since the prevalence of Alzheimer's disease and most other disorders causing dementia increases with age (3,4), the growing number of elderly patients coming into doctors' practices poses additional challenges for primary care providers. Although the recognition, assessment, and management of dementia is difficult in their own right, the presence of dementia also affects the management of coexisting illnesses as well as the types of interventions that are recommended for the physical, psychosocial, and spiritual changes that occur with aging (2). Therefore, the primary care physician must not only be able to recognize that cognitive decline is present but also to determine the cause(s) of the decline either by performing the appropriate evaluation or referring the patient to a consultant.

Each office visit by an elderly person at risk for developing Alzheimer's disease offers opportunities to improve the frequency with which symptoms and signs suggesting Alzheimer's disease can be recognized and to perform the evaluations necessary to establish a diagnosis. In addition, the primary care physician is in a pivotal position to initiate appropriate interventions to slow progression early in the course of the disease and to coordinate the long-term care of patients as the disease progresses. The objectives of the remainder of this chapter are to describe a process whereby primary care providers can (*i*) recognize risk factors and signs and symptoms suggestive of Alzheimer's disease, (*ii*) conduct or coordinate an assessment to establish the diagnosis, and (*iii*) manage Alzheimer's disease by developing a person-centered plan of care.

Recognition

A number of publications suggest that primary care physicians fail to recognize or identify a substantial proportion of their patients who have cognitive impairment or fail to carry out appropriate assessments when they do recognize it (6–11). However, many of these reports focus on whether primary care physicians' screening activities and other processes and practices are consistent with existing clinical practice guidelines on dementia, specifically Alzheimer's disease. The question becomes, then, does the primary care physician fail to recognize and assess the problem or fail to use guidelines? Many of the elderly patients seen in the primary care setting have several medical and neuropsychiatric conditions, and there are potential pitfalls to applying multiple clinical practice guidelines to a single individual (11,12). In addition, many of the guidelines used to address Alzheimer's disease and other dementias were developed by specialists and academic centers and may suffer from limitations described by Kerr White and colleagues almost a half century ago. White's seminal article in the *New England Journal of Medicine* provided an elegant scheme for thinking about medical care from a population-based perspective (13). Using data collected by British general practitioners, White and his coauthors described the ecology of medical care in a population of 1000 adults. In an average month, 750 reported an illness but only 250 visited a physician. Of these 250, nine would be hospitalized, five referred to another physician, and one referred to an academic medical center. An overarching theme in 1961 and again in 2001 when White's medical care ecology construct was revisited (14) is that what is happening in the academic medical center may not be reflective of what is happening in the community. An unintended effect, therefore, may be that medical research and medical education may not provide appropriate guidance for community-based primary care physicians, advance practice nurses, and other clinicians. Primary care practice-based research networks have addressed this potentially incongruent situation and ultimately changed the way common conditions are evaluated and managed (15,16).

Applying the ecology of medical care model to Alzheimer's disease may be instructive. In a hypothetical town of 10,000 people in rural America, about 1500 will be older than 65 years (Figs. 1 and 2). How many of the 1500 have cognitive impairment and what signs and symptoms can be expected? How many of those with cognitive impairment will see a primary care provider? How many with cognitive impairment will be recognized by the primary care provider as having impaired cognition? How many of those recognized as cognitively impaired will be assessed and diagnosed at the primary care level and how many will be referred to academic centers or experts specializing in the diagnosis and treatment of the dementing illnesses? Finally, how many will be treated using a systematic

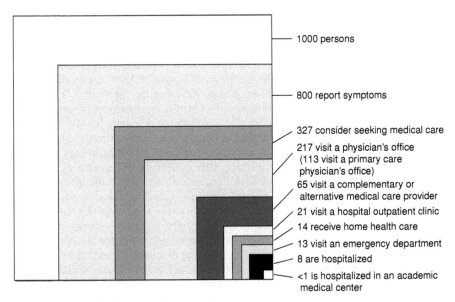

Figure 1 Results of a reanalysis of the monthly prevalence of illness in the community and the roles of various sources of health care. Each box represents a subgroup of the largest box, which comprises 1000 persons. Data are for persons of all ages (14).

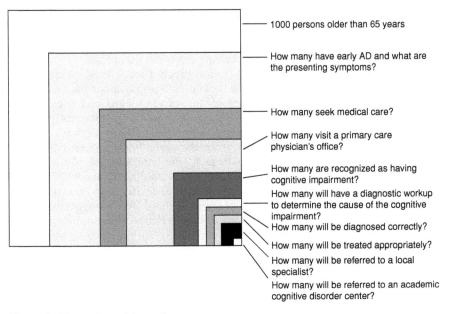

Figure 2 The ecology of dementia care.

care and treatment model? Answers to these questions are important from a public health perspective because of the anticipated increase in the number of people with Alzheimer's disease noted earlier (4).

Given these considerations, what should the primary care physician do to enhance the process of identification of potential cases of Alzheimer's disease? Is screening the answer? The Mini-Mental State Examination (MMSE) (17) has been used for many years and is well validated. The Mini-Cog compares favorably with the MMSE with respect to sensitivity (76% vs. 79%) and specificity (89% vs. 88%) (18). Similarly, the Self-Administered Gerocognitive Examination (SAGE) compares favorably with the MMSE, and its self-administered feature may promote screening by busy clinicians prompting earlier diagnosis and treatment (19).

The U.S. Preventive Services Task Force concludes that there is insufficient evidence to recommend for or against routine screening for dementia in the elderly (20). The Task Force reasoned that while some screening tests have good sensitivity and fair specificity and that while there is good evidence that drug therapy has a beneficial effect on cognitive function, evidence for beneficial effect on instrumental activities of daily living (IADLs) is mixed (20). In addition, little is known about the potential harm of screening such as labeling effect (20). Focus groups of primary care physicians in Michigan provided similar findings with concerns about time and resources, the potential adverse effects of labeling, and the belief that nothing could be done for the patient with Alzheimer's disease (2).

If screening all the elderly people is not recommended, then what can be done to increase the frequency with which primary care physicians recognize risk factors and early signs and symptoms of Alzheimer's disease? Some authors suggest that targeted educational programs and enhanced support for clinical decision making would increase the number of people who are accurately diagnosed and for whom both disease-specific and supportive interventions can be implemented in a timely manner (21). Others have suggested that a constellation of symptoms is associated with early Alzheimer's disease: missing recall items on the MMSE, difficulty doing calculations, repetition, getting lost while driving, forgetting the names of relatives, and having poor judgment (22).

Based on existing literature and clinical practice guidelines, the dementia-prepared primary care practice should be knowledgeable about the risk factors for Alzheimer's disease and be aware of the warning signs and triggers that may suggest dementia (Table 1) (2,23–26). Finally, knowledge about the patient's IADL performance may help the primary care clinician with both recognition of dementia and prognosis. A study from the early 1990s reported that four IADLs correlated with cognitive impairment: telephone use, use of transportation, responsibility for taking medications, and handling finances (27). These correlations were noted to be independent of age, gender, and education (27). Not only was the inability to do one or more of these IADLs suggestive of the presence of dementia but also appeared to be predictive of further decline and health care utilization (27,28).

To summarize his/her role in the recognition phase of Alzheimer's disease, the primary care physician should consider the following questions:

- Does my elderly patient have risk factors for Alzheimer's disease?
- Does my elderly patient have warning signs or triggers that are suggestive of possible early Alzheimer's disease?

Table 1 Primary Care Clues in the Recognition of Alzheimer's Disease

Risk factors

Definite
Age
Family history
Down's syndrome
APOE–E4

Possible
Other genes
Head trauma
Lower educational level
Depression

Warning signs
Memory loss
Difficulty performing familiar tasks
Problems with language
Disorientation to time, place
Poor or decreased judgment
Problems with abstract thought
Misplacing things
Changes in mood, behavior
Changes in personality
Loss of initiative

Triggers
Problems with communication (frequent calls to office, missing
  appointments, difficulty following directions, etc.)
Accidents (falls, motor vehicle accidents, etc.)
Changes in functional status (a move into assisted living, new or increasing
  medication errors, signs of self-neglect, getting lost, etc.)
Changes in medical or neuropsychiatric status (weight loss, delirium,
  depression, etc.)

- Does my elderly patient have difficulty performing one or more of the IADLs correlated with impaired cognition (telephone, transportation, medication, finances)?
- Is the patient, a family member or friend, or a staff member in the primary care office concerned about possible Alzheimer's disease?

If the answer to any of these questions is yes, an assessment to determine the etiology of the cognitive deficits should be initiated as soon as possible.

Assessment and Diagnosis

If Alzheimer's disease is suspected because of the presence of warning signs, triggers, or IADL deficiencies, the primary care physician should consider measuring baseline cognition using the MMSE, Mini-Cog, Seven-Minute Neurocognitive Screen for Alzheimer's disease, or some other standard test of cognitive function that can be administered in the office. The Seven-Minute Screen tests memory, verbal fluency, visuospatial ability, visuoconstruction, and orientation to time (29). Good evidence supports the use of the MMSE (adjusted for age and education) and neuropsychological batteries (30). Evidence is weaker for the Mini-Cog and the Seven-Minute Screen (30).

The National Guideline Clearinghouse (31) lists 38 practice guidelines related to Alzheimer's disease. The American Academy of Neurology (AAN) guideline (30) (published in 2001 and reviewed in 2004) provides a reasonable framework for the primary care practice. The AAN guideline recommends using the DSM-IV criteria to establish the diagnosis of Alzheimer's disease, and the American Association for Geriatric Psychiatry (AAGP) position statement (32) on the principles of care for patients with Alzheimer's disease proposes a similar approach using the criteria in the DSM-IV-TR. The DSM-IV-TR criteria for Alzheimer's disease require the presence of multiple cognitive deficits manifested by memory impairment and aphasia and/or apraxia and/or agnosia, along with disturbances in executive functioning. In addition, the cognitive deficits represent a decline from previous functioning and cause significant impairment in social or occupational functioning with a course that is characterized by gradual onset and continuing decline. To meet criteria for Alzheimer's disease, the cognitive deficits cannot be due to other central nervous system, systemic, or substance-induced conditions that cause progressive deficits in memory and cognition and cannot be better accounted for by another psychiatric disorder (33).

If the patient has evidence of multiple cognitive deficits manifested by memory impairment and aphasia and/or apraxia and/or agnosia, along with disturbances in executive functioning (DSM-IV-TR criteria for Alzheimer's disease), a targeted history and physical examination should be conducted. The history should focus on the following factors:

- Age at onset of any symptom(s) related to possible Alzheimer's disease
- Characteristics and progression of symptoms
- Most prominent cognitive symptoms
- Personality, mood, or behavioral changes
- History of hypertension, lipid disorder, cardiovascular disease, stroke, seizures, or head injury
- Urinary incontinence
- Falls or other injuries requiring medical attention
- Use of prescription and nonprescription drugs, including herbals
- Use of alcohol and other substances
- Family history of dementia
- Problems with driving

In addition to a thorough cardiovascular and pulmonary physical examination, the neurological examination should determine if there are any localizing findings or balance or gait abnormalities.

The presence of multiple cognitive deficits does not necessarily mean Alzheimer's disease. A number of neurodegenerative diseases other than Alzheimer's disease can produce cognitive deficits (vascular dementia, dementia with Lewy bodies, frontotemporal dementia), but they will not be addressed here. Cognitive deficits also can be associated with polypharmacy, mood disorders (especially depression), cerebrovascular disease, and a myriad of medical conditions (2,32). Therefore, a critical early step in the evaluation at the primary care level is to attempt to rule out the most common diseases and conditions that may mimic Alzheimer's disease with appropriate initial actions and tests (Table 2).

Table 2 Initial Primary Care Evaluation for Suspected Alzheimer's Disease

---

Immediate review of medications with consideration of tapering and/or discontinuing drugs that
   may adversely affect cognition (especially the "anti" drugs: anticholinergic, antiemetic,
   antianxiety, antipsychotic, antihistamine, etc.)
Immediate screening test for depression
CBC, chemistries, TSH, vitamin B_{12}
Brain CT or MRI especially if there are localizing neurologic findings, including balance or gait

---

The importance of a thorough review of medications (both prescription and
nonprescription drugs) cannot be overemphasized. Drugs with anticholinergic
activity can have a profound effect on cognition (34–37). Since many of the elderly
persons in the community are on multiple medications, cumulative anticholinergic effect is of increasing concern. Any single drug that an elderly patient is
taking may have only a small anticholinergic effect, but in aggregate, the effect
may be large. In a report on 201 community-dwelling elderly persons who were
randomly selected to undergo testing for serum anticholinergic activity (SAA),
180 (90%) had detectable SAA, and there was a significant association between
SAA and MMSE scores (34). Logistic regression analysis indicated that subjects
with SAA at or above the sample's 90th percentile (SAA $\geq$ 2.80 pmol/mL) were
13 times (odds ratio, 1.08–152.39) more likely than subjects with undetectable SAA
to have an MMSE score of 24 (the sample's 10th percentile) or below (34). The
implications of these findings are that even low SAA activity may be associated
with cognitive impairment.

Depressive symptoms or major depressive disorder (MDD) may either
mimic or accompany Alzheimer's disease; therefore, screening for depression
and crafting a treatment plan for depression are important tasks for the primary
care physician (32,38–40). Two screening tests that are easily administered in the
office setting are the Short-Form Geriatric Depression Scale (GDS) and the Patient
Health Questionnaire-2 (PHQ-2). The Short-Form GDS takes five to seven minutes and can be administered by a provider with minimal training in its use (41).
The PHQ-2 asks about depressed mood and anhedonia over the past 2 weeks
(score 0–3 for each with 0 = "not at all" and 3 = "nearly every day"). A PHQ-2
score $\geq$ 3 has a sensitivity of 83% and a specificity of 92% for major depression
in the primary care setting (42). However, this study involved a younger patient
population.

With regard to laboratory testing, the AAN guideline recommends complete
blood count, glucose, thyroid function tests, serum electrolytes, BUN, creatinine,
liver function tests, and vitamin B_{12} level (30). Table 2 also includes a recommendation for lipid testing because the AAGP emphasizes the importance of
addressing cardiovascular risk factors, including screening for and treating lipid
disorders (32). Controlling cardiovascular risk factors, especially hypertension
and hyperlipidemia, are probably important strategies for preventing or slowing
the progression of mixed dementia (defined as the coexistence of Alzheimer's
disease and vascular dementia), which is likely to increase as the population ages
(43). The AAN guideline does not recommend routine screening for syphilis,
linear or volumetric magnetic resonance or computed tomography measurement strategies, single photon emission computed tomography, apolipoprotein
E (APOE) genotyping, electroencephalogram (EEG), or lumbar puncture (30).

According to the AAN guideline, "structural neuroimaging with either a noncontrast computed tomography or magnetic resonance scan in the initial evaluation of patients with dementia is appropriate" (30). For the most part, the purpose of structural neuroimaging is to provide clues that a process other than Alzheimer's disease may be the cause of the dementia.

If the history, physical examination, and other diagnostic tests are consistent with Alzheimer's disease and if the patient and family are satisfied with the thoroughness of the assessment, a referral to a neurologist, geriatric psychiatrist, or a center specializing in dementia may not be necessary. However, referral for neuropsychological testing should be considered because findings may be helpful when developing the person-centered plan of care (2).

At this stage, the primary care physician should open a discussion with the patient and family about the diagnosis of Alzheimer's disease. Providing information about the diagnosis, how it was made, and why other diagnoses appear unlikely may strengthen the doctor-patient and doctor-family bonds at this critical time (2). An offer to help the patient and family secure a second opinion if they wish and to provide contact information for local community resources is also appropriate at this time (2,44). Open a discussion about safety issues as soon as possible, emphasizing the current living situation and driving. If depression is also suspected, suicide risk must be assessed (45). After these initial steps have been taken, the primary care physician can start to work with the patient and family to develop and implement a more detailed plan of care.

Management

General principles of care

The AAGP position statement about the care of patients with Alzheimer's disease should resonate with primary care physicians (32). The statement contends that while evidence is limited, the existing literature, coupled with clinical experience and common sense, is adequate to produce a set of effective care principles aimed at

- Delaying disease progression,
- Delaying functional decline,
- Improving quality of life,
- Supporting dignity,
- Controlling symptoms, and
- Providing comfort at all stages of Alzheimer's disease (32).

The AAN guideline emphasizes pharmacotherapy for cognitive symptoms, agitation, psychosis, and depression as well as psychosocial support for the person with Alzheimer's disease and the caregiver (30).

Primary care physicians often are best suited to help patients and family members understand Alzheimer's disease, its symptoms and prognosis, and to advise them about community resources. Family members of patients with Alzheimer's disease, especially those who are or will become caregivers, often are devastated when the diagnosis is presented (44). Therefore, spending time with both patient and caregiver at this point can strengthen the relationship between the physician and the patient-caregiver dyad and create a bond that will help all three make the best of the journey ahead. Tailoring disclosure of the diagnosis to the characteristics of the patient and family members is important and may be done best by the physician who has provided primary care prior to the diagnosis (44). Caregivers want physicians to listen and respond to their concerns and to include the patient in discussions even when they may not understand all that is being discussed (44).

There are three resources that are generally available across the country. The Alzheimer's Association is available online (46) or at 800–337–3827 and provides information about local chapters, support groups, 24/7 support line services, education, and safe return programs. Area Agencies on Aging (47) (800–677–1116) offer information and assistance with finding a variety of services, such as care management, home-delivered meals, personal care, and respite or day care. The Family Caregiver Alliance (48) (415–434–3388) is dedicated to working with caregivers and provides fact sheets, research updates, and email-based support groups.

Drugs for Alzheimer's disease

The most obvious and consistent abnormality in the neurochemistry of Alzheimer's disease is a deficiency of acetylcholine. Injury and ultimately death of cholinergic neurons are associated with decreasing activity of acetylcholine in the brain, which in turn leads to some of the clinical manifestations of Alzheimer's disease. This cholinergic hypothesis has focused attention on the development of drugs that prolong activity of any acetylcholine in the brain as long as possible. Acetylcholinesterase inhibitors act by inhibiting acetylcholinesterase, the enzyme that degrades acetylcholine by hydrolysis. The acetylcholinesterase inhibitors are discussed in detail in chapter 3.

Memantine (Namenda, Ebixa) is another drug that is available for the treatment of Alzheimer's disease. Approved for moderate-to-severe disease, memantine is a moderate affinity, uncompetitive glutamate antagonist at the N-methyl-D-aspartate (NMDA) receptor and is also discussed in chapter 3.

The primary care physician is faced with a number of questions when working with patients and their families to make decisions about the drugs approved for Alzheimer's disease. Do any of these drugs offer meaningful clinical benefit? If they do, is one cholinesterase inhibitor preferred over another? When should memantine be used, and should it be added to a cholinesterase inhibitor? How long should pharmacotherapy for Alzheimer's disease be continued? What are the consequences of discontinuing pharmacotherapy, especially a cholinesterase inhibitor for Alzheimer's disease?

Do any of these drugs offer meaningful clinical benefit? Meta-analyses of randomized, controlled trials and systematic reviews of treatment with donepezil, rivastigmine, or galantamine suggest modest benefits on cognitive, behavioral, functional, or global measures and modest benefits with regard to slowing disease progression (49–68). Most guidelines recommend treatment with cholinesterase inhibitors, and the number of prescriptions for these drugs continues to increase (63). A population-based study of cholinesterase inhibitor use among 28,961 patients in Canada found that on average patients had 26 physician visits in the year before cholinesterase inhibitor therapy was started, but only 28% had seen a specialist during that time and over one-third were receiving potentially inappropriate drugs (e.g., benzodiazepines or drugs with anticholinergic effects)

(63). Average length of treatment with a cholinesterase inhibitor was about 2.4 years, 43% remained on the initial dose prescribed, 6% switched to another cholinesterase inhibitor, and 19% died while on cholinesterase inhibitor therapy (63). If these findings are generalizable, they are disturbing on at least two counts. First, primary care physicians may not be doing a very good job of eliminating drugs with anticholinergic effects in patients with Alzheimer's disease. Second, many patients may not be receiving an effective dose of a cholinesterase inhibitor despite being on one of the drugs for well over 2 years. For now, the consensus of expert opinion seems to be that Alzheimer's disease is fatal and that important benefits can be achieved for individual patients and their caregivers by prescribing a cholinesterase inhibitor (69).

Is one cholinesterase inhibitor preferred over another? A number of head-to-head comparisons of cholinesterase inhibitors have been reported, (54,64–68) but these studies are technically difficult because of the different dosing regimens for each of the cholinesterase inhibitors. In addition, most were sponsored by one or another of the manufacturers. At this point, it appears that all three of the cholinesterase inhibitors are efficacious, that donepezil had the advantage of once-a-day dosing (but now galantamine also is supplied in a once-daily extended-release form and there is a rivastigmine patch), and that rivastigmine capsules may have more gastrointestinal side effects (69). For now, the consensus of expert opinion seems to be that the primary care physician should select a cholinesterase inhibitor that seems to fit the person's and caregiver's daily routine the best and titrate to the effective dose as recommended by the manufacturer (69).

When should memantine be used, and should it be added to a cholinesterase inhibitor? Memantine is an important addition to current treatment because it may offer some neuroprotection by partially blocking the excitotoxicity of glutamate (32,70). Symptomatic improvement has been observed in patients with moderate-to-severe Alzheimer's disease and in patients with vascular dementia (69). However, there is insufficient evidence to guide physicians about the best way to use memantine. Further studies are needed and are in progress (69).

How long should pharmacotherapy for Alzheimer's disease be continued? Guidelines are silent about the length of treatment that is optimal, but a Canadian study found that the average time on a cholinesterase inhibitor is well over 2 years (63). For now, the duration of therapy remains a case-by-case, shared decision between the primary care physician and the person with dementia or his/her decision maker.

What are the consequences of discontinuing pharmacotherapy for Alzheimer's disease? Guidelines are likewise silent about when to discontinue cholinesterase inhibitors. One cross-sectional study of outpatients with Alzheimer's disease found that termination of therapy with any cholinesterase inhibitor was associated with a subsequent cognitive decline over 6 to 7 weeks (71). In a study that examined outcomes from three clinical trials involving patients with Alzheimer's disease who prematurely discontinued treatment with placebo or rivastigmine, researchers found that dropouts from rivastigmine-treated groups exhibited less deterioration in cognitive function than dropouts from the placebo-treated groups, suggesting that discontinuation is not necessarily associated with rapid decline (72). For now, discontinuing a cholinesterase inhibitor should be a shared decision between the primary care physician and the person with dementia or his/her decision maker. In practice, by the time the discussion to consider discontinuation comes up, the patient's condition already has deteriorated markedly.

Drugs for depression
Both depressive symptoms and MDD are common among patients with Alzheimer's disease (30,32,38–40). Individual counseling and support groups for the patient and the caregiver may be helpful (45). If medication is needed, a selective serotonin reuptake inhibitor (SSRI) with low anticholinergic effect is a good choice (45,73,74). If the patient is on multiple medications, choosing an SSRI with the fewest drug-drug interactions, given the patient's medication list, is important as well (74).

Drugs for behavioral disturbance
Behavioral symptoms associated with Alzheimer's disease have a substantial negative effect on quality of life of patients and their caregivers (30,32,75). When behavioral problems arise, the caregiver should try to determine if there are triggers for the behaviors and eliminate or modify the triggers if possible. The AAN guideline lists nine strategies to reduce behavioral disturbances, but only the first two have good evidence to support their use: (*i*) music, especially during meals and bathing; (*ii*) walking and other forms of light exercise; (*iii*) simulated presence therapy, e.g., videotapes of family; (*iv*) massage; (*v*) comprehensive psychosocial care programs; (*vi*) pet therapy; (*vii*) commands delivered at the patient's level of comprehension; (*viii*) bright light and white noise; and (*ix*) cognitive remediation (30). Tips for the caregiver from the Alzheimer's Association for managing behavioral disturbances when they do occur include remaining calm and reassuring, being patient and flexible, not arguing or trying to convince the person, acknowledging requests and responding to them, trying not to take behaviors personally, and accepting the behavior as a reality of the disease and trying to work through it (76). When behavioral and environmental approaches do not reduce these disturbances, treatment with cholinesterase inhibitors, alone or in combination with memantine as appropriate for the stage of disease, may be considered as a first-line option in the early pharmacologic management of Alzheimer's disease-related behavioral symptoms (2,76). The use of atypical antipsychotics in patients with behavioral symptoms related to Alzheimer's disease is controversial (2,77). Atypical antipsychotics have been used extensively for treating psychotic symptoms and agitation in the elderly, but have potential complications related to sedation, metabolic disturbances, and anticholinergic effects (77). The Clinical Antipsychotic Trials of Intervention Effectiveness-Alzheimer's Disease (CATIE-AD) found that although these drugs have some efficacy, their adverse effects limit their use in this population (78). The FDA's "black box warning" further complicates the situation (32). Antidepressants, anxiolytics, mood stabilizers, and other classes of drugs have been used as well and a discussion of these agents can be found in chapter 4.

Key decision points
The three situations that can be particularly difficult for the primary care physician when working with the patient with dementia and his/her family are driving, living arrangements, and end-of-life issues. Each of these situations may require

a great deal of time, but anticipating them and addressing them prior to an urgent or crisis situation can be beneficial for the patient, caregiver, and physician.

Driving

Driving is a complex skill that requires sound judgment and the ability to assess a situation quickly and, at times, make a series of rapid responses to changes in road conditions or traffic patterns. The Alzheimer's Association offers the following warning signs of unsafe driving (79):

- Forgetting how to locate familiar places
- Failing to observe traffic signals
- Making slow or poor decisions
- Driving at inappropriate speeds
- Becoming angry and confused while driving
- Hitting curbs
- Poor lane control
- Confusing the brake and gas pedals
- Returning from a routine drive later than usual—the person may be wandering and getting lost driving

A diagnosis of Alzheimer's disease alone does not mean that a person should stop driving, but it is often difficult to determine when the person's cognitive impairment reaches the point that he/she should no longer drive. Office-based cognitive tests recommended in various guidelines do not have validated cutoff scores and are, therefore, not very useful (80). Clinical judgment or testing by the Department of Motor Vehicles (or the equivalent state agency) is generally used to determine the fitness to drive. Primary care physicians who attend patients with Alzheimer's disease should be familiar with their state's rules, regulations, and reporting mechanisms concerning potentially impaired drivers. Once it has been determined that the person with Alzheimer's disease can no longer drive safely, the Alzheimer's Association suggests that the physician write the person a "do not drive" prescription and that the family or caregiver use some of the following approaches to address driving (79):

- Control access to the car keys
- Disable the car by removing the distributor cap or battery
- Park the car on another block or in a neighbor's driveway
- Have the person tested by the Department of Motor Vehicles
- Arrange for another mode of transportation
- Substitute the person's driver's license with a photo identification card in addition to making the car inaccessible

Living arrangements

Most elderly people, including those with Alzheimer's disease, want to live in their own homes. As Alzheimer's disease progresses, home safety and wandering can become areas of concern for the caregiver and the primary care physician. Just as for driving, determining where along the continuum of cognitive decline that a person can no longer live alone or be left alone is difficult and requires open and frank discussions in the office. Sometimes, a referral to a geriatrician, neurologist, psychiatrist, or neuropsychologist or a referral to a center that specializes in dementia is the best way to gauge the person's need for supervision. The Alzheimer's Association provides some useful safety tips about protecting the person with Alzheimer's disease from potentially dangerous situations (81):

- Lock or disguise hazardous areas by covering doors and locks with a painted mural or cloth and using swinging or folding doors to hide entrances to the kitchen, stairwell, or garage.
- Install locks out of sight. Place deadbolts either high or low on exterior doors to make it difficult for the person to wander out of the house.
- Remove locks in bathrooms or bedrooms so the person cannot get locked inside.
- Use child-proof locks and door knob covers to limit access to places where knives, appliances, and poisonous cleaning fluids are stored.
- Use appliances that have an auto shut-off feature. Some brands of irons, toaster ovens, and coffee makers have this feature.

Likewise, tips to reduce wandering behavior may also be helpful (82):

- Encourage movement and exercise to reduce anxiety, agitation, and restlessness.
- Ensure all basic needs are met (toileting, nutrition, thirst).
- Involve the person in daily activities, such as folding laundry or preparing dinner.
- Place color-matching cloth over doorknobs to camouflage.
- Redirect pacing or restless behavior.
- Place a mirror near doorways. The reflection of a person's own face will often stop him or her from exiting the door.
- Reassure the person if he/she feels lost, abandoned, or disoriented.

Tips to protect the person who may wander and get lost are also provided at the Alzheimer's Association website (82):

- Consider enrolling the person in *Safe Return*, the nationwide Alzheimer's Association ID program assisting in the safe return of individuals who wander and become lost.
- Inform neighbors and local emergency responders of the person's condition and keep a list of their names and telephone numbers.
- Keep the home safe and secure by installing deadbolt or slide-bolt locks on exterior doors and limiting access to potentially dangerous areas.
- Never lock the person with dementia in a home without supervision.
- Be aware that the person may not only wander by foot but also by car or by other modes of transportation.

The *Safe Return* is a nationwide identification and support program that is administered by the Alzheimer's Association and provides assistance if a person with Alzheimer's disease wanders and becomes lost. The enrollment fee is reasonable, and assistance is available 24 hours a day, 365 days a year. If an enrollee is missing, one call immediately activates a community support network to help find the lost person.

End-of-life issues

Soon after the diagnosis is made, the physician should open a discussion about advance care directives to ascertain from the patient what interventions he/she wants and does not want as the disease progresses. This discussion should take place early in the course of the disease, thus allowing direct input from the patient. In order to have an informed discussion, however, some estimate of life expectancy is helpful. Life expectancy following the diagnosis of Alzheimer's disease is important not only for meaningful dialog among patients, their families and caregivers, and clinicians, but also for health planners and policy makers (83,84). A study of participants in the Baltimore Longitudinal Study of Aging found that median survival time ranged from 8.3 years for persons diagnosed with Alzheimer's disease at age 65 to 3.4 years for persons diagnosed at age 90 with no significant differences in survival noted between men and women (83). Having a diagnosis of Alzheimer's disease reduced median survival by 67% for 65-year olds and 39% for 90-year olds (83). A prospective observational study using an Alzheimer's disease registry from a base population of 23,000 community-dwelling elders aged 60 and older in the Seattle area reported a median survival of 4.2 years for men and 5.7 years for women following the diagnosis of Alzheimer's disease (84). Features associated with reduced survival at diagnosis were increased severity of cognitive impairment, decreased functional level, history of falls, the presence of frontal release signs, and abnormal gait (84). Both of these studies report a longer mean survival than findings of 3.3 years reported in a 2001 New England Journal of Medicine article (85) and emphasize the importance of age and severity of symptoms at the time of diagnosis.

The message from the Baltimore and Seattle studies for patients and their families is that the median survival may be as long as 7 to 10 years for patients who are diagnosed in their 60s and early 70s (83,84). Given such a prediction, the treatment recommendations outlined above should be discussed in detail with the patient and the family and a care plan outlined taking the person's advance care directive into account. The care plan should be reviewed and revised periodically with the frequency of review and revision determined in a shared way between the primary care physician and the patient and caregiver. In addition, the care plan should also be reviewed and possibly revised whenever there is a change in the patient's condition. A change in condition for a person with Alzheimer's disease may be manifested by a decline in physical function, cognition, or change in mood or behavior. When such a change occurs, it may be helpful for the primary care physician and the caregiver to use the mnemonic shown in Table 3 to work through potential causes of the change in the person's condition. KISSES is easy to remember and provides a systematic approach that can allow the caregiver to provide useful information to the physician and can give the physician and the caregiver a mechanism for reviewing and revising the care plan.

At some point in the course of Alzheimer's disease, the patient's condition will decline to the point that the caregiver and other people who are important in the person's life conclude that treatment targeted at Alzheimer's disease is no longer warranted. Ideally, discussions about this eventuality should have been discussed all along, and the care plan should have focused on function and quality of life as well as disease-driven processes of care. New goals of care should be set and a new care plan established. Depending on the patient's medication list, most of them can either be stopped right away or tapered and stopped. The plan

Table 3 KISSES Mnemonic

Whenever a patient with Alzheimer's disease has a change in mood, behavior, or functional status or a further decline in cognition, he/she should be showered with KISSES.

K. What are the **K**nown medical and neuropsychiatric conditions and are they stable or optimally treated?

I. Is there evidence of an **I**nfection or some other new medical or neuropsychiatric condition?

S. Is there a potential medication **S**ide effect?

S. Is there **S**omething to suggest that the person is having pain?

E. Is there **E**nvironmental chaos?

S. Is there **S**ocial upheaval?

---

and rationale for removing medications should be clear to the caregiver. Patients with Alzheimer's disease, especially near the end of life, and their caregivers and family can benefit from hospice care (86).

SUMMARY

The recognition, assessment, and management of Alzheimer's disease necessarily will become the purview of the primary care physician because of the dramatic aging of the U.S. population and the prevalence of Alzheimer's disease among the elderly. Knowledge about risk factors, warning signs, and triggers will help the primary care physician recognize that an elderly person may have the disease. An accurate history and physical examination along with blood tests, a test to measure cognition, a screen for depression, and a brain imaging study along with application of DSM-IV-TR criteria often will establish the diagnosis. Eliminating or reducing the number of drugs with anticholinergic activity is crucial. Treatment with a cholinesterase inhibitor with the addition of memantine at the appropriate time is indicated as is treatment of depression. Care for the caregiver in the form of information about available resources is a fundamental part of the care plan, which needs to be crafted in a shared manner and reviewed and revised as needed. Hospice can be useful for the patient with Alzheimer's disease as well as the patient's caregiver and family and friends when the disease enters its final stages.

REFERENCES

1. Lawhorne L. Care of the older adult in the office setting. Prim Care Clin Office Pract 2005; 32:11–14.
2. Lawhorne L, Ogle KS. Approaches to the office care of the older adult and the specter of dementia. Prim Care Clin Office Pract 2005; 32:599–618.
3. Hebert LE, Scherr PA, Bienias JL, et al. Alzheimer disease in the US Population. Arch Neurol 2003; 60:1119–1122.
4. Brookmeyer R, Gray S, Kawas C. Projections of Alzheimer's disease in the United States and the public health impact of delaying disease onset. Am J Public Health 1998; 88(9):1337–1342.
5. Federal interagency forum on aging-related statistics. Older Americans update 2006: key indicators of well-being. Federal Interagency Forum on Aging-Related Statistics. Washington, DC: U.S. Government Printing Office, 2006.
6. Ross GW, Abbott RD, Petrovitch H, et al. Frequency and characteristics of silent dementia among elderly Japanese-American men: The Honolulu study. JAMA 1997; 277:800–805.

7. Cranney M, Warren E, Barton S, et al. Why do GPs not implement evidence-based guidelines? A descriptive study. Family Practice 2001; 18(4):359–363.
8. Boise L, Neal M, Kaye J. Dementia assessment in primary care: Results from a study in three managed care systems. J Gerontol A Biol Sci Med Sci 2004; 59A(6):621–626.
9. Turner S, Iliffe S, Downs M, et al. General practitioners' knowledge, confidence and attitudes in the diagnosis and management of dementia. Age Ageing 2004; 33(5):461–467.
10. Dwolatzky T, Clarfield AM. Assessment of dementia in the primary care setting. Expert Rev Neurother 2004; 4(2):317–325.
11. Boyd CM, Darer J, Boult C, et al. Clinical practice guidelines and quality of care for older patients with multiple comorbid diseases: Implications for pay for performance. JAMA 2005; 294(6):716–724.
12. Tinetti ME, Bogardus ST, Agostini JV. Potential pitfalls of disease-specific guidelines for patients with multiple conditions. N Engl J Med 2004; 351(27):2870–2874.
13. White KL, Williams TF, Greenberg BG. The ecology of medical care. N Engl J Med 1961; 265:885–892.
14. Green LA, Yawn BP, Lanier D, et al. The ecology of medical care revisited. N Engl J Med, 2001; 344(26):2021–2025.
15. Nutting PA, Beasley JW, Werner JJ. Practice-based research networks answer primary care questions. JAMA 1999; 281:686–688.
16. Thomas P, Griffiths F, Kai J, et al. Networks for research in primary health care. BMJ 2001; 322:588–590.
17. Folstein M, Folstein SE, McHugh PR. "Mini-Mental State" a practical method for grading the cognitive state of patients for the clinician. J Psych Res 1975; 12(3):189–198.
18. Borson S, Scanlan JM, Chen P, et al. The mini-cog as a screen for dementia: Validation in a population-based sample. JAGS 2003; 51:1451–1454.
19. Scharre DW, Chang SI, Murden RA, et al. Self-administered Gerocognitive Examination (SAGE): A brief cognitive assessment instrument for Mild Cognitive Impairment (MCI) and early dementia. Alzheimer Dis Assoc Disord 2010; 24:64–71.
20. http://www.ahrq.gov/clinic/uspstf/uspsdeme.htm#summary. Accessed October 16, 2006.
21. Down M, Turner S, Bryans M, et al. Effectiveness of educational interventions in improving detection and management of dementia in primary care: Cluster randomized controlled study. BMJ 2006; 332(7543):692–696.
22. Holzer C, Warshaw G. Clues to early Alzheimer dementia in the outpatient setting. Arch Fam Med 2000; 9:1066–1070.
23. http://www.alz.org/Resources/FactSheets/FSADFacts.pdf. Accessed September 26, 2007.
24. Lindsay J. Laurin D, Verreault R, et al. Risk factors for Alzheimer's disease: A prospective analysis from the Canadian study of health and aging. Am J Epidemiol 2002; 156:444–453.
25. Carr DB, Goate A, Phil D, et al. Current concepts in the pathogenesis of Alzheimer's disease. Am J Med 1997; 103(suppl 3A):3S–10S.
26. http://www.alz.org/alzheimers_disease_symptoms_of_alzheimers.asp. Accessed November 1, 2007.
27. Barberger-Gateau P, Commenges D, Gagnon M, et al. Instrumental activities of daily living as a screening tool for cognitive impairment and dementia in elderly community dwellers. JAGS 1992; 40(11):1129–1134.
28. Hill J, Fillit H, Thomas SK, et al. Functional impairment, healthcare costs and the prevalence of institutionalization in patients with Alzheimer's disease and other dementias. Pharmacoeconomics 2006; 24(3):268–280.
29. Solomon PR, Hirschoff A, Kelly B, et al. A 7 minute neurocognitive screening battery highly sensitive to Alzheimer's disease. Arch Neurol 1998; 55:349–355.
30. Knopman DS, DeKosky ST, Cummings JL, et al. Practice parameter: Diagnosis of dementia (an evidence-based review): Report of the quality standards subcommittee of the American Academy of Neurology. Neurology 2001; 56(9):1143–1153.

31. www.guideline.gov. Accessed September 9, 2009.
32. Lyketsos CG, Colenda CC, Beck C, et al. Position statement of the American Association for Geriatric Psychiatry regarding principles of care for patients with dementia resulting from Alzheimer Disease. Am J Geriatr Psychiatry 2006; 14:7.
33. Diagnostic and Statistical Manual of Mental Disorders. 4th ed. with Text Revision. Washington, DC: American Psychiatric Association, 2003.
34. Mulsant BH, Pollock BG, Kirshner M, et al. Serum anticholinergic activity in a community-based sample of older adults: Relationship with cognitive performance. Arch Gen Psychiatry 2003; 60:198–203.
35. Ancelin ML, Artero S, Portet F, et al. Non-degenerative mild cognitive impairment in elderly people and use of anticholinergic drugs: Longitudinal cohort study. BMJ 2006; 332:455–459.
36. Mintzer J, Burns A. Anticholinergic side-effects of drugs in elderly people. J R Soc Med 2000; 93:457–462.
37. Fick DM, Cooper JW, Wade WE, et al. Updating the Beers criteria for potentially inappropriate medication use in older adults: Results of a US consensus panel of experts. Arch Intern Med 2003; 163:2716–2724.
38. Solfrizzi V, D'Introno A, Colacicco AM, et. al. Incident occurrence of depressive symptoms among patients with mild cognitive impairment–the Italian longitudinal study on aging. Dement Geriatr Cogn Disord 2007; 24(1):55–64.
39. Ganguli M, Du Y, Dodge HH, Ratcliff GG, Chang CC. Depressive symptoms and cognitive decline in late life: A prospective epidemiological study. Arch Gen Psychiatry 2006; 63(2):153–160.
40. Lyketsos CG, Lee HB. Depression and treatment of depression in Alzheimer's disease: A practical update for the clinician. Dement Geriatr Cogn Disord 2004; 17:55–64.
41. Geenberg SA. How to try this: The geriatric depression scale: Short form. Am J Nurs 2007; 107(10):60–69.
42. Kroeneke K, Spitzer RL, Williams JB. The patient health questionnaire-2: Validity of a two-item depression screener. Med Care 2003; 41(11):1284–1292.
43. Langa KM, Foster NL, Larson EB. Mixed dementia: Emerging concepts and therapeutic implications. JAMA 2004; 292(23):2901–2908.
44. Holmes SB, Adler D. Dementia care: Critical interactions among primary care physicians, patients, and caregivers. Prim Care Clin Office Pract 2005; 32:671–682.
45. Lawhorne L. Depression in the older adult. Prim Care Clin Office Pract 2005; 32:777–792
46. http://www.alz.org. Accessed September 9, 2009.
47. http://www.aoa.gov/AoARoot/AoA_Programs/OAA/Aging_Network/Index.aspx. Accessed 6/9/2009.
48. http://www.caregiver.org. Accessed September 9, 2009.
49. Farlow MR, Small GW, Quarg P, et al. Efficacy of rivastigmine in Alzheimer's disease patients with rapid disease progression: Results of a meta-analysis. Dement Geriatr Cogn Disord 2005; 20:192–197.
50. Kaduszkiewicz H, Zimmerman T, Beck-Bornholdt HP, et al. Cholinesterase inhibitors for patients with Alzheimer's disease: Systematic review of randomized clinical trials. BMJ 2005; 331:321–327.
51. Lingler JH, Martire LM, Schulz R. Caregiver-specific outcomes in antidementia clinical drug trials: A systematic review and meta-analysis. J Am Geriatr Soc 2005; 53:983–990.
52. Gauthier S, Wirth Y, Mobius HJ. Effects of memantine on behavioural symptoms in Alzheimer's disease patients: Analysis of the Neuropsychiatry Inventory (NPI) data of two randomized, controlled studies. Int J Geriatr Psychiatry 2005; 20:459–464.
53. Passmore AP, Bayer AJ, Steinhagen-Thiessen E. Cognitive, global, and functional benefits of donepezil in Alzheimer's disease and vascular dementia: Results from large scale clinical trials. J Neurol Sci 2005; 229–230:141–146.
54. Harry Rd, Zakzanis KK. A comparison of Donepezil and galantamine in the treatment of cognitive symptoms of Alzheimer's disease: A meta-analysis. Hum Psychopharmacol 2005; 20:183–187.

55. Ritchie CW, Ames D, Clayton T, et al. Metaanlaysis of randomized trials of the efficacy and safety of donepezil, galantamine, and rivastigmine for the treatment of Alzheimer's disease. Am J Geriatr Psychiatry 2004; 12:358–369.
56. Whitehead A, Perdomo C, Pratt RD, et al. Donepezil for the symptomatic treatment of patients with mild to moderate Alzheimer's disease: A meta-analysis of individual patient data from randomized controlled trials. Int J Geriatr Psychiatry 2004; 19:624–633.
57. Lanctot KL, Herrmann N, Yau KK, et al. Efficacy and safety of cholinesterase inhibitors in Alzheimer's disease: A meta-analysis. Can Med Assoc J 200;169:557–564.
58. Trinh NH, Hoblyn J, Mohanty S, et al. Efficacy of cholinesterase inhibitors in the treatment of neuropsychiatric symptoms and functional impairment in Alzheimer's disease: A meta-analysis. JAMA 2003; 289:210–216.
59. Birks J, Harvey RJ. Donepezil for dementia due to Alzheimer's disease. Cochrane Database Syst Rev 2006; 1:CD001190.
60. Loy C, Schneider L. Galantamine for Alzheimer's disease and mild cognitive impairment. Cochrane Database Syst Rev 2006; 1:CD001747.
61. Birks J, Grimley EJ, Iakovidou V, et al. Rivastigmine for Alzheimer's disease. Cochrane Database Syst Rev 2006; 1:CD001191.
62. Takeda A, Loveman E, Clegg A, et al. A systematic review of the clinical effectiveness of donepezil, rivastigmine and galantamine on cognition, quality of life and adverse events in Alzheimer's disease. Int J Geriatr Psychiatry 2006; 21:17–28.
63. Herrmann N, Gill S, Bell C, et al. A population-based study of cholinesterase inhibitor use for dementia. J Am Geriatr Soc 2007; 55(10):1517–1523.
64. Jones RW, Soininen H, Hager K, et al. A multinational, randomized 12-week study comparing the effects of donepezil and galantamine in patients with mild to moderate Alzheimer's disease. Int J Geriatr Psychiatry 2004; 19:58–67.
65. Wilcock G, Howe I, Coles H, et al. A long term comparison of galantamine and donepezil in the treatment of Alzheimer's disease. Drugs Aging 2003; 20:771–789.
66. Hogan DB, Goldlist B, Naglie G, et al. Comparison studies of cholinesterase inhibitors for Alzheimer's disease. Lancet Neurol 2004; 3:622–626.
67. Wilkinson DG, Passmore AP, Bullock R, et al. A multinational, randozmied, 12-week comparative study of donepezil and rivastigmine in patients with mild to moderate Alzheimer's disease. Int J Clin Pract 2002; 56:441–446.
68. Bullock R, Touchon J, Bergman H, et al. Rivastigmine and donepezil treatment in moderate to moderately-severe Alzheimer's disease over a 2-year period. Curr Med Res Opin 2005; 21:1317–1327.
69. Ritchie CW, Ames D, Masters CL, et al (eds.). Therapeutic Strategies in Dementia. Oxford, UK: Clinical Publishing, 2007.
70. Parsons CG, Stöffler A, Danysz W. Memantine: A NMDA receptor antagonist that improves memory by restoration of homeostasis in the glutamatergic system—too little activation is bad, too much is even worse. Neuropharmacology 2007; 53(6):699–723.
71. Rainer M, Mucke HA, Kruger-Rainer C, et al. Cognitive relapse after discontinuation of drug therapy in Alzheimer's disease: Cholinesterase inhibitors versus nootropics. J Neural Transm 2001; 108(11):1327–1333.
72. Farlow M, Potkin S, Koumaras B, et al. Analysis of outcome in retrieved dropout patients in a rivastigmine vs placebo, 26-week, Alzheimer disease trial. Arch Neurol 2003; 60(6):843–848.
73. Alexopoulos GS, Katz IR, Reynolds CF 3rd, et al. The expert consensus guideline series. Pharmacotherapy of depressive disorders in older patients. Postgrad Med 2001; (Spec Report):1–86.
74. Lebert F. Serotonin reuptake inhibitors in depression of Alzheimer's disease and other dementias. Presse Med 2003; 32(25):1181–1186.
75. Beier MT. Treatment strategies for the behavioral symptoms of Alzheimer's disease: Focus on early pharmacologic intervention. Pharmacotherapy 2007; 27(3):399–411.

76. http://www.alz.org/professionals_and_researchers_behaviors_pr.asp. Accessed November 1, 2007.
77. Beier MT. Pharmacotherapy for behavioral and psychological symptoms of dementia in the elderly. Am J Health Syst Pharm 2007; 64(2 suppl 1):S9–S17.
78. Schneider LS, Tariot PN, Dagerman KS, et al. Effectiveness of atypical antipsychotic drugs in patients with Alzheimer's disease. N Engl J Med 2006; 355(15):1525–1538.
79. http://www.alz.org/living_with_alzheimers_driving.asp. Accessed November 1, 2007.
80. Molnar FJ, Patel A, Marshall SC, et al. Clinical utility of office-based cognitive predictors of fitness to drive in persons with dementia: A systematic review. JAGS 2006; 54(12):1809–1824.
81. http://www.alz.org/living_with_alzheimers_home_safety.asp. Accessed November 1, 2007.
82. http://www.alz.org/living_with_alzheimers_wandering.asp. Accessed November 1, 2007.
83. Brookmeyer R, Corrada MM, Curriero FC, et al. Survival following a diagnosis of Alzheimer's disease. Arch Neurol 2002; 59:1764–1967.
84. Larson EB, Shadlen MW, Wang L, et al. Survival after initial diagnosis of Alzheimer disease. Ann Intern Med 2004; 140:501–509.
85. Wolfson C, Wolfson DB, Asgharian M, et al. A reevaluation of the duration of survival after the onset of dementia. N Engl J Med 2001; 344:1111–1116.
86. Ogle KS, Hopper K. End-of-life care for older adults. Prim Care Clin Office Pract 2005; 32:811–828.

9 Ethical issues in dementia

Caroline N. Harada and Greg A. Sachs

INTRODUCTION

Ethical dilemmas arise frequently in the course of caring for a person with dementia. Some of these issues are specific to dementia, while others are general issues in medical ethics that become more complex when a patient has dementia. We will begin with a discussion of ethical issues at the time of diagnosis, followed by a summary of issues that arise during the course of the disease, and then an overview of those that occur at the end of life. We will conclude with a discussion of selected ethical issues pertinent to dementia that operate at the societal level.

DIAGNOSIS

Three areas with potential for ethical questions related to the diagnosis of dementia will be discussed here: diagnostic disclosure, genetic testing, and mild cognitive impairment (MCI).

Diagnostic Disclosure

Many challenging ethical issues can arise at the time a person is diagnosed with dementia. In particular, there can be conflict with regard to who is informed about a new diagnosis of dementia and how this is done. Three diagnostic disclosure issues will be discussed here: disclosing a diagnosis of dementia to patients, disclosing a diagnosis to a patient's family, and the process of disclosure itself.

Disclosure to patients

Families may request that the diagnosis of dementia be withheld from the patient. This raises a difficult question: does the clinician have an ethical obligation to tell the patient his/her diagnosis? We will address this question by outlining the arguments for and against disclosure, reviewing data on attitudes toward diagnostic disclosure, and presenting data describing current practices.

There are both theoretical and practical reasons to support diagnostic disclosure. Some argue that implicit in the clinician–patient contract is the obligation of the clinician to disclose all medical diagnoses. To withhold a diagnosis would be a breach of patient trust. In addition, some argue that in order for patients to be fully autonomous, they must be fully informed of their health status, and that withholding a diagnosis of dementia is, in effect, denying patient autonomy (1). On a more practical note, diagnostic disclosure can be emotionally helpful for persons with dementia: those who retain insight may be relieved to have an explanation for their symptoms, or to have confirmation of a diagnosis they already suspect (2). Knowledge of the diagnosis also provides an opportunity to express emotions and address unresolved relationship issues before patients are unable to do so due to disease progression. Awareness of dementia allows patients to plan for the future, settle their affairs, make specific and appropriate advance directives, seek a second opinion, and consent to participate in research. In cases where insight is preserved, knowledge of the diagnosis also may encourage people to understand their limitations and accept assistance when necessary.

Theoretical arguments against disclosure are based on the concept that disclosure should not take place if it may be harmful to a person with dementia. Some argue that this therapeutic privilege even gives clinicians the responsibility to withhold a diagnosis of dementia, if necessary, to protect patients. Receiving a diagnosis of dementia can cause shock, anxiety, increased confusion, depression, and sometimes even suicidal ideation (2). Unfortunately, studies of the impact of learning a diagnosis of dementia are difficult to interpret as it is usually unclear whether a given emotional response is due to learning the diagnosis or a symptom of the dementia itself (3). As treatment options are limited, disclosing a diagnosis of dementia exposes a person to distress without the offer of cure or impressive reduction of symptoms. Most agree that when a patient does not want to be told of a diagnosis of dementia, his/her wishes should be respected. When a person with advanced dementia cannot understand the diagnosis, and therefore would be unable to benefit from the knowledge, it also is generally agreed that disclosure is no longer warranted (1,4).

After becoming familiar with the theoretical arguments on either side of the debate, one might turn to empirical evidence of the attitudes of the patients and caregivers themselves with regard to receiving a diagnosis of dementia. Unfortunately, this does not provide an easy answer to the question either. There is great variability in survey results of patient and caregiver preferences: 33% to 96% of patients and 17% to 100% of caregivers favor diagnostic disclosure (3). The majority of these studies included only cognitively intact subjects, asking them to speculate about their future preferences in the event of developing dementia. One study that did include patients with dementia found that 21 out of 30 patients with dementia wanted to know what was wrong with them (2). In some studies, there is evidence of a kind of double standard when it comes to disclosure: one study found that 80% of family members said they would want to be told of their diagnosis, whereas only 66% said they would want their family member with dementia to be made aware of the diagnosis (5). In another study, 83% of family members said that if they had dementia, they would want to be told their diagnosis, whereas only 17% wanted their family member with dementia to be made aware of the diagnosis (6).

In actual practice, diagnostic disclosure to patients occurs only about 50% of the time according to physician self-reports, although it seems that geriatricians and geriatric psychiatrists are more likely to disclose than physicians in other specialties (4). Clinicians find it difficult and time consuming to disclose the diagnosis of dementia (3). Caregivers are more often told of a diagnosis than patients themselves. For example, one study reports that 93% of caregivers had been told of the diagnosis, compared to only 49% of patients (7). Clinicians appear to disclose a diagnosis of dementia more often when dementia is less severe (4). Belief in the advantages of early diagnosis also affects disclosure rates: clinicians who believe that it is better to diagnose dementia early tend to tell patients the diagnosis more frequently (3).

Therefore, while there are arguments on each side of the debate, full disclosure is supported by studies of patient preferences, as well as by clinical guidelines (such as those from the Alzheimer's Association) (8). Actual practice seems to lag behind, however, and routine disclosure to patients is not yet a standard practice for many clinicians.

Disclosure to family members

Occasionally, a patient with mild dementia asks that this diagnosis be withheld from family members. This is an area less commonly discussed in the literature than the issue of disclosure to patients. Patients may be motivated by a desire to protect family members from anxiety or depression caused by knowing the diagnosis and what the future might hold, or they may also fear stigmatization, abuse, or abandonment by family members. Since clinicians are obligated to maintain patient confidentiality, the American Medical Association suggests that clinicians respect this request as long as the patient has decision-making capacity (9). On the other hand, informing family members of a person's dementia allows them to plan more realistically, and may encourage them to provide more support (both emotional and practical) to the patient. Patients who request their diagnosis be withheld from family members also delay opportunities for family members to seek genetic counseling to learn about their own risk of developing dementia. In this uncomfortable situation, patients should be encouraged to share their diagnosis with family, but as long as the patient retains the capacity to decide, clinicians should respect his/her request for confidentiality. The difficult issue of how to protect a person with dementia while maximizing his autonomy is addressed in more detail later in this chapter.

Process of disclosure

Studies of the process of diagnostic disclosure have found wide variability and significant room for improvement. Clinicians vary in their definition of disclosure: many use euphemisms such as "memory problems" or "brain aging" (4). As these terms are ambiguous, they represent a less complete form of disclosure than when more specific terms such as "dementia" or "Alzheimer's disease" (AD) are used. There is debate over whether patients and family should be told of the diagnosis together or in separate meetings (4). The way in which patients and family are told of the diagnosis has been criticized in surveys of caregivers, who were sometimes frustrated by lack of sensitivity among clinicians, insufficiencies in information provided, and clinicians who were reluctant to be precise or to explain terminology (3,7). In addition, caregivers wanted more opportunity to address emotional reactions to learning the diagnosis (3).

Conclusions

Despite the fact that diagnostic disclosure to patients is not yet routinely performed, most agree, based on both theoretical arguments and data on patient preferences, that it should be a standard practice. In cases where patients request their diagnosis be concealed from family members, their wishes should be respected as long as they are competent. There is reason to believe that the process through which clinicians disclose a diagnosis of dementia could be improved. As better biologic markers and treatments for dementia become available, early diagnosis will become more common, and it will be important for clinicians to master the technique of accurate yet compassionate disclosure.

Genetic Testing

While the complexities of genetic testing are too extensive to be discussed in detail here, there are several issues worthy of brief discussion. Early onset AD (onset prior to age 65) accounts for 2% to 5% of cases of AD, and has been linked to three determinative genes that predict disease (these are autosomal dominant genes with very high penetrance): PSEN1 (coding for the presenilin-1 protein), PSEN2 (coding for presenilin-2 protein), and APP (coding for amyloid precursor protein). Testing for these genes is available for persons with AD and for the children or siblings of persons with early onset AD and a known gene mutation. When genetic testing is performed in this context, genetic counseling should be provided by experts both before and after testing. Late onset AD, which affects a great majority of patients with AD, presents a much more complicated situation. The gene most definitively associated with late onset AD is the APOE ε4 allele; this is a predictive (rather than determinative) gene, meaning that carriers do not necessarily develop the disease, and noncarriers can still develop the disease. It is also very common: 15% of the population carry this allele. We will first discuss this test's application for asymptomatic individuals and then for those with dementia.

Because this gene marker is so inaccurate at predicting AD, it is not recommended for susceptibility testing in asymptomatic persons, even if they are family members of people susceptible with late onset AD (10). Knowledge of a strong family history of AD is likely more helpful than knowledge of APOE genotype (11). Focus groups of caregivers indicate that few are interested in undergoing susceptibility testing because of the low accuracy of the marker and the lack of therapeutic options available (10). In addition, other potential harms of pre-symptomatic testing include the potential for employment discrimination, increased insurance costs, and psychological distress. Nonetheless, knowledge of a predisposition to AD might allow an individual to make advance directives, arrange for long-term care insurance, participate in research, and, although no options are yet available, receive therapy to delay or prevent development of AD.

Although not recommended currently, there is debate over whether or not patients with known AD should be tested for APOE ε4, either to confirm the diagnosis or to allow family members to be tested. Since APOE testing is not determinative, a negative test is not helpful, although a positive test adds diagnostic confidence (12). Nonetheless, because of the low predictive accuracy of the test, the diagnosis of dementia continues to depend on clinical, not genetic, criteria. At present, APOE testing is only performed routinely for AD patients participating in research, and results are typically available only to the investigators, not to the patients or families.

The issue of using surrogates, who are often family members, to consent to genetic testing of patients with AD raises the potential for conflicts of interest, as test results could have significant personal impact for family caregivers (13).

In summary, predictive genetic testing for AD is at present available (and likely appropriately so) only for patients or family members with early onset AD, and genetic counseling should be available to all those considering testing. APOE testing is used only in the research arena, as its predictive accuracy is so low that it is not clinically useful.

Mild Cognitive Impairment

Making a diagnosis of MCI raises many of the same issues as genetic testing for AD, as MCI is a condition associated with higher than average risk of developing AD. Like APOE testing, there is much uncertainty associated with the significance of MCI. First, diagnostic criteria for MCI are not yet as useful as hoped for, partly because of confusion over nonamnestic forms of MCI and reliance on neuropsychological testing profiles instead of clinical criteria (14,15). Second, prognosis is not predictable: many people with MCI remain stable or convert back to normal cognitive function, and so a diagnosis of MCI does not necessarily predict progression to dementia (14). Third, limited treatment options are available to prevent or delay progression from MCI to AD. The largest study using donepezil for this indication found significant delay in progression of cognitive impairment over the first 12 months, but no delay was seen at the end of 36 months (16). Fourth, the diagnostic label of MCI might expose patients to the same social discrimination as is feared with genetic testing, not to mention the psychological stress of the knowledge of having an increased risk of developing dementia. Given these limitations, some have questioned the usefulness of MCI as a clinical entity. Although it is sometimes helpful to have a diagnosis that can improve communication between clinicians and patients as well as among clinicians (17), there is little yet that can be offered to MCI patients in terms of prognostic information or treatment. The empirical study of MCI is still in its formative stages, and there is even less evidence than in the area of genetic testing to guide clinicians. The concept of MCI originated in the research arena, where it is still a useful concept, but until better definitions, prognostic information, and treatment options are available, clinical application of the term may not be helpful to patients.

ONGOING CARE OF THE PERSON WITH DEMENTIA

During the course of caring for a person with dementia, multiple ethical issues may arise. These may involve the role of the caregiver, decision-making capacity and surrogate decision making, balancing respect for patient autonomy with the need to protect the patient and others, managing difficult behaviors, nursing home life, and management of nondementia illnesses.

Role of the Caregiver

Caregivers play an essential role in the life of a person with dementia. Their presence fundamentally alters the traditional clinician–patient relationship, and it often becomes necessary for clinicians to address the needs of the caregiver in the course of caring for the patient.

The traditional clinician–patient dyad is necessarily expanded to (at minimum) a triad: clinician–patient–caregiver. Because people with advancing dementia experience a decline in memory, communication skills, and decision-making capacity, caregivers should be included in most clinical interactions because they can provide information, discuss recommendations, help with decision making, and execute changes in the treatment plan. Rules for strict clinician–patient confidentiality are altered, as the presence of the caregiver is necessary in most discussions.

Clinicians also find themselves dealing with the needs of the caregivers of their patients. This is important because addressing a caregiver's burdens, both psychological and physical, can improve quality of life for the patient with dementia (18). Resources available to help caregivers range from caregiver support groups, education, and adult day care to bedside commodes and assistants to help with bathing. Failing to attend to a caregiver's needs can result in worsening caregiver stress, which can put the patient with dementia at higher risk for elder abuse and neglect (19). Clinicians should make every effort to ensure that caregivers receive adequate education, counseling, and support, as well as referrals to the appropriate social services.

Balancing the needs of the patient with dementia with those of the caregiver can be difficult. Although caring for the caregiver is important, the needs of the patient are a clinician's priority, and in some cases conflicts of interest can arise. One problem we have encountered occurs when the patient's increasing care needs make nursing home placement necessary, but the caregiver lives in the patient's home. In this situation, families with limited financial resources often have to sell the home in order to pay for the nursing home, thus forcing the caregiver to move. When the caregiver resists nursing home placement for the patient, it is not surprising that clinicians are then forced to second-guess the motivations of the caregiver. This situation is best handled by an interdisciplinary team that can mediate and try to find solutions that are satisfactory to all.

Research shows that caregivers of people with dementia are concerned about these conflicts of interest, as well as a large number of other ethical issues (20), many of which are covered in other sections of this chapter.

In summary, then, the clinician–patient–caregiver relationship presents a significant shift in traditional medical interactions, and requires clinicians to attend to caregiver needs as well as to deal with potentially complex conflict of interest situations. In addition to the physical and emotional burdens of caring for a person with dementia, caregivers themselves also struggle with many of the ethical issues discussed in this chapter.

Decision-Making Capacity

As dementia progresses, questions may arise regarding a patient's ability to make decisions. Assessment of decision-making capacity can be complex, and a determination of incapacity can have serious implications for patients and families.

Definition of terms

Assessment of capacity is distinct from determination of competence. *Competence* is a legal term, generally referring to a global inability to make personal decisions; it is determined by a judge. *Capacity*, on the other hand, is assessed by clinicians, and is task-specific, meaning that a person may have the capacity to make some decisions but not others. Decision-making capacity should be thought of as being on a sliding scale: the more important or irreversible the consequences of a decision, the higher the standard to which patients with dementia should be held (21). Another important point to recognize is that decision-making capacity is dynamic—as a patient's mental status fluctuates, so does his/her capacity to understand, store, and manipulate information. Thus, each time medical decisions are made, decision-making capacity should be re-evaluated. Most clinicians rely on a clinical "gestalt" to make these assessments; however, formal standards and recommendations for the assessment process exist and will be reviewed here.

The process of assessing decision-making capacity

In order to be able to make a medical decision competently, patients must first be given sufficient information to understand their current clinical situation, the proposed interventions (including the risks and benefits), the risks and benefits of the alternatives (including no intervention), and the recommendation of the clinician (22). After this information is conveyed to the patient, it is essential that the clinician ask the patient to rephrase, in his/her own words, what has just been said. This allows the clinician to evaluate the patient's level of understanding and ability to recall. The assessment is an iterative process: if the patient has misunderstood or failed to remember certain points, the clinician should rephrase the clinical information until he/she is satisfied that the patient has been given every opportunity to maximize his/her understanding (23). Patients should be given the best possible chance to demonstrate capacity (24). Environmental and psychosocial issues (such as time of day, stressors in the environment, depression, anxiety, or delirium) should be addressed and optimized prior to the assessment interview. Discussion with family members and more than one meeting may be required in order to give a person the fairest evaluation.

Appelbaum and Grisso have outlined a set of abilities that are widely used to guide clinicians in assessing decision-making capacity (23). First, to have decision-making capacity, patients must be able to communicate a choice and exhibit reasonable stability of that choice. Second, patients must be able to understand the relevant information. Third, patients must appreciate the implications of their situation and apply this information to themselves. Fourth, patients must be able to manipulate the information rationally, and reach conclusions that are logically consistent with the starting premises.

Several instruments have been developed to assess decision-making capacity. One example is Appelbaum and Grisso's MacArthur Competence Assessment Tool for Treatment (MacCAT-T), a structured interview tool with a standardized rating system designed around the four abilities outlined earlier (24). These instruments have not been widely adopted for general use, likely due to the time required for administration. Instead, expert opinion is relied on by many for determining decision-making capacity; unfortunately, these expert opinions may not always be consistent, as demonstrated by one study showing very poor agreement between expert evaluators (25). In a follow-up study, however, expert evaluators were trained to assess competency using specific legal standards, resulting in much improved inter-rater agreement (26). This success with a more structured interview style and use of uniform standards suggests that clinicians could be taught to assess decision-making capacity in a more consistent manner (27). Refusal to participate in the assessment of decision-making capacity does not imply that a person lacks capacity. In this situation, clinicians should investigate the reasons for refusal and schedule a follow-up interview; in emergencies, it is probably acceptable to rely on family members to use substituted judgment (23).

Surrogate decision making

If a patient is determined to lack capacity to make a given decision, a proxy decision maker must be appointed. This often is done informally, without legal proceedings. In selecting the proxy, it is very helpful if the patient designated a surrogate decision maker while he/she was still competent. If there is no designated health care power of attorney, then state law often dictates a hierarchy of people to serve as surrogate—often starting with the patient's spouse, then adult children, and so on. If there is no state law to provide guidance, then clinicians should look to the person most likely to know the patient's values and preferences. If there is no one available to act as surrogate decision maker, then petitioning the courts to appoint a guardian may be necessary. Surrogate decision making should be based on one of three standards: last competent preference, substituted judgment, or best interests. First, the patient's last competent expression of preferences should be used to guide decision making. If the patient completed an advance directive, this can be very helpful. If, as in many cases, the current clinical situation was never explicitly discussed with the patient, the surrogate should use the second standard: substituted judgment. This means that the proxy should use his/her knowledge of the patient's values and preferences to guide decision making. Unfortunately, this can be difficult to do, and there is some evidence that proxies tend to rely on their own values more than those of the patient when making decisions (24). The third standard, basing decisions on what the surrogate believes is in the best interests of the patient, is an alternative to substituted judgment. Some states use this standard in the event that substituted judgment is impossible because a patient's prior values and preferences are not known. In our clinical experience, most surrogates incorporate both elements of substituted judgment and consideration of the patient's best interests when making decisions as a proxy. This is likely the most appropriate and practical method for surrogate decision making.

Competency and guardianship

Although not routinely used, legal procedures are available for determining whether a person with dementia lacks competence (this refers to global functioning, it is not task-specific), and designating a guardian to act as surrogate decision maker. Specifics of these laws vary from state to state, but in most cases declaration of incompetence results in considerable loss of autonomy and basic rights, including the right to vote.

Autonomy Versus Beneficence

As with decision-making capacity, other abilities are lost with the progression of dementia, and task-specific assessments may need to be made to ensure a patient's safety. A difficult balancing act develops between restricting a person's autonomy due to a desire to protect the person with dementia (and others in his/her community) and allowing him/her to perform tasks that are essential to the individual's sense of personhood. Much has been written about tasks such as driving, voting, wandering, sexual activity, possession of firearms, and managing personal finances—both with regard to how to assess capacity to perform these tasks and the impact of restricting a person's participation (10,28–33). Driving, in particular, has received much attention in medical literature from the United States. Because of diminished visuospatial skills, executive function, processing speed, and memory, drivers with dementia can present a significant danger. Given these concerns, many feel that the clinician has an obligation to report unsafe drivers both for the protection of the driver and that of others in the community. Mandatory reporting of dementia to departments of motor vehicles is advocated by some. Because many people with dementia can continue to drive safely for the first few years of the disease, others argue that the issue of driving safety can create unnecessary barriers between patients and clinicians. Opponents of mandatory reporting argue that it results in compromise of confidentiality and may also deter people with dementia from seeking medical attention (34). In our experience, discussing restricting driving privileges against a patient's will has been very stressful for patients, families, and clinicians, and has damaged the clinician–patient relationship in some cases.

Voting is another area with potential for debate: a mildly demented person with capacity to vote could be unfairly deprived of his/her rights because of a diagnostic label, or, alternatively, a demented person lacking capacity to vote could be allowed to do so. Needed are uniform methods for assessing capacity to vote, programs to assist demented persons with capacity to vote, and policies to guide voting in long-term care settings (28). There are many more examples of tasks that become impossible for persons suffering from dementia, and it is an ongoing struggle to protect patients while allowing them as much autonomy as possible. One guiding principle is that, when possible, alternatives should be offered whenever privileges are restricted in order to allow patients to achieve the same goals (34).

A new twist to the autonomy versus beneficence struggle is the development of electronic surveillance systems, which, in many cases, are designed to allow a person to maintain some degree of autonomy, for example, to live alone, while also protecting him/her from harm. People with dementia can be tagged (given bracelets that signal when they have left a certain area) or tracked (fitted with devices that report their location) or even watched through cameras in the home. But many argue that these technologies deny patients privacy and freedom, treating them as criminals under house arrest (35). In addition, these technologies may result in decreased human contact for persons with dementia, the very thing some argue is needed most. Much more discussion and research is needed before these technologies come into widespread use.

Management of Difficult Behaviors

Physical restraints

The ethical implications of the use of physical restraints are important to consider. Outside of medical, psychiatric, and criminal justice settings, it is considered morally and legally unacceptable to tie someone down against their wishes. Many feel that even in medical settings, this practice also is troubling and should be minimized. There are health-related reasons to avoid the use of physical restraints in older patients. Research has shown that there is great potential for harm, both physical and psychological, including deconditioning, pressure ulcers, asphyxiation, skin trauma, intestinal obstruction, nerve compression, incontinence, nosocomial infections, premature death, increased agitation, social isolation, humiliation, and loss of dignity (36).

Although with decreased frequency than in the past, use of physical restraints persists, usually with the well-intentioned aim of protecting the demented individual from harming himself or others. In the setting of acute agitation, when a person is truly endangering himself or others, it is acceptable for restraints to be used for a short time, but medical evaluation for the cause of agitation and frequent reassessment of the need for restraints is essential.

Guidelines recommend use of the least restrictive restraint possible for the shortest amount of time possible (37). Like any medical intervention, especially one with significant risks, a patient's family should be made aware of the risks and benefits of restraints when they are applied. Some argue that informed consent should be obtained from the demented person or a proxy when restraints are applied (37,38), although this can be impractical and is rarely done.

Restraints are unethical when used for the convenience of others, as a substitute for close supervision, or as punishment for certain behaviors. They are also unethical when incompatible with the goals of care. For example, in a person who is actively dying, the goals should be to prevent suffering. Since restraints used to prevent this person from pulling out his/her feeding tube will cause suffering, they are incompatible with these goals. Instead, caregivers should reassess the need for the feeding tube (38).

Chemical restraints

Use of medications to sedate patients significantly restricts their autonomy, and thus brings up many of the same issues as physical restraints. This is not to say that all sedating medications are chemical restraints—the distinction lies in the intent with which the medication is used. If used to treat symptoms that are upsetting to the patient (e.g., frightening hallucinations) or to prevent potential harm to the patient (e.g., when a patient refuses to eat because of a belief the food is poisoned), then these drugs are therapeutic, not restraining. If, on the other hand, these medications are used to prevent a person from wandering in the nursing home or from hitting a nurse who is drawing a blood sample, they are chemical restraints.

As with physical restraints, there are significant risks associated with these medications, which are discussed in detail in chapter 4. For example, certain antipsychotics, like haloperidol, are associated with tremor and other potentially serious movement disorders (39). In addition, chemical restraints can result in decreased ability to interact with others due to sedation, thus resulting in increased social isolation, loneliness, and potentially depression. Finally, a concerning issue is the evidence that antipsychotics, both typical and atypical, may be associated with increased risk of stroke and death (40,41).

Given these risks, chemical restraints, like physical restraints, should be used only when absolutely necessary to protect a person from harm. They should be used with great caution, in the lowest possible doses, and for the shortest time possible (34). In the nursing home, these guidelines are mandated in federal regulations. Chemical restraints are never a substitute for close surveillance and their use should always prompt a medical evaluation for underlying causes of agitation (37).

Ethics and the Nursing Home

Many nursing home residents have dementia; one recent study reported that 48% of new nursing home admissions had dementia (42). Nursing home life is usually geared toward providing basic health, hygiene, and safety for a group of individuals who are highly heterogeneous in terms of cognitive and functional abilities, reasons for being in the nursing home, and educational, cultural, and religious background (43). Unfortunately, individual autonomy is difficult to maintain because of the need to maintain resident safety and health, the desire to protect the rights and preferences of other residents, and the many regulatory and financial constraints on the nursing home. Simple things taken for granted outside the nursing home, like deciding when to take a shower or how late to stay up, tend to be regulated by strict routine in the nursing home. In one interview study of nursing home residents, most residents were frustrated by the lack of control they had over everyday life matters such as roommates and use of the telephone (44). Autonomy also requires that there be opportunities and options available to a person; these are frequently absent in the nursing home (45). For example, a person with dementia may want to eat junk food, and even though there is no rule against it at the nursing home, if the resident has no way of obtaining potato chips and chocolate bars, she will not have full autonomy.

Privacy and individuality are also difficult to maintain (43). Shared rooms and limited space for entertaining visitors make it difficult to maintain a private life. Telephones are often in common spaces. Minimal storage space and concerns for theft make it difficult to keep personal effects that might remind residents and caregivers of a person's background, tastes, and identity. Because residents are often dependent on nursing home staff for activities of daily living such as bathing, there is little room for personal preference as to when or how an event occurs: bath versus shower, morning versus evening, and so on. Many of the simple things that define a person as an individual may be lost in the nursing home.

Because opportunities for autonomy, individuality, and privacy are limited, it behooves nursing home staff and administrators to respect the seemingly trivial matters that arise in nursing homes: roommate selection, meal choice, bedtimes, and so on, as these small things can make an enormous difference in a resident's quality of life (45). Allowing a resident to switch roommates or stay up late to watch a certain television show can mean significant improvement in a person's everyday experience, and may also have tremendous symbolic value in permitting autonomy and individuality.

Nondementia Illnesses

The idea that dementia occurs in people who are otherwise completely healthy is a misconception. In fact, because dementia is a chronic condition that becomes more common with advancing age, patients with dementia are likely to have coexisting medical conditions. When making decisions about preventive measures and management of comorbid conditions, the presence of dementia is both ethically and clinically relevant for many reasons.

First, because life expectancy is shortened in patients with dementia, the risks of many preventive measures and diagnostic tests may outweigh the benefits. For example, mortality benefits from yearly mammography are not apparent for the first four years, so a person who is not expected to live longer than four years would not benefit (46). The increased mortality seen in persons with dementia does not mean that they do not have a right to active medical care, however. Clinicians and family can unconsciously discriminate against persons with dementia because of their own biases and fears about living a life with cognitive impairment and, as a result, fail to provide adequate care to demented persons. For example, while a clinician may forgo mammography in a person with dementia who is expected to live only two to three more years, a flu shot may be appropriate to prevent mortality and morbidity in the coming months.

Because of the complexities of many of these decisions, and concerns for both over-treatment and under-treatment, it is essential to establish clear goals of care with the patient and family (47). This can be done by discussing realistic goals for patients with dementia, and then deciding which are appropriate for a specific individual (48).

A second reason that dementia is relevant in the management of comorbid conditions is the fact that the cognitive symptoms of dementia can make many aspects of care difficult. Patients may not be able to report or describe symptoms, thus creating challenges for diagnosis of disease and detection of adverse effects of therapy (49). Patients may not understand the purpose of a given test, and in these circumstances even a seemingly innocuous test like an x-ray may be extremely stressful or frightening (50). When considering cancer screening tests, many patients report that the greatest benefit from a negative screening test is the reassurance it offers—patients with dementia who do not understand the purpose of the testing will not benefit in this way.

When patients lack decision-making capacity, decisions that were once simply a matter of eliciting the patient's preference become more complex. These decisions, unlike those about end of life, do not tend to be ones that patients have discussed in the past with family members (46). Adherence to therapy can also be a problem in patients who forget or refuse treatment due to dementia.

One final point worthy of mention is that studies show that patients with dementia have poor outcomes compared to those without dementia (51). For example, one study of outcomes among patients with pneumonia reported that 53% of patients with end-stage dementia died within 6 months, compared to only 13% of patients without cognitive impairment (52). Another study showed that men with AD hospitalized for gastrointestinal bleeding, congestive heart failure, acute myocardial infarction, and hip fracture were at greater risk of death than men who were cognitively intact (53). It is not yet known exactly why this difference exists, although it is likely due to the progressive, neurodegenerative nature of dementia, in combination with a number of other factors such as multiple comorbidities, conscious decisions to forgo aggressive interventions, delays in diagnosis of comorbid diseases, higher complication rates, or nonadherence with treatment (51).

Unfortunately, there is very little evidence to guide clinical decision making with regard to comorbid disease, and each decision must be made with a clear set of goals in mind, and with full consideration of the patient's clinical state, prognosis, and the characteristics of the test or treatment. In the case of preventive measures or diagnostic tests, there should also be consideration of whether one would treat a condition if it were discovered (47). If this framework is used, we believe it is possible to successfully navigate management of the often complicated medical problems of patients with dementia.

END OF LIFE

The most striking ethical issue at the end of life is the concerning fact that people with dementia are not always offered excellent end-of-life care (54,55). We will discuss the problems associated with recognizing dementia as a terminal condition, the role of advance directives, and, finally, we will describe palliative care and some of the issues specific to palliative care for patients with dementia.

Dementia as a Terminal Condition

Although dementia is generally considered to be a terminal condition, many professionals, patients, and families do not perceive it as such (55). The fact that the proximal cause of death in many cases is infection, heart attack, or stroke makes it easy to overlook the fact that dementia is the underlying condition that ultimately results in death (34). Like many other chronic conditions, death from dementia does not usually occur soon after diagnosis; rather, patients can live for years with dementia. As a consequence, it is a challenge for many to think of dementia as a terminal disease, and so patients with dementia are sometimes deprived of the comfort-oriented care and services available to those with diseases more generally accepted as terminal, such as cancer (54,55).

The prognosis in dementia is hard to predict: patients tend to have a downward trajectory punctuated by multiple acute illnesses (e.g., infections or hip fractures) followed by subsequent partial recovery (rarely do patients return to previous levels of health). Unfortunately, it is usually difficult to predict which acute illness will result in death, so clinicians accustomed to the cancer model have difficulty preparing patients and their families for death (54). Most U.S. hospice programs require a six-month life expectancy for patient enrollment, and this can be very hard to establish in patients with dementia. The result is that a smaller proportion of patients with dementia end up using and benefiting from hospice care services compared to patients with cancer (55,56).

Advance Directives

As dementia progresses, surrogates are asked to make more and more decisions on behalf of patients. Often, the most difficult decisions arise around health care at the end of a demented person's life: decisions about feeding tubes, treatment of infections, resuscitation, and hospice care. Advance directives can help clinicians and family members make these decisions, many of which are choices between life-prolonging treatments that may increase discomfort versus comfort care that might have the potential to hasten death. In the interests of maximizing patient autonomy, discussions about end-of-life preferences ideally should be held early in the disease course, when patients still have the capacity to make decisions about their medical care. Creating advance directives that document a patient's preferences also may lessen some of the emotional burden of surrogate decision making experienced by caregivers.

Advance directives can take multiple forms. Designating a power of attorney for health care, a surrogate decision maker, is often the simplest form of advance directive for patients to perform and often the easiest for clinicians to utilize. A second form of advance directive is the living will: a document that can vary in its content but is intended to address specific wishes for end-of-life care. Unfortunately, living wills are often vague, and it is difficult to know whether or not the preferences outlined really apply to a given situation as it presents itself. A person with mild dementia cannot truly understand what life is like with severe dementia until he/she develops severe dementia, at which point decision-making capacity will have been lost. Thus, sometimes clinicians and family members are forced to balance respect for precedent autonomy with the need to provide beneficent care, which may result in an overruling of a patient's previously stated preferences (10). Some urge that this practice should not be encouraged, for if preferences as expressed in advance directives are disregarded, the entire concept of advance directives will become meaningless, and patients will be deprived of the autonomy and reassurance they can provide (10).

A third specific form of advance directive is the "do not resuscitate" (DNR) order. This can be agreed to by a competent patient at any point in their disease, but many fear that signing such a document is tantamount to signing away all rights to medical care. Patients and family members should understand that completing a DNR only means that they do not wish to undergo resuscitation attempts at the end of life, but that all other appropriate care will continue.

A fourth advance directive is the "do not hospitalize" order, sometimes used in long-term care settings. This can be completed when patients or their proxies feel that the burdens of hospitalization (transportation, frequent phlebotomy, and the unfamiliar and often uninviting physical environment) outweigh the potential benefits.

Palliative Care

Definition
Patients with advanced dementia should receive palliative care, which "aims to relieve suffering and improve the quality of life for patients with advanced illnesses" (57). Palliative care is distinct from euthanasia or physician-assisted suicide. In voluntary, active euthanasia, the clinician intentionally ends the patient's life at his/her request. In physician-assisted suicide, the patient intentionally ends his/her own life using medications prescribed by the physician. Neither of these concepts is practical for use with patients with advanced dementia as they both require decision-making capacity at the time of the event.

Palliative care is also distinct from hospice, which refers to a program of care designed for patients who are likely to die within six months of enrollment. There is little medical significance to the six-month time frame, but it has become an important benchmark for end of life because it was the cutoff established by Medicare when the federal hospice program was adopted. In hospice, patients forgo life-prolonging or curative treatment, and treatment is instead focused on maintaining comfort. Hospice is often appropriate for persons with advanced dementia, but because it is so difficult to predict death in dementia, palliative care is more helpful, as it can be administered in conjunction with curative treatment and initiated long before a six-month life expectancy is reached (54). In this model of care, both curative and palliative treatments are available to a person, but as dementia progresses, the majority of care should shift from curative to palliative therapy. This can be a very natural shift in many cases, when it becomes apparent that curative therapy is no longer effective. On the other hand, many clinicians and family members find it difficult to withhold or withdraw life-sustaining treatments. This can be made easier if clinicians and family members conduct ongoing discussions throughout the course of the disease with regard to prognosis and goals of care (48).

Specific palliative care issues in dementia
There are numerous ethical dilemmas in palliative care for dementia patients. Especially challenging issues surround management of pain, artificial nutrition and hydration, and treatment of infections

Cognitive impairment can sometimes make it difficult to recognize pain in patients with dementia. Research has shown that patients with dementia suffering from conditions generally felt to cause pain, such as hip fracture, are at greater risk of not receiving pain medications when compared to those with intact cognition (58). It is often recommended that patients with dementia who are unable to express themselves or describe their pain be treated empirically with pain medication if there is reason to suspect the patient has pain (59).

Another complicated issue in pain management arises when a clinician is uncomfortable with "the rule of double effect," in which certain therapies necessary for achieving patient comfort have the unintended effect of hastening death. Morphine, for example, is effective at treating pain, but also can have the unintended effect of suppressing respiration and lowering blood pressure. There is a general consensus that if such treatments are necessary to achieve comfort for a patient with a terminal illness, they should be administered (60).

A second challenging issue is artificial nutrition and hydration. At the end of life, patients with dementia sometimes refuse to eat, or alternatively, aspirate oral contents into their lungs due to lack of coordination of the pharyngeal muscles. In these situations, well-meaning family members and physicians sometimes think placement of a feeding tube will help. In fact, in advanced dementia, tube feeding has no real benefits, and as a medical therapy, can be withheld if the risks outweigh the benefits (61). Research has shown that tube feeding does not prevent aspiration pneumonia, prevent the consequences of malnutrition, or improve wound healing (62). Tube feeding does not, when compared to feeding patients by hand, improve survival for patients at terminal stages of dementia (61). This is likely because patients are in the final stages of life, and tube feeding is unable to change the course of the underlying disease. The final and most compelling argument against feeding tubes in palliative care is that placement of a feeding tube fails to increase patient comfort. Extrapolating from data on patients dying with cancer, it is clear that most patients who are close to death do not experience hunger, and those that do, experience it only initially (63). This maybe due to release of endorphins that create a sensation of comfort and well-being that can be lost if feeding recurs. Thirst was more common, but easily treated with small sips of liquids, ice chips, and mouth care (63). Dehydration seems to make the dying process more comfortable, for patients are less likely to choke on secretions, have gastric distension, or suffer from pulmonary or peripheral edema (10). Tube feeding, on the other hand, is associated with many complications resulting in discomfort: diarrhea; tube malfunction, leakage, or clogging; infections at the insertion site; peritonitis; and discomfort caused by the tube itself. Patients with dementia often try to pull out the tube, perhaps because of discomfort, and this sometimes prompts caregivers to use restraints (10).

Treatment of infections is another issue that can become controversial at the end of life. Although less invasive than feeding tubes, antibiotics may be ineffective in preventing death in patients with end-stage dementia (56,64). In making the decision to use antibiotics in a dying patient, the goals of care must be considered: discomfort caused by infections can be treated with morphine and antipyretics, and antibiotics may only prolong the dying process (56).

Concerns about pain management, artificial nutrition and hydration, and treatment of infections can make administering palliative care to patients with advanced dementia challenging. The key is that the goals of medical care in

advanced dementia should be focused on achievable goals, such as pallia-
tion of symptoms and avoidance of nonbeneficial therapies, rather than life
prolongation.

ETHICAL ISSUES AT THE SOCIETAL LEVEL
In discussing the ethical issues affecting people with dementia that extend beyond
the clinical encounter, two areas are important to mention. Research involving
people with dementia is an area of much debate; we will discuss issues of consent,
protecting research subjects, and industry-sponsored research. Cultural issues
also come into play when discussing ethical issues in dementia.

Research Involving People with Dementia

Capacity to consent to research, proxy consent, subject assent
Because of the nature of dementia, the process of obtaining informed consent
from subjects with dementia is more complex than in typical research endeavors.
Because of the lack of federal regulations addressing the special issues arising in
research involving this population, organizations such as the National Bioethics
Advisory Commission, the Alzheimer's Association, and the American Geriatrics
Society have published statements and specific recommendations in an effort to
ensure that this process proceeds in an ethical manner (65–68). The following is a
synthesis and summary of these recommendations.

The capacity to consent to research must be assessed, as some subjects will
still be capable of making research enrollment decisions despite the presence
of dementia (69). As with other health care decisions, a sliding scale should be
applied: the higher the risks or burdens associated with a study procedure or
medication, the higher the standard should be to determine competence (21). In
competent subjects, if there is a significant decline in cognitive abilities during
the course of a study, reassessment of the capacity to consent is recommended.
Competent subjects also should appoint a proxy decision maker at the beginning
of a study in the event that they become incapable of decision making during
the course of the study. It also is strongly recommended that the procedure
for assessing decision-making capacity be described in research protocols, and
that standardized tools such as the MacArthur Competence Assessment Tool for
Clinical Research be employed routinely (67,70).

If a person is found to lack capacity, then advance directives for research,
if available, may be used to determine the willingness to participate. In our
experience, patients with dementia rarely complete research advance directives,
and in cases when they have been completed, they are not always useful due to
concerns that the person did not anticipate all the burdens associated with the
study in question when he/she agreed to participate in research. In addition,
there are concerns that with the progression of dementia, cognitive ability and
personality change so much that perhaps advance directives no longer apply
to this being who is now, effectively, a different person (71). Although not yet
subjected to the same degree of study and scrutiny as advance directives for
health care, we are concerned that research advance directives similarly may
prove to be not as helpful as originally hoped.

When research advance directives are unavailable, then proxy consent is
acceptable. Plans for how proxies are identified should, ideally, be clearly detailed

in research protocols ahead of time (70). Proxies may enroll subjects or withdraw them from studies if they believe it to be in the best interests of the person with dementia (even if this decision is in conflict with the patient's advance directive) (66,72). Use of proxies to consent for research participation involves many of the same issues as when they are used for surrogate medical decision making, as outlined earlier in this chapter.

In addition to subject or proxy consent, subject assent is required; even if decision-making capacity is absent, the subject should display a willingness to participate in the research protocol (73). A subject's resistance to study-related procedures such as phlebotomy or taking pills should be respected, and consistent dissent may require withdrawal from the study (66).

Two important caveats to the above discussion are important to note. First, legal standards for research advance directives and the use of proxies are still evolving, and there are still many questions that remain to be answered. Second, while decision making with regard to research is similar to clinical decision making, there is an important difference: participation in research is optional. In clinical situations, the patient is already a participant, and the patient or his/her proxy has no choice but to proceed with the process of care, trying to do what is in the patient's best interests. For example, when the proxy for a nursing home resident with dementia chooses not to make a DNR order, this patient will undergo resuscitation attempts. In other words, choosing not to do something is, in effect, choosing to do something else. There is no option to avoid participation in most clinical situations. In research, on the other hand, participation is never mandatory, and this is most strikingly illustrated in research protocols in which there is no reasonable expectation of direct benefit to the subject. It can be, thus, difficult to argue that participation is in the best interests of the subject, and yet, whether out of a desire to help future subjects or out of unrealistic optimism, many subjects are enrolled in research protocols every year. It is because of this optional aspect of research participation that standards for subject consent are necessarily more stringent than those for clinical decision making.

Protecting subjects with dementia versus seeking new knowledge

As a society, we have a responsibility to protect vulnerable people from exploitative research, and because those with dementia often are unable to give informed consent, this responsibility is all the greater. These concerns have prompted additional safeguards for people with dementia above and beyond those already in place to protect research subjects (67). Most guidelines state that subjects unable to give informed consent can, with proxy consent, participate in studies associated with minimal risk to subjects or in those with greater than minimal risk if there is a reasonable potential for the subject to directly benefit from the research (66,67). If there is no reasonable prospect of direct benefit, participation should not be offered to those who lack decision-making capacity. In addition, studies without prospect of direct benefit to individuals should not be performed unless justified by the knowledge to be gained from the research (67,70).

On the other hand, without research on dementia, patients and families will continue to suffer from this disease. Research is the only hope for preventing or treating dementia, and it would thus be a disservice to those with dementia to prohibit it. In fact, one recent study of older adults reports that the majority of subjects were willing to consent in advance to Alzheimer's research that presented no direct benefit to subjects, suggesting that Americans may recognize the importance of this type of research (74). Some also have argued that, once enrolled in a research protocol, subjects receive extra human contact and attention, thereby profiting from these indirect benefits of the research process itself (71). Clearly, a balance must be achieved between protecting patients with dementia from the risks of participation in research and encouraging research that has potential to help them or others with this disease.

Industry and research
Many complex ethical issues arise when clinical research is performed by companies with obligations not only to patients but also to their stockholders. Many of these issues are not specific to research on dementia, and will not be discussed here. However, it is important to note that because dementia and MCI affect such large numbers of people, dementia research, especially drug development, is potentially highly lucrative. As a result, many companies in the health care industry are involved in research on dementia, and potential issues such as academic scientists with conflicts of interest, failure to report negative studies, and failure to reveal complete details about adverse events are highly relevant (75).

Culture and Dementia
Dementia affects people of all races and cultures and, as such, takes on different meanings (and therefore has different implications) for different people. It could be argued that the approach taken in this chapter on ethics is a "Western" approach, and that there are many other sets of ethical issues that arise for people with different cultural beliefs. These are too numerous to discuss in this chapter, but one example is helpful to illustrate the ethical issues that can arise in different cultures. A recent study described the variety of explanatory models employed by caregivers of demented people in two cities in the United States (76). Asian-American caregivers were more likely to adhere to folk models to explain a loved one's dementia, attributing their symptoms to psychosocial stress, normal aging, or even spirit possession. Anglo-European-American caregivers were more likely to rely on biomedical models, using terms such as Alzheimer's disease, brain deterioration, and mini-strokes to explain dementia symptoms. This difference has several ethical implications. First, when disclosing a diagnosis of dementia, patients and caregivers may prefer to reinterpret biomedical terminology into folk models of disease. This brings up the issue of whether clinicians should attempt to "educate" families to try to convince them of the superiority of the biomedical model. Second, a family who attributes dementia to normal aging or psychosocial stressors may be less interested in pharmacologic treatment for dementia and may also be less likely to take advantage of social services designed to relieve caregiver stress such as day programs and Alzheimer's support groups. These cultural differences in explanatory models mean that clinicians adhering to a biomedical model have less to offer patients who adhere to folk models, and thus it could be argued that these differences result in a mismatch between what the patient and family needs and what the clinician has to offer. Third, folk models of dementia can have especially significant implications for end-of-life care. For example, one African-American caregiver in the study cited earlier felt that his wife's symptoms were due to the stress of having children who were using drugs, and hoped that she would "snap out of it." The belief that this condition

is reversible may cause him to refuse palliative care when his spouse reaches the end stages of life, a decision that clinicians employing biomedical models may find incomprehensible. Clearly, ethnicity and culture may play enormous roles in the medical care of the patient with dementia, and cultural "mismatches" can result in ineffective care (77).

CONCLUSION

We have attempted to review some of the most frequently encountered ethical issues that occur in the course of caring for a person with dementia. Both clinicians and caregivers struggle with many of these issues daily and often make decisions on how to proceed without even recognizing that they are facing ethical dilemmas. It is our hope that by presenting these issues and summarizing the work of ethicists and researchers in these areas, clinicians and caregivers will be better prepared to recognize the issues they face and to benefit from guidance already available.

REFERENCES

1. Drickamer MA, Lachs MS. Should patients with Alzheimer's disease be told their diagnosis? N Engl J Med 1992; 326(14):947–951.
2. Marzanski M. Would you like to know what is wrong with you? On telling the truth to patients with dementia. J Med Ethics 2000; 26(2):108–113.
3. Bamford C, Lamont S, Eccles M, et al. Disclosing a diagnosis of dementia: A systematic review. Int J Geriatr Psychiatry 2004; 19(2):151–169.
4. Carpenter B, Dave J. Disclosing a dementia diagnosis: A review of opinion and practice, and a proposed research agenda. Gerontologist 2004; 44(2):149–158.
5. Holroyd S, Snustad DG, Chalifoux ZL. Attitudes of older adults on being told the diagnosis of Alzheimer's disease. J Am Geriatr Soc 1996; 44(4):400–403.
6. Maguire CP, Kirby M, Coen R, et al. Family members' attitudes toward telling the patient with Alzheimer's disease their diagnosis. BMJ 1996; 313(7056):529–530.
7. Holroyd S, Turnbull Q, Wolf AM. What are patients and their families told about the diagnosis of dementia? Results of a family survey. Int J Geriatr Psychiatry 2002; 17(3):218–221.
8. http://www.alz.org/professionals_and_researchers_diagnostic_disclosure.asp. Accessed October 5, 2010.
9. Guttman R, Seleski M, eds. Diagnosis, Management, and Treatment of Dementia. Chicago, IL: American Medical Association, 1999.
10. Post SG. Key issues in the ethics of dementia care. Neurol Clin 2000; 18(4):1011–1022.
11. Post SG. Genetics, ethics, and Alzheimer disease. J Am Geriatr Soc 1994; 42(7):782–786.
12. Roses AD. A new paradigm for clinical evaluations of dementia: Alzheimer disease and apolipoprotein E genotypes. In: Post SG, Whitehouse PJ, eds. Genetic Testing for Alzheimer Disease. Baltimore, MD: The Johns Hopkins University Press, 1998:37–65.
13. Ciarleglio LJ, Bennett RL, Williamson J, et al. Genetic counseling throughout the life cycle. J Clin Invest 2003; 112(9):1280–1286.
14. Gauthier S, Touchon J. Mild cognitive impairment is not a clinical entity and should not be treated. Arch Neurol 2005; 62(7):1164–1166; discussion 1167.
15. Petersen RC, Morris JC. Mild cognitive impairment as a clinical entity and treatment target. Arch Neurol 2005; 62(7):1160–1163; discussion 1167.
16. Petersen RC, Thomas RG, Grundman M, et al. Vitamin E and donepezil for the treatment of mild cognitive impairment. N Engl J Med 2005; 352(23):2379–2388.
17. Petersen RC, Doody R, Kurz A, et al. Current concepts in mild cognitive impairment. Arch Neurol 2001; 58(12):1985–1992.

18. Gitlin LN, Winter L, Dennis MP, et al. A biobehavioral home-based intervention and the well-being of patients with dementia and their caregivers: the COPE randomized trial. JAMA 2010; 304(9):983–991.
19. Lacks MS, Pillemer K. Abuse and neglect of elderly persons. N Engl J Med 1995; 332(7):437–443.
20. Hughes JC, Hope T, Savulescu J, et al. Carers, ethics and dementia: A survey and review of the literature. Int J Geriatr Psychiatry 2002; 17(1):35–40.
21. Drape JF. Competency to give an informed consent. A model for making clinical assessments. JAMA 1984; 252(7):925–927.
22. Geriatrics at Your Fingertips, Online Edition. http://www.geriatricsatyourfinger tips.org/ebook/gayf_2.asp#c2s4_INFORMED_DECISION_MAKING. Accessed January 9, 2006.
23. Appelbaum PS, Grisso T. Assessing patients' capacities to consent to treatment. N Engl J Med 1988; 319(25):1635–1638.
24. Appelbaum PS, Grisso T. Assessing Competence to Consent to Treatment: A Guide for Physicians and Other Health Professionals. New York: Oxford University Press, 1998:31–60, 77–126.
25. Marson DC, McInturff B, Hawkins L, et al. Consistency of physician judgments of capacity to consent in mild Alzheimer's disease. J Am Geriatr Soc 1997; 45(4):453–457.
26. Marson DC, Earnst KS, Jamil F, et al. Consistency of physicians' legal standard and personal judgments of competency in patients with Alzheimer's disease. J Am Geriatr Soc 2000; 48(8):911–918.
27. Kim SY, Karlawish JH, Caine ED. Current state of research on decision-making competence of cognitively impaired elderly persons. Am J Geriatr Psychiatry 2002; 10(2):151–165.
28. Karlawish JH, Bonnie RJ, Appelbaum PS, et al. Addressing the ethical, legal, and social issues raised by voting by persons with dementia. JAMA 2004; 292(11):1345–1350.
29. Mendez MF. Dementia and guns. J Am Geriatr Soc 1996; 44(4):409–410.
30. Hughes JC, Louw SJ. Electronic tagging of people with dementia who wander. BMJ 2002; 325(7369):847–848.
31. Kamel HK, Hajjar RR. Sexuality in the nursing home, part 2: Managing abnormal behavior—legal and ethical issues. J Am Med Dir Assoc 2003; 4(4):203–206.
32. Freedman ML, Freedman DL. Should Alzheimer's disease patients be allowed to drive? A medical, legal, and ethical dilemma. J Am Geriatr Soc 1996; 44(7):876–877.
33. Wadley VG, Harrell LE, Marson DC. Self- and informant report of financial abilities in patients with Alzheimer's disease: Reliable and valid? J Am Geriatr Soc 2003; 51(11):1621–1626.
34. Post SG, Whitehouse PJ. Fairhill guidelines on ethics of the care of people with Alzheimer's disease: A clinical summary. J Am Geriatr Soc 1995; 43(12):1423–1429.
35. Welsh S, Hassiotis A, O'Mahoney G, et al. Big brother is watching you—the ethical implications of electronic surveillance measures in the elderly with dementia and in adults with learning difficulties. Aging Merit Health 2003; 7(5):372–375.
36. Miles SH, Meyers R. Untying the elderly: 1989 to 1993 update. Clin Geriatr Med 1994; 10(3):513–525.
37. The American Academy of Neurology Ethics and Humanities Subcommittee. Ethical issues in the management of the demented patient. Neurology 1996; 46(4):1180–1183.
38. Moss RJ, La Puma J. The ethics of mechanical restraints. Hastings Cent Rep 1991; 21(1):22–25.
39. Sink KM, Holden KF, Yaffe K. Pharmacological treatment of neuropsychiatric symptoms of dementia: A review of the evidence. JAMA 2005; 293(5):596–608.
40. Schneider LS, Dagennan KS, Insel P. Risk of death with atypical antipsychotic drug treatment for dementia: Meta-analysis of randomized placebo-controlled trials. JAMA 2005; 294(15):1934–1943.
41. Wang PS, Schneeweiss S, Avorn J, et al. Risk of death in elderly users of conventional vs. atypical antipsychotic medications. N Engl J Med 2005; 353(22):2335–2341.

42. Magaziner J, German P, Zimmerman SI, et al. The prevalence of dementia in a statewide sample of new nursing home admissions aged 65 and older: diagnosis by expert panel. Epidemiology of Dementia in Nursing Homes Research Group. Gerontologist 2000; 40(6):663–672.

43. Kane RA. Everyday life in nursing homes: The way things are. In: Kane RA, Caplan AL, eds. Everyday Ethics: Resolving Dilemmas in Nursing Home Life. New York: Springer Publishing Company, 1990:3–20.

44. Kane RA. Ethics and long-term care: Everyday considerations. Clin Geriatr Med 1994; 10(3):489–499.

45. Caplan AL. The morality of the mundane: Ethical issues in the daily lives of nursing home residents. In: Kane RA, Caplan AL, eds. Everyday Ethics: Resolving Dilemmas in Nursing Home Life. New York: Springer Publishing Company, 1990:37–50.

46. Raik BL, Miller FG, Fins JJ. Screening and cognitive impairment: Ethics of forgoing mammography in older women. J Am Geriatr Soc 2004; 52(3):440–444.

47. Sachs GA. Flu shots, mammograms, and Alzheimer's disease: Ethics of preventive medicine and dementia. Alzheimer Dis Assoc Disord 1994; 8(1):8–14.

48. Sachs GA. Dementia and the goals of care. J Am Geriatr Soc 1998; 46(6):782–783.

49. Brauner DJ, Muir JC, Sachs GA. Treating nondementia illnesses in patients with dementia. JAMA 2000; 283(24):3230–3235.

50. American Geriatrics Society Ethics Committee. Health screening decisions for older adults: AGS position paper. J Am Geriatr Soc 2003; 51(2):270–271.

51. Larson EB, Shadlen MF, Wang L, et al. Survival after initial diagnosis of Alzheimer disease. Ann Intern Med 2004; 140(7):501–509.

52. Morrison RS, Siu AL. Mortality from pneumonia and hip fractures in patients with advanced dementia. JAMA 2000; 284(19):2447–2448.

53. Laditka JN, Laditka SB, Cornmeal CB. Evaluating hospital care for individuals with Alzheimer's disease using inpatient quality indicators. Am J Alzheimers Dis Other Demen 2005; 20(1):27–36.

54. Sachs GA, Shega JW, Cox-Hayley D. Barriers to excellent end-of-life care for patients with dementia. J Gen Intern Med 2004; 19(10):1057–1063.

55. Mitchell SL, Teno J, Kiely DK, et al. The clinical course of advanced dementia. N Engl J Med 2009; 361:1529–1538.

56. Hurley AC, Volker L. Alzheimer Disease: "It's okay, Mama, if you want to go, it's okay." JAMA 2002; 288(18):2324–2331.

57. Morrison RS, Meier DE. Clinical practice. Palliative care. N Engl J Med 2004; 350(25):2582–2590.

58. Morrison RS, Siu AL. A comparison of pain and its treatment in advanced dementia and cognitively intact patients with hip fracture. J Pain Symptom Manage 2000; 19(4):240–248.

59. AGS Panel on Persistent Pain in Older Persons. The management of persistent pain in older persons. J Am Geriatr Soc 2002; 50(6 Suppl):S205–S224.

60. Quill TE, Dresser R, Brock DW. The rule of double effect—a critique of its role in end-of-life decision making. N Engl J Med 1997; 337(24):1768–1771.

61. Gillick MR. Rethinking the role of tube feeding in patients with advanced dementia. N Engl J Med 2000; 342(3):206–210.

62. Finucane TE, Christmas C, Travis K. Tube feeding in patients with advanced dementia: A review of the evidence. JAMA 1999; 282(14):1365–1370.

63. McCann RM, Hall WJ, Groth-Juncker A. Comfort care for terminally ill patients: The appropriate use of nutrition and hydration. JAMA 1994; 272(16):1263–1266.

64. Fabiszewski KJ, Volicer B, Volicer L. Effect of antibiotic treatment on outcome of fevers in institutionalized Alzheimer patients. JAMA 1990; 263(23):3168–3172.

65. Stocking CB, Hougham GW, Baron AR, et al. Are the rules for research with subjects with dementia changing? Views from the field. Neurology 2003; 61(12):1649–1651.

66. American Geriatrics Society Ethics Committee. Informed consent for research on human subjects with dementia. J Am Geriatr Soc 1998; 46(10):1308–1310.

67. Alzheimer's Association. Research consent for cognitively impaired adults: Recommendations for institutional review boards and investigators. Alzheimer Dis Assoc Disord 2004; 18(3):171–175.
68. National Bioethics Advisory Commission. Report and recommendations of the National Bioethics Advisory Commission. In: Research involving persons with mental disorders that may affect decision-making capacity. Rockville: US Government Printing Office, 1998:88.
69. Karlawish JH, Casarett DJ, James BD. Alzheimer's disease patients' and caregivers' capacity, competency, and reasons to enroll in an early-phase Alzheimer's disease clinical trial. J Am Geriatr Soc 2002; 50(12):2019–2024.
70. Karlawish JH. Research involving cognitively impaired adults. N Engl J Med 2003; 348(14):1389–1392.
71. Sachs GA, Cassel CK. Ethical aspects of dementia. Neurol Clin 1989; 7(4):845–858.
72. Kim SY, Kim HM, Langa KM, et al. Surrogate consent for dementia research: a national survey of older Americans. Neurology 2009; 72(2):149–155.
73. Sachs GA, Cohen HJ. Ethical challenges to research in geriatric medicine. In: Cassel CK, Leipzig RM, Cohen HJ, Larson EB, Meier DE, eds. Geriatric Medicine: An Evidence Based Approach. 4th edition. New York: Springer-Verlag. 2003:1253–1261.
74. Karlawish J, Rubright J, Casarett D, et al. Older adults' attitudes toward noncompetent subjects participating in Alzheimer's research. Am J Psychiatry 2009; 166:182–188.
75. Whitehouse PJ. Lessons and responses in Alzheimer disease research. JAMA 2003; 290(1):115.
76. Hinton L, Franz CE, Yeo G, et al. Conceptions of dementia in a multiethnic sample of family caregivers. J Am Geriatr Soc 2005; 53(8):1405–1410.
77. Blackhall LJ, Murphy ST, Frank G, et al. Ethnicity and attitudes toward patient autonomy. JAMA 1995; 274(10):820–825.

Legal issues in dementia

Marshall B. Kapp

INTRODUCTION

Cognitively impaired individuals may encounter a variety of serious problems in the course of obtaining appropriate medical care for both their cognitive medical conditions and medical issues they may have that are wholly unconnected to their cognitive impairments (1). These problems may include difficulties in making appointments, remembering appointments, and getting lost en route to appointments. They include failing to fill prescriptions, forgetting to take medications, or taking an excess of medications. Cognitively impaired elderly people may also ignore important symptoms with the result that their most significant problems may not be treated (2).

The presence of medically significant cognitive impairment in patients is not recognized in a timely way sometimes by clinicians (3,4). A delay in the diagnosis of dementia may entail legal repercussions for the physician. For the purposes of this chapter, however, it is assumed that a correct diagnosis of dementia has been made and the challenges faced are those of long-term patient management.

The professional care of patients with varying degrees of dementia over time may implicate a variety of legal (as well as ethical) considerations (5). Important legal issues arise in the context of medical decision making concerning diagnostic tests (for non-dementia-related purposes), therapeutic treatments, and research participation. Questions about informed consent, decisional capacity, advance planning, and the extent and limits of surrogate decision makers' authority to speak on behalf of incapacitated patients are implicated. This chapter outlines the most salient aspects of these legal issues as they pertain to the long-term management of persons with dementia.

INFORMED DECISION MAKING FOR DIAGNOSIS AND TREATMENT

Informed Consent

In caring for any patient over a period of time, a number of medical decisions may arise regarding diagnostic and therapeutic interventions. Ordinarily (in the case of adult patients), for legal purposes, the patient ultimately is the one who gets to make decisions about undergoing or declining particular recommended interventions ranging from surgery to the taking of drugs. The doctrine of informed choice, popularly but incompletely referred to as the right of informed consent, is the legal embodiment of the fundamental ethical principle of autonomy or self-determination (6).

In order for a medical choice to be considered legally valid, the choice must be made voluntarily, without coercion or undue influence exerted on the decision maker. Additionally, the health care provider who will be performing a particular medical intervention (e.g., doing a diagnostic procedure or prescribing a medication) has an obligation to assure that the patient's decision is properly informed. Required informational items include a description in understandable lay language, of at least: the nature of the problem for which the medical intervention is recommended, the prognosis with and without the proposed intervention, reasonably foreseeable risks associated with the proposed intervention, and reasonable alternatives (including non-intervention) and their anticipated risks and benefits.

Decisional Capacity

The third essential element of legally valid medical decision making is sufficient cognitive and emotional capacity on the part of the decision maker to engage in a rational process, resulting in an autonomous, informed, voluntary choice. As a general rule, the law starts with the presumption that every adult patient possesses that minimum required level of decisional capacity. This is a rebuttable presumption, however, meaning that it may be overcome by the presentation of sufficient evidence to the contrary. Sometimes, because of mental disability, the patient is not capable of comprehending relevant information and self-sufficiently engaging in a rational, authentic (i.e., consistent with previously held values), voluntary, and informed decision-making process (7).

Accurately assessing decisional capacity in older individuals may be a complex and difficult job (8), especially when a patient in the early stage of dementia is involved. No simple, reliable instrument or tool exists to make the task quick and easy (9), although continuing attempts to develop measurement instruments to assist in this task persist. Many of these various standardized instruments are quite useful for measuring mental status for purposes of assisting in making a diagnosis or structuring a therapeutic research plan for the individual, but the instruments are not specifically designed to take the place of clinical judgment in assessing cognition for the legal and ethical purposes of judging decision-making capacity.

Nevertheless, there are some general guidelines that the clinician should keep in mind when conducting this type of assessment. The primary point is that decisional capacity should not be evaluated on the basis of the patient's diagnostic label or category, such as dementia, nor solely predicated on the physician's view of the wisdom of the patient's particular choice. Instead, the focus should be placed on the patient's functional ability—that is, on the thought processes used in arriving at a "good" or a "bad" decision. This approach would take into account the patient's clinical diagnosis of dementia, but recognize that a diagnosis, by itself, tells us little about the current severity of the patient's condition or the ways in which that diagnosis actually affects the current cognitive and emotional capacity of the individual.

In conducting a functional inquiry, the following sort of basic questions should be explored: (*i*) Can the patient make and communicate any decisions at all? (*ii*) Does the patient have the ability to present any reasons for the choices made that illustrate at least some degree of reflection and serious consideration about the choices? (*iii*) Are the reasons presented by the patient in support of the choices made based on factually accurate suppositions that are logically applied? For instance, in one case an older woman who refused to consent to amputation of her gangrenous leg because she denied the presence of any medical problem other than dirt on her leg that could easily be washed off was properly deemed by the court to be decisionally incapacitated (10). (*iv*) Is the patient able to comprehend the implications (the likely risks and benefits) of the available alternatives and the choices expressed, as well as the fact that these ramifications apply to that specific patient? and (*v*) Does the patient actually understand the ramifications of the choices made for himself/herself?

Capacity needs to be examined on a decision-specific basis; put differently, an individual with dementia may be able to rationally make some kinds of decisions (e.g., whether or not to follow a low salt diet) but not others, such as whether to undergo bypass surgery. Therefore, capacity should not necessarily be envisioned as a global matter pertaining to all decisions, although some patients (particularly those in advanced stages of dementia) in fact may be globally incapacitated. For others, though, partial capacity (the ability to make some kinds, but not all kinds, of decisions) is possible. The inquiry should be whether the patient is capable "enough" to make the particular decision in question.

Moreover, capacity may fluctuate for a particular patient with dementia according to such variables as time of day, day of the week, physical location of the assessment, co-morbidities (especially acute and transient medical problems), other persons available to interact with the patient and support or coerce his/her choice (11), and reactions to medications. Some of these factors may be sufficiently susceptible to manipulation by the physician that discussions with the patient about the care plan can take place in reasonably lucid circumstances. Whenever possible, physicians should try to maximize the patient's ability to participate in medical decisions before they look to a surrogate to act on behalf of the patient. (Surrogates are discussed below.)

ADVANCE HEALTH CARE PLANNING

General

An adult may use a variety of legal mechanisms of advance planning to take action, while still mentally capable, to anticipate and prepare for eventual incapacity by voluntarily delegating or directing future authority concerning medical decision making (12). The advance planning opportunity is available to persons in the early stages of dementia, although ideally individuals should be encouraged to avail themselves of these legal mechanisms when they are young and healthy, before the prospect of dementia ever becomes a real issue.

Congressional enactment of the federal Patient Self-Determination Act (PSDA) (13) in 1990 was intended to function as a catalyst to encourage more adults to execute advance medical directives in a timely fashion. Hospitals, nursing facilities, hospices, managed care organizations, and home health agencies that receive any Medicare or Medicaid funding are obligated by this statute to, among other things, adopt and make available to patients and their surrogates a written organizational policy on medical decision making, ask patients (at or before the time of their admission or enrollment) whether or not they have previously executed an advance directive, and offer presently capable patients an opportunity to execute an advance directive if they wish to but have not done so earlier.

Proponents of advance directives claim that formal advance care planning may help individuals and their families avoid the human and financial costs of court involvement in future medical treatment decisions in a way that is consistent with patient autonomy or self-determination, and may reduce the emotional or psychological stress on family and friends in difficult crisis situations. These goals are especially important for patients and families who are dealing with the ravages of a dementia diagnosis. It must be added, however, that a growing number of health care practitioners and observers have expressed skepticism, based on disappointing experience, about just how well advance directives effectively achieve their goals.

In the United States, legal mechanisms for individuals to engage in prospective (before-the-fact) planning about their own health care have their foundations in various statutes enacted by state legislatures. A number of state statutes are modeled on the Uniform Health Care Decisions Act adopted by the National Conference of Commissioners on Uniform State Laws in 1993. In some other countries (e.g., Great Britain), advance directives have been recognized by the courts even though they have not been codified in statutory form. Advance directives may be utilized by competent persons to either limit future medical treatment or, conversely, demand the provision of specific interventions (such as artificial feeding and hydration) in the future.

Consistently, courts and state legislatures have indicated that state advance directive statutes are not intended to be the only means by which patients may exercise their right to make decisions about future medical interventions. For instance, a patient might convey preferences regarding future medical treatment orally to the physician during an office visit, with the physician documenting the patient's words in the medical chart. If that patient later becomes unable to make contemporaneous medical decisions personally, the patient's oral advance instructions are just as legally valid as would be a written document executed in compliance with all of the statutory formalities contained in the state's advance directive statute.

State advance directive statutes all specifically excuse a health care provider who decides, for reasons of personal conscience, not to fulfill the clearly stated treatment wishes of a patient or surrogate, as long as the provider does not impede efforts to have the patient transferred to the care of another provider who agrees to implement the patient's advance directive. In the same vein, courts generally have not held health care providers liable for monetary damages for failure to follow the instructions of a patient or surrogate to withdraw or withhold particular forms of treatment, on the grounds that providing life-prolonging intervention cannot cause the type of injury or harm against which the civil justice system is supposed to protect.

Durable Powers of Attorney

The durable power of attorney (DPOA) is a proxy directive, a written legal document in which an individual (the principal) may appoint an agent, or "attorney-in-fact," to conduct transactions and make future decisions for the principal. Depending on the specific jurisdiction, the agent so appointed may be termed a proxy, a surrogate, or a representative. Unlike the situation created with an ordinary power of attorney, the authority of an agent under a DPOA is not ended when the principal subsequently becomes decisionally incapacitated.

Every state has enacted a statute that explicitly permits the use of a DPOA to empower the appointed agent to make medical decisions on the patient's behalf.

The agent's decision-making authority may become effective immediately (an immediate DPOA) upon execution of the document or may "spring" into action only when a specifically delineated event (such as, "when my physician certifies that I am unable to make my own medical decisions") has taken place. The DPOA would then endure beyond that triggering event. The principal may terminate or revoke the arrangement at any time, as long as the principal remains mentally competent to do so.

A designated agent is supposed to make decisions on the incapacitated patient's behalf based on the patient's substituted judgment (i.e., what the patient personally would choose if presently able to make and express autonomous choices). If application of the substituted judgment principle is not realistic in a particular situation because the surrogate honestly does not know what the individual would have wanted to do under the circumstances, then the surrogate, as the patient's fiduciary, is required to act according to the surrogate's careful judgment about the patient's best interests. The DPOA provides the advantage, for both patients and their caregivers, of legally empowering a live advocate for the principal who can enter into discussions and make decisions regarding the principal based on the most current information and other considerations, most importantly the agent's interpretation of the principal's previously expressed and implied wishes.

In most states, to prevent a real or apparent conflict of interest from materializing, the health care providers for the principal who has executed a DPOA are disqualified from serving as agents under the DPOA. The agent may be, but does not have to be, a family member of the principal. An obvious limitation of the DPOA device is the legal and practical requirement that the person who would like to delegate certain decision-making authority to an agent actually have available a suitable, willing, and able person to whom to delegate that authority. The DPOA does not help people (the "unbefriended" population) who do not have available to name as a potential agent someone else whom they can trust to make future personal decisions for them.

Living Wills

The DPOA, as a proxy directive, is distinguishable from a living will (in some jurisdictions called a "health care directive"), which is an instruction type of advance directive. In a living will, a mentally capable person documents his/her general or specific desires regarding future medical treatment, rather than naming an agent, to make future treatment decisions in the eventuality of the patient's later incapacity. The DPOA and living will are not mutually exclusive, and patients may be encouraged to execute them in tandem because the instructions specified in the living will may help the agent named under a DPOA to exercise the patient's substituted judgment more accurately. If there is a direct conflict between the instructions in a presently incapacitated patient's living will and the decision of the agent, applicable state law governs which directive takes precedence.

Mentally capable adults are empowered to execute living wills by state statutes that often are termed "natural death" acts. Compliance with the provisions of such a directive protects or immunizes involved health care professionals and treatment facilities against possible civil or criminal liability for withholding or withdrawing medical treatments under the conditions specified in the directive.

The person executing a living will must be decisionally capable at the time the document is created. The legal force of the living will goes into effect only when the patient, after signing the document, subsequently becomes cognitively and/or emotionally incapable of making and expressing medical choices personally. In most situations, it is left to the individual's personal physician to clinically determine when that person has become incapable of engaging in a rational decision-making process any longer and, therefore, when the living will should be relied on for guidance. Until such a determination is made, the contemporaneously expressed choices of the capable patient himself/herself should be followed.

One criticism of living wills is that they frequently express the patient's prospective treatment wishes in a way that is too general and vague to provide much actual guidance to those who ultimately must figure out how to implement those wishes in clinical practice. A variety of models have been suggested regarding the composition of living wills. Some of these proposed models concentrate on specific clinical scenarios and medical interventions (containing statements such as, "Do not resuscitate me if I suffer cardiac arrest when I am permanently and severely demented"). Other models, by contrast, rely on provisions that focus more on identifying the patient's key values and goals (like, "I want to avoid pain and indignity more than I desire to live forever") (14). In the best-case scenario, prior to the patient actually writing down instructions in a legal document, there would have been an unpressured conversation during which the physician attempted to get the patient to clarify his/her future treatment preferences; in reality, though, such discussions (to the extent they occur at all) take place in the crisis context of the bedside after the patient has already become critically ill. With patients who have a condition such as dementia associated with a steady and irreversible cognitive decline, the timeliness of advance planning discussions, as well as execution of advance planning documents, is especially important.

There is a growing body of evidence that, frequently, patients' wishes as stated in their living wills concerning future medical interventions, particularly life-sustaining medical treatments, are not respected and implemented by families and/or health care providers at the crucial juncture (15). Proof of this common disregard for living will instructions has influenced a substantial number of legal and ethical commentators to question the practical value of living wills and their continuing viability as part of the advance health care planning process.

"Do Not" Orders

A "do not" order is another kind of advance directive. It is an order written by the physician, based on discussions with the patient and/or the patient's decision-making surrogate, if applicable. The order instructs other health care providers that, in the event of a medical emergency, certain specified interventions (such as cardiopulmonary resuscitation, intubation, or hospitalization) are to be withheld. Most states have regulations pertaining to the writing and implementation of "do not" orders, and many of these regulatory schemes distinguish in their procedural requirements between orders to take effect within hospital walls and those pertaining to out-of-hospital contingencies.

SURROGATE DECISION MAKING

When a patient lacks sufficient cognitive and emotional capacity to make decisions personally, the physician may not dispense with the requirement to obtain informed consent prior to initiating a medical intervention. Instead, in that situation, the physician must deal with someone else who acts as a surrogate or proxy on the patient's behalf (16). Surrogate decision making for a decisionally incapacitated person may occur through either a planned or unplanned process.

Planned

The primary mechanism of planned surrogate decision making is the execution of a DPOA, as discussed above. State statutes empower decisionally capable adults (such as those in the early stages of dementia) to plan ahead for their possible future incapacity and maintain some degree of prospective autonomy by naming a person of their own choosing to act as a decision-making surrogate when the need later arises. The DPOA relies heavily on the principal's trust that the surrogate will act according to the principal's substituted judgment or, if that is not feasible, the principal's best interests. Timely creation of a DPOA allows for transfer of decision-making power from the patient to the surrogate, if needed, without any involvement of the courts or other external bodies, with all the time, expense, and hassle that such external legal involvement routinely entails.

The other available, although not often utilized, legal mechanism for accomplishing surrogate decision making in a planned fashion is voluntary guardianship. (The topic of involuntary guardianship is discussed below.) State statutes permit a decisionally capable individual to petition a court to appoint a guardian of that person's own choice, but authority to make decisions shifts from the individual to the guardian only if the court subsequently finds that the initiating person has become decisionally incapable. The advantage of the voluntary guardianship approach, compared with the inexpensive and non-time-consuming alternative of executing a DPOA, is that, once empowered, the guardian would be subject to routine monitoring of his/her fiduciary performance by the court to assure that decisions are being made properly.

Unplanned

Family consent statutes

To whom can the physician turn if a patient is decisionally incapable but has not previously executed a DPOA or living will or initiated a voluntary guardianship? One answer is that a majority of states have enacted statutes authorizing family members or others close to the patient to make medical decisions for incapacitated persons without decision-making agents appointed by the person himself/herself or a court as part of a guardianship proceeding. In states that have such statutes (generally generically labeled "family consent statutes"), ordinarily interventions may be initiated upon achievement and documentation of unanimous agreement among the attending physician, the highest priority surrogate decision maker specified in the family consent statute who is available at the time, and sometimes also consultant physicians.

The legislative trend in this direction was fueled by the U.S. Supreme Court's decision in *Cruzan v. Director* (17) holding that the extent and conditions of proxy decision-making authority is a matter of state legislative, rather than

federal constitutional, policy. Even in the few states still without family consent
legislation, courts nonetheless pretty universally recognize the family's authority
(either as a matter of common law or under the state's own constitution) to exercise the incapacitated patient's decision-making rights on behalf of the patient.
The small number of litigated cases in this arena establishes legal precedent for
families to act in other, future cases without the need for prior judicial approval.

In its *Cruzan* decision, the Supreme Court held that a state could constitu-
tionally mandate that surrogate decision makers prove the incapacitated patient's
desire to limit aggressive medical intervention by "clear and convincing" evidence, if the surrogate wanted to overcome the legal presumption that maximum
treatment ought to proceed. Several states (e.g., New York and Missouri) currently appear to require this demanding standard of proof. The Supreme Court
left ambiguous exactly what kind of evidence would be necessary to meet the
"clear and convincing" test, although almost certainly some written, witnessed
documentation of the patient's preferences, made while the patient was still decisionally capable, would be sufficient. What proof, short of a precisely worded,
written instruction directive, may be adequate would be determined on a case-
by-case basis, and the outcome may vary among different jurisdictions.

Guardianship/conservatorship
In situations involving a decisionally incapacitated person and no valid advance
directive, family consent statute, or applicable judicial precedent empowering
the family to act, creation of a guardianship (in some jurisdictions, notably
California, called instead a conservatorship) may be advisable to formally transfer decision-making power from an incapacitated patient to a surrogate. This
process entails appointment by a state court (in most jurisdictions situated in
the probate division) of a surrogate (the "guardian" or "conservator"), who is
explicitly empowered to make either all or specified decisions on behalf of the
decisionally incapable person (the "ward") whom the court declares to be legally
incompetent. As noted in the previous section, a voluntary guardianship may
be initiated by the ward, while he/she is still decisionally capable, to take effect
in the future. In the overwhelming number of cases, however, courts appoint
guardians for an incompetent ward in response to a petition filed by the family, a
caregiver, or an Adult Protective Services (APS) program. In contested guardianship proceedings, adjudication of the ward's incompetence is supported by the
sworn affidavit or live testimony of physicians and/or psychologists who are
familiar with the patient's mental condition (18).

State guardianship statutes contain a two-step definition of competence.
First, the person must fall within a specific diagnostic category, such as dementia.
Next, the individual needs to be found impaired functionally—in other words,
actually unable to care appropriately for his/her person or property—as a result
of being within that first clinical category. The criterion of substantial functional
impairment is emphasized in those states, such as California, whose statutes limit
eligibility for guardianship/conservatorship to individuals who are "gravely disabled" or the equivalent.

Guardianship usually is a benevolently inspired exercise of the state's *parens
patriae* power to protect especially vulnerable persons from the consequences of
inability to fend for themselves. The origins of some sort of guardianship based
on the state's benevolent intentions toward the dependent and vulnerable can be

traced back beyond thirteenth-century England. Nevertheless, because creating total or plenary guardianship ordinarily involves extensive intrusion into an individual's basic personal and property rights, the "least restrictive/least intrusive alternative" doctrine makes a limited guardianship preferred whenever possible (19). The idea is that if the state must impose limits on someone's rights, those restrictions should go no further than is necessary to accomplish the legitimate goal of protecting the individual against harm. Probate courts have the statutory authority to limit the guardian's power to make only those particular types of decisions that the ward personally is unable to handle rationally.

Traditionally, guardians have been required to make decisions predicated on the guardian's belief about the patient's best interests. This is still the standard in some jurisdictions. However, here as elsewhere in the realm of surrogate decision making, the modern trend has been toward a substituted judgment standard, under which the guardian is required to make those choices that the patient, if able to express personal preferences and values, would have made by himself/herself. The performance of the guardian/conservator as a fiduciary or trust agent of the ward remains subject to ongoing oversight by the appointing court (20).

The individual or entity appointed to act as a guardian/conservator ordinarily is a private person (a relative, friend, or attorney of the ward), financial institution (bank or trust company), or agency. The majority of guardians/conservators are related to the ward in some way, although (especially when there is substantial money in the individual's estate) professional guardians are available for a fee (21). Almost all the states have developed some form of public guardianship, under which a governmental agency, acting either directly or through contract with a private, not-for-profit, or for-profit organization, functions in the guardian/conservator role for a ward who has no one else willing and able to act in that capacity (22). Additionally, some private corporations and organizations (often but not necessarily sectarian) offer their services as guardians/conservators directly to the courts, either for a fee or on a voluntary, pro bono (charitable) basis.

INVOLUNTARY COMMITMENT

Every state has enacted legislation authorizing the state, under its inherent police power to protect and promote the general health, safety, welfare, and morals of the community, to involuntarily (civilly) commit to a public or publicly licensed mental health facility persons who have been adjudicated mentally ill and dangerous to others. The same statutes, relying on the state's *parens patriae* authority to protect individuals who are unable to protect themselves, also empower states to civilly commit mentally ill individuals who pose a serious danger only to themselves. Persons with dementia sometimes are the subject of involuntary commitment proceedings if their conduct has become unmanageable, in terms of assuring safety to the individual or others, within the setting of a private residence, assisted living, or a nursing facility.

In most jurisdictions, anyone may initiate a petition starting the civil commitment process. Usually, this proceeding is conducted in a state probate court, with the state as moving party bearing the burden of proving by at least clear and convincing evidence the mental illness and dangerousness of the person to be committed. This is a higher burden than the preponderance of the evidence test that usually applies in civil cases. Some states go even further and require proof beyond a reasonable doubt, as in criminal prosecutions.

The physician's role in the civil commitment process, once a case gets to court, is as a provider of evidence, through a sworn affidavit or live testimony, on the issue of the patient's mental condition. Before the situation gets to that juncture, though, the physician may contribute positively by helping the patient, family, and other caregivers to explore less restrictive alternatives that might keep the matter away from the probate court system altogether.

For a growing number of older persons whose cognitive impairments would technically qualify them for plenary or limited guardianship, the most pressing practical problem is the unavailability of relatives or close friends who are willing and able to take on guardianship responsibilities. When there is no available local public guardianship system, local volunteer guardianship program, or sufficient assets to hire a private, professional guardian, a cognitively incapacitated individual with no willing and available family and friends (the "unbefriended") often literally "falls between the cracks." Important decisions about medical treatment and other matters may be made, or not made, by default until an emergency situation has developed and caregivers are able to rely on the doctrine of presumed consent to proceed.

A guardianship/conservatorship may be discontinued when it is no longer needed. In many jurisdictions, the continued appropriateness of a guardianship must be reviewed periodically according to a set schedule. The party arguing for termination of the guardianship bears the burden of proving that the ward's competence has been adequately restored.

INFORMED DECISION MAKING FOR RESEARCH PARTICIPATION

The generic legal aspects of conducting biomedical or behavioral research involving human participants are governed by extensive federal (23) and state (24) regulations, and have been described at length elsewhere (25,26). However, given the disproportionate prevalence of dementias (Alzheimer's, vascular, frontal lobe, and Lewy body) and other severe mental disabilities [such as depression (27), Huntington's disease, schizophrenia, and Wernicke–Korsakoff syndrome] among the elderly, the legal and ethical Catch-22 of conducting biomedical and behavioral research using elderly human participants who are severely demented or otherwise too cognitively compromised to make their own decisions presents a particular dilemma (28). On the one hand, progress in developing new interventions that can eventually become part of standard clinical practice (29) for the diagnosis and treatment of medical and psychological problems associated with dementia requires that research projects be done in which individuals suffering from the precise problems of interest be the basic units of study. At the same time, though, those very conditions that qualify a person for eligibility as a participant in such a research project frequently make it impossible for that person to take part in a rational, autonomous decision-making process about his/her own participation as a research subject (30). This paradox is exacerbated by the fact that research participants ordinarily are more vulnerable to possible exploitation, and therefore need more protection, than patients in therapeutic circumstances because of, among other factors, the researchers' potential conflicts of interest (31).

Thus, research protocols that anticipate the enrollment of participants with severe cognitive impairment, or that want to avoid enrolling those persons, must contain procedures for assessing the decision-making capacity of potential subjects. Specific assessment methods should be expressly built into the initial enrollment phase of the protocol, and therefore subject to review by an institutional review board (IRB), so that individuals lacking sufficient decision-making capacity can either be excluded at the outset or else have surrogates identified for them. Moreover, periodic reassessment may be necessary over the course of a long-term research project to be certain that a participant having adequate cognitive capacity when enrolled at the beginning of the protocol still maintains enough capacity throughout the protocol, such that he/she could exercise the right to withdraw if that option were desired (32). Several formal screening devices have been developed to aid, but not displace the vital role of professional judgment of, researchers in the capacity assessment process (33,34).

Federal regulations covering biomedical and behavioral research mandate that informed consent for participation be obtained from the "subject or the subject's legally authorized representative" (35). One problem is that a subject's legally authorized representative is defined in a circular way to mean an "individual or judicial or other body authorized under applicable [presumably state] law to consent on behalf of a prospective subject" (36). Hence, state law, even when unclear, controls in this sphere.

Several alternative possibilities for accomplishing acceptable surrogate decision making in the research context have been suggested. These mechanisms include: a durable power of attorney for research participation, research living wills (37), reliance on family consent statutes for research as well as diagnostic and therapeutic interventions, informal (i.e., without explicit legal authorization) reliance on available family members as surrogate decision makers, guardianship orders with express authorization for the guardian to make research decisions, specific prior court orders authorizing the incapacitated subject's participation in research protocols on a case-by-case basis, an independent patient advocate supplied by the organization sponsoring the research or by a government agency, and identification of a surrogate by the IRB or a long-term care facility's resident council. The American Geriatrics Society has taken the position that surrogates should be permitted to deviate from subjects' research advance directives based on the surrogate's own assessment of the subject's best interests or intent (38).

Some legal and ethical commentators have recommended that special, additional procedural safeguards are needed to protect vulnerable, cognitively impaired human volunteers from injury as a result of research participation. These safeguards might encompass heightened IRB involvement in the protocol approval process, enhanced IRB activity in the postapproval continuous monitoring and supervision phase of the research (including the IRB serving as a venue for appeals and objections by the investigator), and requiring assent by individual participants (in other words, giving participants a veto power) even when informed proxy consent to research participation has been obtained already. An obvious and important question, especially because the research participants of interest are mentally impaired, concerns the definition of assent to be used, namely, whether a failure to actively object to participation in a protocol is enough to be interpreted as a tacit or implied form of assent or whether some more affirmative indication of agreement is necessary.

The National Bioethics Advisory Commission proposed in 1998 that the federal Department of Health and Human Services promulgate regulations and that states adopt legislation specifically targeted at biomedical and behavioral research involving participants with serious cognitive impairments (39). Thus far, however, such specifically targeted regulations have not been promulgated nor, in most states, legislation enacted. Severely cognitively impaired potential research participants, therefore, must continue to rely on the legal protections provided in generic federal and state laws pertaining to human subjects' research.

CONFIDENTIALITY
Whether acting in the diagnostic, therapeutic, or research context, health care providers must respect the rights of patients regarding the privacy of their personal health information. The ethical fiduciary, or trust, obligation of professionals to hold in confidence all intimate patient information entrusted to them may be legally enforced through civil damage suits based on both statutes and common law (judge-made precedent), and is embodied in the licensing provisions of virtually all state professional practice acts and accompanying regulations.

Federal regulations that became effective in 2003 (40) to implement the Health Insurance Portability and Accountability Act (HIPAA) of 1996 (41) impose on covered health care entities and their business associates very specific requirements regarding the handling of personally identifiable medical information contained in patient records. These regulations impose severe criminal and civil sanctions for unauthorized disclosures of personal health information (PHI), such as a patient's name, address, or identification number of any sort. Any health plan, health care clearinghouse, or health care provider that transmits individually identifiable health care information electronically is a covered entity required to comply with HIPAA.

One major exception to the general confidentiality rule and the state and federal statutes supplementing it occurs when a patient voluntarily and knowingly waives, or gives up, the right to confidentiality concerning particular information. Such waivers are done by patients daily in medical offices and health care facilities to make information available to third-party payers, quality-of-care auditors, and other public and private entities. When, because of significant cognitive and/or emotional deficits, the patient is personally incapable of making his/her own health care decisions, this incapacity also applies to decisions about waiving one's right to confidentiality of PHI. In those circumstances, the same party who functions as the patient's surrogate for purposes of giving or withholding informed consent for diagnostic, therapeutic, or research interventions also must decide in what circumstances, if any, to waive the patient's right to confidentiality.

More generally, when the patient personally lacks decision-making capacity, the health care provider should share with the decision-making surrogate all information that usually would be shared with the patient himself/herself. This rule is consistent with the dictates of the informed consent doctrine (discussed above); the surrogate stands in the incapacitated patient's shoes and, in order to make informed decisions on the patient's behalf, needs access to the same information as would otherwise be provided directly to the patient as part of the informed consent process.

The patient's expectation of privacy also must yield when the health care provider is mandated by state statute to report to specified public health or law enforcement authorities the health care provider's reasonable suspicion that certain conditions or activities (e.g., elder mistreatment or neglect, domestic violence, or dementia or other disorder that would interfere with the patient's ability to operate a motor vehicle safely) are present or have occurred. Mandatory reporting statutes embody the state's exercise of its inherent police power to protect and promote the general health, safety, welfare, and morals of the community or its *parens patriae* authority to protect individuals (such as severely cognitively or emotionally impaired persons) who are not capable of protecting themselves.

Further, a health care professional may be compelled to reveal otherwise confidential information about particular patients by the force of legal process, that is, by a judge's issuance of a court order requiring such release. This is a possibility in any lawsuit or administrative proceeding (e.g., a guardianship or civil commitment hearing, or a will contest challenging the testamentary capacity of the deceased at the time the will was executed) involving a factual dispute about a patient's present or past physical or mental condition. A court order requiring one to produce personally identifiable patient information may overrule the state's provider/patient testimonial privilege statute. Every testimonial privilege statute provides for court-ordered testimony and production of records by the health care provider when, for instance, the patient has placed his/her own health condition and medical treatment in issue in a lawsuit.

The delivery of health care today ordinarily involves a team effort. Thus, every patient implicitly gives permission for the sharing of certain otherwise private information among members of the treatment or research team. Information sharing of this sort is necessary to provide optimal care. However, only information that is clearly pertinent and needed to facilitate the contribution of each team member ought to be made available to the various team members. Additionally, each team member who has access to PHI is fully obligated to abide by all relevant legal constraints on the inappropriate release of such information.

REFERENCES

1. Brauner DJ, Muir JC, Sachs GA. Treating nondementia illnesses in patients with dementia. JAMA 2000; 283(24):3230–3235.
2. Olness K, Loue S. Coping with daily living: Housing, finances, transportation, medical care. J Long Term Home Health Care 2004; 5(4):221–227.
3. Chodosh J, Petitti DB, Elliott M, et al. Physician recognition of cognitive impairment: Evaluating the need for improvement. J Am Geriatr Soc 2004; 52(7):1051–1059.
4. Boustani M, Callahan CM, Unverzagt FW, et al. Implementing a screening and diagnosis program for dementia in primary care. J Gen Intern Med 2005; 20(7):572–577.
5. Gilchrist BJ. Legal and ethical issues. In: Hay DP, Klein DT, Hay LK, et al., eds. Agitation in Patients with Dementia: A Practical Guide to Diagnosis and Management. Washington, DC: American Psychiatric Publishers 2003:221–229.
6. Faden RR, Beauchamp TL. A History and Theory of Informed Consent. New York: Oxford University Press, 1986.
7. Grisso T, Appelbaum PS. Assessing Competence to Consent to Treatment. New York: Oxford University Press, 1998.
8. Kapp MB, ed. Decision-Making Capacity and Older Persons. New York: Springer Publishing Company, 2004.

9. Kapp MB, Mossman D. Measuring decisional capacity: Cautions on the construction of a "capacimeter." Psychol Public Policy Law 1996; 2(1):73–95.
10. *State Department of Human Services v. Northern,* 563 S.W.2d 197 (Tenn. Ct. App. 1978).
11. Woods B, Pratt R. Awareness in dementia: Ethical and legal issues in relation to people with dementia. Aging Ment Health 2005; 9(5):423–429.
12. Lowder JL, Buzney SJ, French CM, et al. The importance of planning for the future. J Long Term Home Health Care 2004; 5(4):235–244.
13. Ulrich LP. The Patient Self-Determination Act—Meeting the Challenges in Patient Care. Washington, DC: Georgetown University Press, 1999.
14. Kolarik RC, Arnold RM, Fischer GS, et al. Advance care planning: A comparison of value statements and treatment preferences. J Gen Intern Med 2002; 17(8):618–624.
15. Hardin SB, Yusufaly YA. Difficult end-of-life treatment decisions. Arch Intern Med 2004; 164(14):1531–1533.
16. Dubler NN, symposium ed. The doctor-proxy relationship. J Law Med Ethics 1999; 27(1):5–86.
17. *Cruzan v. Director, Missouri Department of Health,* 110 S. Ct. 2841 (1990).
18. Quinn MJ. Guardianship of Adults. New York, NY: Springer Publishing Company, 2004.
19. Frolik LA. Promoting judicial acceptance and use of limited guardianship. Stetson Law Rev 2002; 31(3):735–755.
20. Hurme SB, Wood E. Guardian accountability then and now: Tracing tenets for an active court role. Stetson Law Rev 2002; 31(3):867–940.
21. Barnes A. The virtues of corporate and professional guardians. Stetson Law Rev 2002; 31(3):941–1026.
22. Schmidt WC Jr. The Wingspan of Wingspread: What is known and not known about the state of the guardianship and public guardianship system thirteen years after the Wingspread national guardianship symposium. Stetson Law Rev 2002; 31(3):1027–1046.
23. 42 Code of Federal Regulations Part 46.
24. Kapp MB. Protecting human participants in long-term care research: The role of state law and policy. J Aging Soc Policy 2004; 16(3):13–33.
25. Kapp MB. Regulating hematology/oncology research involving human participants. Hematol Oncol Clin North Am 2002; 16(6):1449–1461.
26. Coleman CH, Menikoff JA, Dubler NN, et al. The Ethics and Regulation of Research with Human Subjects. Newark, NJ: Matthew Bender & Company, 2005.
27. Elliott C. Caring about risks: Are severely depressed patients competent to consent to research? Arch Gen Psychiatry 1997; 54(2):113–116.
28. Kapp MB, ed. Issues in Conducting Research with and About Older Persons: Ethics, Law & Aging Review, vol. 8. New York: Springer Publishing Company, 2002.
29. Kapp MB. Legal standards for the medical diagnosis and treatment of dementia. J Legal Med 2002; 23(3):359–402.
30. Dresser R. Dementia research: Ethics and policy for the twenty-first century. Georgia Law Rev 2001; 35(2):661–690.
31. Gatter R. Walking the talk of trust in human subjects research: The challenge of regulating financial conflicts of interest. Emory Law J 2003; 52(1):327–401.
32. Loue S. The participation of cognitively impaired elderly in research. J Long Term Home Health Care 2004; 5(4):245–257.
33. Palmer BW, Dunn LB, Appelbaum PS, et al. Assessment of capacity to consent to research among older persons with schizophrenia, Alzheimer disease, or diabetes mellitus. Arch Gen Psychiatry 2005; 62(7):726–733.
34. Buckles VD, Powlishta KK, Palmer JL, et al. Understanding of informed consent by demented individuals. Neurology 2003; 61(12):1662–1666.
35. 45 Code of Federal Regulations § 46.116 and 21 Code of Federal Regulations § 50.20.
36. 45 Code of Federal Regulations § 46.102(d) and 21 Code of Federal Regulations § 50.3(m).

37. Dresser R. Mentally disabled research subjects: The enduring policy issues. JAMA 1996; 276(1):67–72.
38. American Geriatrics Society. Position Statement: Informed Consent for Research on Human Subjects with Dementia. 1998.
39. National Bioethics Advisory Commission. Research Involving Persons with Mental Disorders That May Affect Decision-making Capacity: Report and Recommendations. Washington, DC: U.S. Government Printing Office 1998.
40. 45 Code of Federal Regulations Parts 160 and 164.
41. Public Law No. 104–191, title XI, Part C.

11 Caregiver stress and possible solutions

Mary D. Dodge and Janice K. Kiecolt-Glaser

INTRODUCTION

Providing care for a relative with Alzheimer's disease or another progressive dementia is associated with many hardships. The course of the illness is largely uncontrollable and unpredictable, and eventual death is the only certainty. Patients may live from a few years to over a decade after the onset of dementia. Caregivers often describe their experience as one of living bereavement, as they watch the personality and intellect of their loved one disintegrate. While grieving their loved ones, caregivers also face great challenges maintaining their own quality of life. Caregiving is encompassing, requiring time, energy, and resources that place tremendous strain on an individual.

There are several different theories about peoples' response to the strains of chronic dementia caregiving (1,2). The "wear-and-tear hypothesis" suggests that, over time, caregivers' functioning will steadily decline as a result of prolonged stress. In contrast, the adaptation hypothesis posits that people will adapt to the demands of caregiving over time; their physical and mental health may ultimately stabilize or improve under strenuous circumstances. A third model, the trait hypothesis, suggests that in spite of dementia progression, caregivers may function well because of individual characteristics like personal resources, coping skills, and social supports (1).

Although the adaptation theory has received the most support, a dementia patient's symptoms cannot be defined as "worsening" or increasing; the severity and type of impairments do not proceed in a linear fashion (1). For example, patients may lose the ability to work and manage finances early on, disruptive personality and behavioral problems may appear later, and basic self-care issues are typically problematic later in illness (1). Various illness manifestations affect caregivers differently, with significant personal and social consequences. Thus, caregiver stress, commonly called burden, cannot be tied strictly to the severity of a dementia patient's illness or length of time someone has provided care. Burden is also greatly affected by factors beyond the patient's condition. A person's response to caregiving depends on their ability to manage present symptoms, their support systems, and ways of coping (3–5). The individual's perception of the larger implications and emotional meaning of their loved one's deficits, and conflicts external to their relationship with the patient also play a substantial role in caregiver well-being. By assessing both difficult aspects of caregiving and the protective effects of personal and external resources, we can better understand how caregiver stress evolves.

This chapter addresses a number of issues pertaining to dementia caregivers. First, we discuss caregiver burden, beginning with an overview of key stressful points in dementia. Next, we describe other contributors to burden, including family conflict and social isolation. We explore how variations in family relationships, gender, and race may affect stress and coping. Finally, we focus on the evidence behind caregiver interventions, including respite care. We conclude by looking at the feasibility of individualizing caregiver assessments and interventions, and the role of primary care clinicians in helping caregivers.

CAREGIVER ISSUES OVER THE COURSE OF ALZHEIMER'S DISEASE

Caregivers face different issues throughout Alzheimer's disease, and these vary over the course of illness. In this section, we provide an outline of common dementia patient symptoms in the early, middle, and late stages of illness, and caregivers' responses. Dementia is a dynamic process, and the caregiver must adapt to many alterations in their day-to-day routine, responsibilities, and emotions throughout illness.

Alzheimer's disease may initially appear as short-term memory disturbances or personality changes long before formal diagnosis is made (6). These early symptoms often concern caregivers; in fact, the initial diagnosis may provide some relief. However, an Alzheimer's diagnosis is also stressful, raising many difficult questions for caregivers and patients.

As cognitive changes continue, patients may have difficulty dealing with money or performing tasks like shopping, causing frustrating mistakes. Caregivers may also worry about the patient's safety while driving or using household appliances. Patients often want to continue doing activities, which may be potentially harmful, to retain independence. Meanwhile, caregivers often prefer that patients avoid certain tasks to prevent accidents.

Differing perspectives related to patient activities are common sources of conflict in early illness, and finding solutions that satisfy both parties can be difficult. In addition to addressing immediate concerns, caregivers and patients need to think about the future. Approaching topics such as the possibility of the patient's eventual nursing home placement and advanced directives may be stressful, but discussions would ideally occur while the patient has only mild mental deficits.

In middle phases of illness, patients have poorer short-term memory and communication abilities, greater personality changes, and impairments in abstract thinking and judgment (6,7). These deficits lead to patient confusion and repetitive questioning, which caregivers commonly describe as very burdensome. Patients may also exhibit anger and agitation, which may be more distressing to caregivers than cognitive changes (8,9). Depression, which is also common in dementia patients, greatly worries caregivers (8). As dementia symptoms become more complex, a cycle of negative emotions may begin in both the caregiver and patient.

In addition to contributing to burden, both patient and caregiver depression are risk factors for physical aggression directed toward the caregiver. Indeed, nearly 25% of female caregivers experience some form of aggression from their partner in the middle stages of illness (10). Women should be aware that physical aggression may accompany dementia, so they can feel prepared to assert themselves if needed, preventing harm of themselves or the patient. However, patients may also be victims; as functioning decreases, they are at increased risk for physical or verbal mistreatment (11). Caregivers are more likely to yell at or insult their loved ones if they are depressed or anxious, actions that may lead to feelings of guilt, thus increasing burden.

By the middle to late stages of dementia, many caregivers decide that using respite care or nursing home placement is the best choice to provide optimal care to their loved one and to preserve their own health. Although it would seem that nursing home placement would ultimately decrease caregiver burden, this does not necessarily occur. For example, a recent multi-site study looked at caregiver mental health immediately and 1 year following dementia patient placement into an extended care facility (12). The researchers found that while caregiver anxiety decreased after placement, depression did not. Anxiety was higher in cohabiting caregivers at baseline; improvement may occur when the individual no longer had to deal with unpredictable behavior issues and the patient's poor health status on a daily basis. In contrast, depression may have persisted after placement because of new financial strains, the loss of companionship, and concerns about the quality of nursing home care.

As the patient approaches terminal stages, it is helpful if end-of-life medical care has been discussed. One survey of advanced directives showed that dementia patients were more likely to have a durable power of attorney for health care and living will than other ill elderly patients. By having advanced directives in place, caregivers can be sure that their decisions about life-sustaining measures are aligned with their loved one's wishes (13). Moreover, caregivers who are uncertain about health care decisions have higher rates of depression, and preemptive discussions may reduce future burden (14).

Despite the many difficulties of caregiving, the death of the dementia patient does not reliably ease burden. The year following death, depression often declines, but may remain at a significant level for several years (15,16). More burdened caregivers may be particularly susceptible to depression, and may find that their social networks have deteriorated, leaving them without an important coping resource (15,16).

If available, the support of family and friends can truly make a difference during grieving; caregivers who have social support show reduced risk for depression (15,16). Throughout illness, positive interactions with family may serve as a source of strength and peace. However, in the presence of conflict, family involvement may also hinder caregiver health (17,18).

ADDITIONAL CAREGIVER CHALLENGES: CONFLICTS WITH FAMILY AND FRIENDS

Family conflict may begin with the patient's initial diagnosis. Logically, individuals living with dementia patients, typically spouses, are the first parties to notice memory loss or personality change. Often, these individuals will not share their concerns with others, hoping that these alterations are temporary. However, this silence may be problematic when a dementia diagnosis finally occurs: other family members may then deny that symptoms are significant even when problems may have been present for years. Differing perceptions of disease severity may cause families to clash over the course of their loved one's illness.

Multiple aspects of dementia may induce family controversy, including sharing caregiving and financial responsibilities. Also, it may be challenging for caregivers who are already strained to mediate family disagreements. Families may have difficulty finding practical solutions to problems. Trouble communicating within families may actually increase burden (19,20). Individual or group counseling may help to improve problem solving, collaboration, and conflict resolution, thereby decreasing associated burden (21). Granted, times of stress may not be the most conducive for working toward better communication, but changing negative patterns may significantly lower stress.

Friendships may be less likely to raise conflict and often provide another important source of support for caregivers (4). However, as the patient's cognitive and functional abilities decline, many caregivers lose contact with friends, contributing to social isolation (16,22). While discussing taking care of her husband, one woman said "The hardest part was losing all of our friends. He couldn't play cards anymore, didn't enjoy dinner conversation anymore eventually they stopped calling." Caregivers often report that friends are generally kind and forgiving of patient behaviors when provided with clear explanation in advance. However, combined with potential difficulties in orientation, walking, and continence, behavioral outbursts may contribute to fewer social outings and isolation.

Support groups are one place caregivers may feel comfortable outside their homes. Many groups allow dementia patients to attend, eliminating the caregiver's need for respite care. Thus, support groups are a good way for caregivers to decrease social isolation, in addition to gaining knowledge and receiving emotional support.

THE ROLE OF RELATIONSHIPS, GENDER, AND ETHNICITY IN CAREGIVER STRESS

Dementia patients are most often cared for by their spouses or children. Although burden is a relevant issue for all caregivers, spousal care is more prevalent, and married caregivers seem to be studied more in the literature. Certain elements of caregiving particularly affect spouses, who cope with losses in their intimate relationship while managing the challenges of cohabitation and providing daily care.

Spousal caregivers often take over domestic responsibilities, such as cooking, shopping, and managing finances, that were previously assumed by their partner. As changes in household functioning occur, strain may result. Additionally, spouses may be stressed while adapting to differences in the emotional workings of their relationship. For example, the caregiver might need to adjust their expressions of logic, emotion, or affection to maintain balance within the marriage. Even if relationship changes are desired, adjustments may be stressful. Some spouses have even commented that having a partner with Alzheimer's "is like living with someone new."

Spouses may also be negatively affected as dementia upsets their partner's sleep patterns. Dementia patients' sleep cycles are commonly abnormal, resulting in odd hours of rest and wakefulness (6,23). Incontinence and yelling may also disrupt the patient's sleep, and in turn, their spouse's. Whether spouses share a bed or sleep separately, these disturbances can decrease the quantity and quality of caregivers' rest, affecting their mood, energy, and health.

Adult children caring for their parents may not always experience the strains of cohabitation, but are stressed in other ways. Filial caregivers, while caring for their own children, may feel guilt that they are not doing enough for their parents (22). In addition to being torn by family responsibilities, sons and daughters may also continue working while managing caregiving.

Due to competing obligations, employment can become increasingly difficult, and many caregivers report voluntarily cutting back work hours (24). Employees may also be late or absent, and work tensions may contribute to burden (25). Despite difficulties balancing work and caregiving, many people say that their employers have been quite flexible and understanding. Still, lost work time may lead to financial strain, contributing to burden.

Regardless of their relationship to the care recipient, women are more commonly caregivers, and they typically spend more hours providing care than men (26,27). Across cultures, women report the most burden and are at greater risk for depression and anxiety as the patient's health worsens (26–29). The physical health of women also declines while caregiving, whereas men pay more attention to their own health and are less likely to have health decrements.

In holding themselves to internal and societal expectations, women may feel that they should be able to independently provide support to an ill relative. Consequently, they may experience feelings of guilt in taking time for themselves or asking for help (30). In their roles as wives, mothers, and daughters, women may take sole responsibility for caregiving; if family members do not offer assistance, women may not ask for it, even under great stress. One spousal caregiver described caregiving for her husband as a nuptial and maternal duty saying "He's not the kids' responsibility. I don't want him to be a burden to them."

Although husbands or wives may take on the role of household money manager, greater attention has recently been given to helping elderly women manage finances (31). Elderly women may experience both gender and age discrimination in handling business matters, which may have been previously reduced by their spouse's involvement (30,31). For both women and men who lack experience, instruction in financial management may help to prevent stress by decreasing actual difficulties and anxiety related to potential problems.

Racial differences may also affect how individuals handle caregiving stress. African-American caregivers may feel more positively about caregiving, and may have different ways of coping. For example, they report more reliance on religion, including prayer and attending formal services, and may place greater importance on religion in general (32). Additionally, African-American caregivers are less distressed by memory and behavior problems (33).

Latino caregivers place a similar emphasis on religion and may be more likely to use spiritual coping (34,35). Religious values may influence Latino caregivers' acceptance of the role, viewing challenges as fate from God to enhance spiritual growth (35). Latinos also view caregiving more positively than Caucasians. It has been suggested that differences in satisfaction may arise from the cultural emphasis on family and the benefits of caregiving to the larger family unit. Cultural values may translate into a greater acceptance of caregiving from the beginning: Mexican Americans take on the caregiver role earlier than Caucasians, even when their relatives are less impaired (35).

Like Latinos, African Americans may also more readily accept caregiving, due to the expectation that children will take care of their parents in old age, as well as a greater traditional respect for elders in black culture. In contrast, caregiving may be seen as a process that is unexpected and interruptive of plans for retirement in white culture; feelings of loss that accompany caregiving may extend to personal goals that an individual may have had for later life (36). The aforementioned differences highlight only a few of many cultural variations that may exist in caregiver beliefs, stress, and coping. It is increasingly important for clinicians and researchers to acknowledge cultural differences to effectively intervene in problems facing people of all backgrounds.

As we have shown, burden is affected not only by behaviors of the dementia patient, but characteristics of the caregiver and the context of their life. Stress affects the individual, their relationships with their family and friends, work abilities, and the patient's health. If these are not reasons enough to be concerned with stress, we turn to another consequence of caregiving: the negative effects of burden on the caregiver's physical health.

HEALTH OUTCOMES OF CAREGIVING: STRESS, IMMUNE DYSFUNCTION, AND INFLAMMATION

How significant is the caregiver's response to stress? To illustrate this point with the most dramatic example, one prospective longitudinal study found that, over a 4-year period, the relative risk for all-cause mortality among strained caregivers was 63% higher than non-caregiving controls (37). The causes of increased mortality are many, but research on stress and the immune system provides important insights about the interplay between stress and health, and the dangers of chronic stress for older adults.

The immunological decrements associated with the stress of caregiving are of particular concern because older individuals already have age-related reductions in cellular immune function with important health consequences. Older adults are generally more susceptible to infectious diseases such as influenza and pneumonia which are major causes of death in this age group (38). Furthermore, caregivers appear to be at even greater risk for these illnesses. For example, dementia caregivers exhibit significant deficits relative to well-matched non-caregivers in their immune responses to an influenza virus vaccine (39,40). Caregivers also may have poorer immune responses to pneumococcal vaccines than age-matched non-caregivers (41). Adults who show poorer responses to vaccines also experience higher rates of clinical illness, and these vaccine data suggest that caregivers have increased vulnerability to influenza and pneumonia infections, as well as other infectious agents (38).

The immune system also has a central role in wound healing, and caregiving-related distress provokes substantial delays in wound healing (42). Clinically, differences in wound healing leave caregivers susceptible to prolonged pain and recovery post-surgery or injury and higher rates of infection. Repeated, chronic, or slow-resolving infections or wounds enhance secretion of proinflammatory cytokines, important chemical mediators in the immune system.

Some of the key evidence about caregiver physical health risks comes from studies on proinflammatory cytokines, and their secondary effects on stress hormones and immune response. Cytokines modulate the body's immune response by attracting immune cells to sites of infection or injury, and priming them to become activated to respond (43). Interleukin-6 (IL-6) is one cytokine of particular relevance. Epidemiological studies of individuals 65 years or older have found that the highest quartile of serum IL-6, values greater than 3.19 pg/mL, was associated with twofold greater risk of death compared to the lowest quartile (44,45).

The production of proinflammatory cytokines is stimulated by both depression and stress (46–50). Some of the strongest data have come from studies of caregivers. One longitudinal community study assessed IL-6 production over six years in 119 spousal dementia caregivers and 106 non-caregivers who were matched for chronic health problems, medications, and health behaviors (51). Caregivers' average rate of increase in IL-6 was about four times as large as that of non-caregivers. Moreover, the mean annual changes in IL-6 among former caregivers did not differ from that of current caregivers even several years after the death of the impaired spouse. In this study, the data suggested that spousal caregivers would have reached the upper quartile for IL-6 levels around age 75; this level would not be reached by average non-caregiving controls until after age 90 (51).

The risks associated with increased IL-6 and proinflammatory cytokines have been highlighted in recent medical literature. The link to cardiovascular disease, the leading cause of death, has attracted the greatest attention; the association with IL-6 is related in part to the central role that this cytokine plays in promoting the production of C-reactive protein (CRP), an important risk factor for myocardial infarction (52–54).

In addition to cardiovascular disease, inflammation has been linked to a spectrum of other major health problems associated with aging, including osteoporosis, arthritis, type 2 diabetes, certain lymphoproliferative diseases or cancers (including multiple myeloma, non-Hodgkin's lymphoma, and chronic lymphocytic leukemia), Alzheimer's disease, and periodontal disease (55). More globally, chronic inflammation has been suggested as one key biological mechanism that may fuel declines in physical function leading to frailty, disability, and, ultimately, death (56–57).

For clinicians, these data highlight the importance of assessing both psychosocial and biomedical risk factors in caregivers. Scientifically, the data provide insight about the interplay between stress and health, and the dangers of chronic stress for the elderly.

POSITIVE ASPECTS OF CAREGIVING

Although it is important to understand the significance of burden, the positive aspects of caregiving must not be overlooked. Amidst the challenges, many individuals find enhanced spirituality, self-efficacy, and personal growth through caring for a loved one. Companionship and a sense of purpose are parts of caregiving that many individuals appreciate (58). The majority of caregivers report that they feel needed and good about themselves, and have a greater appreciation of life since they have been caring for their loved one (59). Many people say that caregiving has strengthened their relationships with others, and has improved their attitude toward life (59).

People who find positive elements in their experience are less depressed and burdened than those who do not (58). Also, individuals who focus on gains, rather than losses, rate their quality of life higher than those who do not (60). The caregiver's outlook may change throughout the patient's illness, and positive perceptions may be a useful indicator of mental health in addition to negative measures, such as depression and burden (58).

CAREGIVER INTERVENTIONS

The many factors contributing to burden make it difficult to identify specific interventions, even after decades of caregiver research. Typically, educating caregivers on disease course, managing dementia behaviors, and addressing legal and financial issues does not appear to reduce burden alone (61,62). Combining educational interventions with another type of support may be more helpful (63). Unfortunately, the evidence thus far is that individual counseling and caregiver support groups often show only short-term effectiveness. Thus, caregivers may find psychosocial interventions useful in crisis; however, they have shown little success in the long-term reduction of burden and depression. Respite care, assistance provided by formal, paid personnel, or unpaid family and friends, has been researched more extensively than other non-pharmacologic interventions; however, the results have been mixed.

Some studies show that respite care decreases burden, while others do not (64–67). Differences may be due to difficulties accessing care, or increases in caregiver guilt associated with the use of respite care. Many caregivers also use respite time for work, which may contribute to stress during non-caregiving time (64). Despite gaps in evidence as to its efficacy in decreasing caregiver burden, respite care remains a cornerstone of caregiver support.

Adult day centers are the largest growing segment of respite care, ideally providing meaningful activities and social interaction for dementia patients, and a break for caregivers (68). Some care centers also provide meals and transportation. In spite of these benefits, respite care is often underutilized due to costs, convenience, and the dementia patient's response to the care environment. When asked why they do not use respite services, 48% of caregivers cite inconvenience associated with hours and location, and program styles not matching their needs (69). Health care and social service professionals can look to area Alzheimer's associations, senior organizations, long-term care facilities, and adult day care programs to make appropriate recommendations to their clients.

Adult day care costs currently averaged around $46 per day in 2004 (68). Possibly due to the cost, day care is utilized over three times more frequently by households with an income over $50,000 per year (68). Even though government programs may subsidize the costs of day care for low-income families, barriers still remain. Racial disparities exist as with many community resources in that a smaller proportion of minorities use respite care than non-minorities (70).

Approximately one-third of caregivers do not use respite care because of the dementia patient's negative response (69). Early stage Alzheimer's patients often become depressed or irritated after day care as they are surrounded by others whom they recognize as more ill than themselves. Late stage patients often become agitated in any new environment, which can cause additional home stress after a session at day care. Caregivers who do not use formal respite care may not need it if they receive unpaid assistance from family and friends; however, if people believe they have a greater duty to independently provide care, they are also less likely to use respite care (70). Therefore, caregivers should be assisted in finding programs that suit their needs, and encouraged to use respite care if they think it would be helpful.

Home health is the most preferred form of respite care and may be more highly utilized if available. Caregivers report greater trust with the safety and quality of home health care compared with nursing home care (71). Caregivers are also more likely to use respite time for patient self-care if it occurs in the home. Still, conflicting research exists regarding the effects of home health on burden.

For example, caregiver depression and subjective burden did not decrease over a 3-month period of home health assistance (72). Nevertheless, the authors suggest that care provision by personnel who could also provide patient education, such as nurses or social workers, may be more likely to reduce depression and burden (72). Although many caregivers prefer home health, respite care outside the home may be more beneficial. One excellent study showed that caregivers' feelings of depression, anger, and strain decreased significantly following use of adult day care for 3 months (67).

Research designed to isolate one type of intervention may not necessarily capture circumstances that are true to life. For instance, most support groups are both emotionally supportive and educational, and many people may participate in these while they utilize respite care. These realistic situations are not always reflected in study design. Also, researchers do not typically screen caregivers for specific problems before testing the usefulness of particular interventions (73). Therefore, problem-specific interventions may have better results if applied to people with related needs.

Reviewers of caregiving literature say that multi-component interventions, which include education, social support, respite, and psychotherapy, most effectively reduce negative outcomes of caregiving (61,62,73). Multi-component interventions decrease depression and burden while improving knowledge and overall well-being.

ADDRESSING CAREGIVER NEEDS IN PRIMARY CARE

The implementation of multi-component, individualized caregiver interventions provides a challenge: who has the time, money, and knowledge needed to work with caregivers in this way? Specialized groups like the Alzheimer's Association do an excellent job providing services to those with whom they come in contact. However, research illustrates differences in the utilization of caregiver resources related to gender, race, socioeconomic status, and geographic location. Although many health care providers make referrals to these resources, many caregivers do not or cannot access them.

The majority of caregivers report that, aside from family, physicians are their primary source of support (74). Routine contact with health professionals may alone improve caregiver health, by increasing social support and reducing isolation (75). Specialists may provide expert advice in dementia management, but family practice clinicians, including physicians, physician's assistants (PAs), and nurse practitioners (NPs), may see caregivers and dementia patients more frequently. Indeed, primary care providers (PCPs) may serve as the main professional support for some caregivers, particularly to families with limited access to health care and social services (76).

A greater awareness of caregiver needs will help clinicians serve this population. Caregivers summarize their concerns as both emotional and practical (76,77). They report needing help with dealing with change, managing competing responsibilities and stressors, and experiencing emotional responses to care provision. As stated previously, an individual's perspective on illness and their role can affect their mental health. In addition to providing emotional support and screening for depression and anxiety, PCPs should encourage caregivers to seek help from friends and family, and counseling or spiritual support if appropriate.

Local resources often include 24-hour helplines for caregivers or the elderly; caregivers should be aware of these and also be encouraged to seek help if they ever feel like hurting the patient or themselves.

Caregivers additionally seek advice about providing care, and finding and using resources, concerns which PCPs should be prepared to address (76,77). As patients' functioning decreases, a wider range of skills may be needed to provide care and caregivers will likely need guidance. In addition to discussing management of activities of daily living/instrumental activities of daily living during appointments, PCPs should also consider referral to outside agencies for assistance, including home nursing care, and physical and occupational therapy (78). Eventually, respite care and adult day facilities, and long-term care or hospice may be necessary (78,79).

By asking caregivers specifically about their own concerns with caregiving, and screening for common problems such as depression, anxiety, sleep disturbance, and fatigue, clinicians can begin to assess caregiver issues. After identifying a particular problem, understanding the effects of patient behaviors on a caregiver's condition may be important in finding effective treatment for the caregiver. For example, caregiver sleep disturbance is one common problem that may have multiple causes, including incontinence or patient-related issues. In this case, triggers and management of patient-related behaviors should be addressed. However, caregiver sleep may be additionally affected by psychological factors like depression or anxiety, or poor sleep hygiene.

True solutions to caregiver problems may involve interventions for both patient and caregiver, and clinicians must provide treatment that caregivers will actually follow. For instance, many caregivers refuse to take sleeping pills for fear that they will not hear the dementia patient in need, so adherence to sedating medications may be low. Although less-sedating alternatives may be available, some patients may strongly prefer non-pharmacologic interventions.

Many clinicians may not be able to schedule time to talk extensively with patients and caregivers. However, longer appointments may be cost effective due to the potential resultant decreases in medication and health care utilization (80). For example, the results of one study showed that caregivers with detailed verbal and written instructions related to sleep hygiene and regular exercise had significantly higher compliance than those with written information only (80). The group with more instruction also showed greater declines in depression, anxiety, and health care utilization.

One large multi-site study compared interventions to be implemented during a primary care office visit (63). One included only dementia-focused education and another included the same patient education with an additional stress management component. The stress management portion of the intervention included discussions of coping with negative thoughts and feelings, dealing with grief and improving communication, and teaching anger management and relaxation techniques. The combined educational and stress management intervention lasted 60 minutes per session. The inclusion of stress management assistance resulted in significantly lower depression 6 and 18 months later. While these sessions were "brief" with respect to some, they were not reflective of a typical 15-minute office visit in primary care today. Although components of these examples of primary care interventions may be useful in certain clinical settings, greater attention is needed toward the feasibility of these interventions. By designing and testing interventions that are widely useable, we will be better able to treat caregiver stress on a clinical level.

Multi-component interventions, described as ideal by research, are implemented by large groups like the Alzheimer's Association. Because these coordinated services are unavailable to many caregivers, clinicians should strive to holistically manage caregiver needs by mirroring comprehensive evidence-based interventions to the best of their ability. While health care, mental health, and social service providers cannot remove the causes of burden, they can certainly help the caregiver to manage stressors by working together to improve the quality of life of both the caregiver and the dementia patient.

REFERENCES

1. Haley WE, Pardo M. Relationship of severity of dementia to caregiving stressors. Psychol Aging 1989; 4(4):389–392.
2. Townsend AL, Noelker L, Deimling G, et al. Longitudinal impact of interhousehold caregiving on adult children's mental health. Psychol Aging 1989; 4(4):393–401.
3. Pearlin LI, Mullan JT, Semple SJ, et al. Caregiving and the stress process: An overview of concepts and their measures. Gerontologist 1990; 30(5):583–594.
4. Yates ME, Tennstedt S, Chang B. Contributors to and mediators of psychological well-being for informal caregivers. J Gerontol B Psychol Sci Soc Sci 1999; 54(1):P12–P22.
5. Talkington-Boyer S, Snyder K. Assessing impact on family caregivers to Alzheimer's disease patients. Am J Fam Ther 1994; 22(1):57–66.
6. Griggs RC, Jozefowocz RF, Amenoff MJ. Approach to the patient with neurologic disease. In: Cooper JAD, Pappas PG, eds. Cecil Textbook of Medicine, 22nd ed. Philadelphia, PA: Elsevier Saunders, 2004:2253–2255.
7. Mittelman MS. Community caregiving. Alzheimers Care Q 2003; 4(4):273–285.
8. Mourik JC, Rosso SM, Niermeijer MF, et al. Frontotemporal dementia: Behavioral symptoms and caregiver distress. Dement Geriatr Cogn Disord 2004; 18(3–4):299–306.
9. Donaldson C, Tarrier N, Burns A. Determinants of carer stress in Alzheimer's disease. Int J Geriatr Psychiatry 1998; 13(4):248–256.
10. O'Leary D, Jyringi D, Sedler M. Childhood conduct problems, stages of Alzheimer's disease, and physical aggression against caregivers. International J Geriatr Psychiatry 2005; 20(5):401–405.
11. Beach SR, Schulz R, Williamson G, et al. Risk factors for informal caregiver behavior. J Am Geriatr Soc 2005; 53(2):255–261.
12. Schulz R, Belle SH, Czaja SJ, et al. Long-term care placement of dementia patients and caregiver health and well-being. JAMA 2004; 292(8):961–967.
13. Mezey M, Kluger M, Maislin G, et al. Life sustaining treatment decisions by spouses of patients with Alzheimer's disease. J Am Geriatr Soc 1996; 44:144–150.
14. Smerglia VL, Deimling GT. Care related decision making satisfaction and caregiver well-being. Gerontologist 1997; 37(5):658–665.
15. Aneshensel CS, Botticello AL, Yamamoto-Mitani N. When caregiving ends: The course of depressive symptoms after bereavement. J Health Soc Behav 2004; 45(4):422–440.
16. Robinson-Whelen S, Tada Y, MacCallum RC, et al. Long-term caregiving: What happens when it ends? J Abnorm Psychol 2001; 110(4):573–584.
17. Gaugler JE, Davey A, Pearlin LI, et al. Modeling caregiver adaptation over time: The longitudinal impact of behavior problems. Psychol Aging 2000; 15(3):437–450.
18. Semple SJ. Conflict in Alzheimer's caregiving families: Its dimensions and consequences. Gerontologist 1992; 32(5):648–655.
19. Mitrani VB, Feaster DJ, McCabe BE, et al. Adapting the structural family systems rating to assess patterns of interaction in families of dementia caregivers. Gerontologist 2005; 45(4):445–455.
20. Heru AM, Ryan CE, Iqbal A. Family functioning in the caregivers of patients with dementia. Int J Geriatr Psychiatry 2004; 19(6):533–537.

21. Fisher L, Weihs KL. Can addressing relationships improve outcomes in chronic disease? (Report of the National Working Group on Family-Based Interventions in Chronic Disease.) J Fam Pract 2000; 49(6):561–566.
22. Ankri J, Andrieu S, Beaufils B, et al. Beyond the global score of the Zarit Burden Interview: Useful dimensions for clinicians. Int J Geriatr Psychiatry 2005; 20(3):254–260.
23. Purandare N, Burns A, Burns A. Behavioural and psychological symptoms of dementia. Rev Clin Gerontol 2000; 10:245–260.
24. National Alliance for Caregiving and the American Association of Retired Persons. Family caregiving in the US: findings from a national survey. NAC and AARP, 1997. Web. 21 September 2010.
25. Edwards AB, Zarit SH, Stephens MAP, et al. Employed family caregivers of cognitively impaired elderly: An examination of role strain and depressive symptoms. Aging Ment Health 2002; 6(1):55–61.
26. Barber CE, Pasley K. Family care of Alzheimer's patients: The role of gender and generational relationship on caregiver outcomes. J Appl Gerontol 1995; 14(2):172–192.
27. Yee JL, Schulz R. Gender differences in psychiatric morbidity among family caregivers: A review and analysis. Gerontologist 2000; 40(2):147–164.
28. Adams B, Aranda MP, Kemp B, et al. Ethnic and gender differences in distress among Anglo American, African American, Japanese American, and Mexican American spousal caregivers of persons with dementia. J Clin Gastroenterol 2002; 8:279–301.
29. Bedard M, Kuzik R, Chambers L, et al. Understanding burden differences between men and women caregivers: The contribution of care-recipient problem behaviors. Int Psychogeriatr 2005; 17(1):99–118.
30. Estes CL, Zulman DM. Informalization of caregiving: A gender lens. In: Harrington C, Estes CL, eds. Health Policy: Crisis and Reform in the U.S. Health Care Delivery System, 4th ed. Sudbury, Massachusetts: Jones & Bartlett Publishers, 2004:147–156.
31. Into FH. Older women and financial management: Strategies for maintaining independence. Educ Gerontol 2003; 29(10):825–839.
32. Haley WE, Gitlin LN, Wisniewski SR, et al. Well-being, appraisal, and coping in African-American and Caucasian dementia caregivers: Findings from the REACH study. Aging Ment Health 2004; 8(4):316–329.
33. McClendon MJ, Smyth KA, Neundorfer MM. Survival of persons with Alzheimer's disease: Caregiver coping matters. Gerontologist 2004; 44(4):508–519.
34. Coon DW, Rubert M, Solano N, et al. Well-being, appraisal, and coping in Latina and Caucasian female dementia caregivers: Findings from the REACH study. Aging Ment Health 2004; 8(4):330–345.
35. Phillips LR, Torres de Ardon E, Komnenich P, et al. The Mexican-American caregiving experience. Hisp J Behav Sci 2000; 22(3):296–313.
36. Haley WE, Roth DL, Coleton MI, et al. Appraisal, coping, and social support as mediators of well-being in Black and White family caregivers of patients with Alzheimer's disease. J Consult Clin Psychol 1996; 64(1):121–129.
37. Schulz R, Beach R. Caregiving as a risk factor for mortality: The Caregiver Health Effects Study. JAMA 1999; 282(23):2215–2219.
38. Burns EA, Goodwin JS. Immunodeficiency of aging. Drugs Aging 1997; 11:374–397.
39. Kiecolt-Glaser JK, Glaser R, Gravenstein S, et al. Chronic stress alters the immune response to influenza virus vaccine in older adults. Proc Natl Acad Sci U S A 1996; 93:3043–3047.
40. Vedhara K, Cox NKM, Wilcock GK, et al. Chronic stress in elderly carers of dementia patients and antibody response to influenza vaccination. Lancet 1999; 353:627–631.
41. Glaser R, Sheridan JF, Malarkey WB, et al. Chronic stress modulates the immune response to a pneumococcal pneumonia vaccine. Psychosom Med 2000; 62:804–807.
42. Kiecolt-Glaser JK, Marucha PT, Malarkey WB, et al. Slowing of wound healing by psychological stress. Lancet 1995; 346:1194–1196.
43. Kiecolt-Glaser JK, Glaser R. Depression and immune function: Central pathways to morbidity and mortality. J Psychosom Res 2002; 53:873–876.

44. Harris T, Ferrucci L, Tracy RP, et al. Associations of elevated interleukin-6 and C-reactive protein levels with mortality in the elderly. Am J Med 1999; 106;506–512.
45. Reuben DB, Ferrucci L, Wallace R, et al. The prognostic value of serum albumin in healthy older persons with low and high serum interleukin-6 (IL-6) levels. J Am Geriatr Soc 2000; 48:1404–1407.
46. Miller AH. Neuroendocrine and immune system interactions in stress and depression. Psychiatr Clin North Am 1998; 21;443–463.
47. Dentino AN, Pieper CF, Rao KMK, et al. Association of interleukin-6 and other biologic variables with depression in older people living in the community. J Am Geriatr Soc 1999; 47:6–11.
48. Lutgendorf SK, Garand L, Buckwalter KC, et al. Life stress, mood disturbance, and elevated interleukin-6 in healthy older women. J Gerontol A Biol Sci Med Sci 1999; 54:M434–M439.
49. Penninx BWJH, Leveille S, Ferrucci L, et al. Exploring the effect of depression on physical disability: Longitudinal evidence from the established populations for epidemiologic studies of the elderly. Am J Public Health 1999; 89:1346–1352.
50. Irwin M. Psychoneuroimmunology of depression: Clinical implications. Brain Behav Immun 2002; 16:146.
51. Kiecolt-Glaser JK, Preacher KJ, MacCallum RC, et al. Chronic stress and age-related increases in the proinflammatory cytokine IL-6. Proc Natl Acad Sci U S A 2003; 100;9090–9095.
52. Ridker PM, Cushman M, Stampfer MJ, et al. Inflammation, aspirin, and the risk of cardiovascular disease in apparently healthy men. N Engl J Med 1997; 336:973–979.
53. Papanicolaou DA, Wilder RL, Manolagas SC, et al. The pathophysiologic roles of interleukin-6 in human disease. Ann Intern Med 1998; 128;127–137.
54. Kiechl S, Egger G, Mayr M, et al. Chronic infections and the risk of carotid atherosclerosis: Prospective results from a large population study. Circulation 2001; 103:1064–1070.
55. Ershler W, Keller E. "Age-associated increased interleukin-6 gene expression, late-life diseases, and frailty." Ann Intern Med 2000; 51:245–270.
56. Hamerman D. Toward an understanding of frailty. Ann Intern Med 1999; 130:945–950.
57. Taaffe DR, Harris TB, Ferrucci L, et al. Cross-sectional and prospective relationships of interleukin-6 and C-reactive protein with physical performance in elderly persons: MacArthur Studies of Successful Aging. J Gerontol A Biol Sci Med Sci 2000; 55:M709–M715.
58. Cohen CA, Colanonio A, Vernich L. Positive aspects of caregiving: Rounding out the caregiving experience. Int J Geriatr Psychiatry 2003; 17:184–188.
59. Tarlow BJ, Wisniewski SR, Belle SH, et al. Positive aspects of caregiving: Contributions of the REACH project to the development of new measures for Alzheimer's caregiving. Res Aging 2004; 4(26):429–453.
60. Pinquart M, Sorensen S. Associations of caregiver stressors and uplifts with subjective well-being and depressive mood: A meta-analytic comparison. Aging Ment Health 2004; 8(5):438–449.
61. Sorensen S, Pinquart M, Duberstein P. How effective are interventions with caregivers? An updated meta-analysis. Gerontologist 2002; 42(3):356–372.
62. Brodaty H, Green A, Koschera A. Meta-analysis of psychosocial interventions for caregivers of people with dementia. J Am Geriatr Soc 2003; 51(5):657–664.
63. Burns R, Nichols LO, Martindale-Adams J, et al. Primary care interventions for dementia caregivers: 2-Year outcomes from the REACH study. Gerontologist 2003; 43(4):547–555.
64. Berry GL, Zarit SH, Rabatin VX. Caregiver activity on respite and nonrespite days: A comparison of two service approaches. Gerontologist 1991; 31(6):830–835.
65. Lawton MY, Brody E, Saperstein AR. A multi-service respite program for caregivers of Alzheimer's patients. J Gerontol Soc Work 1989; 14:41–74.
66. Lee H, Cameron M. Respite care for people with dementia and their carers. The Cochrane Database of Systematic Reviews 2004, Issue 1. Art. No.: CD004396.pub2. DOI: 10.1002/14651858.CD004396.pub2.

67. Zarit SH, Stephens MAP, Townsend A, et al. Stress reduction for family caregivers: Effects of adult day care use. J Gerontol B Psychol Sci Soc Sci 1998; 53B(5):s267–s277.
68. Reever KE, Mathieu E, Gitlin LN, et al. Adult day services plus: Augmenting adult day centers with systematic care management for family caregivers. Alzheimers Care Q 2004; 5(4):332–339.
69. Beisecker AE, Wright LJ, Chrisman SK, et al. Family caregiver perceptions of benefits and barriers to the use of adult day care for individuals with Alzheimer's disease. Res Aging 1996; 18(4):430–450.
70. Kosloski K, Montgomery RJV, Youngbauer JG. Utilization of respite services: A comparison of users, seekers, and non-seekers. J Appl Gerontol 2001; 20(1):111–132.
71. Feinberg LF, Whitlatch J. Family caregivers and in-home respite options: The consumer-directed versus agency-based experience. J Gerontol Soc Work 1998; 30 (3–4):9–28.
72. Schwarz KA, Blixen CE. Does home health care affect strain and depressive symptomatology for caregivers of impaired older adults? J Community Health Nurs 1997; 14(1):39–48.
73. Acton GJ, Kang J. Interventions to reduce the burden of caregiving for an adult with dementia: A meta-analysis. Res Nurs Health 2001; 24(5):349–360.
74. Loos C, Bowd A. Caregivers of persons with Alzheimer's disease: Some neglected implications of the experience of personal loss and grief. Death Stud 1997; 21(5):501–514.
75. Castro CM, Wilcox S, O'Sullivan P, et al. An exercise program for women who are caring for relatives with dementia. Psychosom Med 2002; 64(3):458–468.
76. Fortinsky RH. Health care triads and dementia care: Integrative framework and future directions. Aging Ment Health 2001; 5(suppl 1):S35–S48.
77. Farran CJ, Loukissa D, Perraud S, et al. Alzheimer's disease caregiving information and skills. Part II: Family caregiver issues and concerns. Res Nurs Health 2004; 27(1):40–51.
78. Coon DW, Williams MP, Moore RJ, et al. The Northern California Chronic Care Network for Dementia. J Am Geriatr Soc 2004; 52(1):150–156.
79. Gitlin LN, Hauck WW, Dennis MP, et al. Maintenance of effects of the home environmental skill-building program for family caregivers and individuals with Alzheimer's disease and related disorders. J Gerontol A Biol Sci Med Sci 2005; 60(3):368–374.
80. McCurry SM, Gibbons LE, Logsdon RG, et al. Nighttime insomnia treatment and education for Alzheimer's disease: A randomized, controlled trial. J Am Geriatr Soc 2005; 53(5):793.

12 Local and national resource listing

Nancy Theado-Miller

Care options and services	Administration on Aging
	Alzheimer's Association
	Alzheimer's Foundation of America
	American Health Care Association
	Assisted Living Federation of America
	Centers for Medicare and Medicaid
	Eldercare Locator
	National Adult Day Services Association
	National Association of Area Agencies on Aging
	National Association of Geriatric Care Managers
	ParentGiving
Caregiver support	ADEAR
	Administration on Aging
	Alzheimer's Association
	Alzheimer's Disease International
	Alzheimer's Foundation of America
	Alzheimer's Resource Room
	Alzheimer's Society
	Alzheimer's Society of Canada
	AlzOnline
	American Health Assistance Foundation
	Association for Frontotemporal Dementias
	Centers for Medicare and Medicaid
	Children of Aging Parents
	Creutzfeldt–Jakob Foundation
	ElderCare Online
	Ethnic Elders Care
	Family Caregiver Alliance
	Foundation for Health in Aging
	Healing Well
	Lewy Body Dementia Association
	National Family Caregivers Association
	ParentGiving
Caregiving products	Alzheimer's Store
	Caregivers World
	ParentGiving
Chat rooms and Message boards	Alzheimer's Association
	AlzOnline
	Children of Aging Parents
	ElderCare Online
	Healing Well
	National Family Caregivers Association
	ParentGiving

Congressional advocacy	AARP
	Alzheimer's Association
	Alzheimer's Foundation of America
	American Health Care Association
	Creutzfeldt–Jakob Foundation
	Family Caregiver Alliance
	Foundation for Health in Aging
	National Association of Area Agencies on Aging
	National Family Caregivers Association
Consumer education materials	ADEAR
	Administration on Aging
	Alzheimer's Association
	Alzheimer's Disease International
	Alzheimer's Foundation of America
	Alzheimer's Society
	American Geriatrics Society (education link)
	American Health Assistance Foundation
	Centers for Medicare and Medicaid
	Eldercare Locator
	Family Caregiver Alliance
	Geriatric Resources
	Healing Well
End-of-life care	National Hospice and Palliative Care Organization
Financial planning	AARP
	Financial Planning Association
Fundraising	Alzheimer's Association
	Alzheimer's Society
	Alzheimer's Society of Canada
	Foundation for Health in Aging
General Alzheimer's disease and related dementias information	ADEAR
	Alzheimer's Association
	Alzheimer's Disease International
	Alzheimer's Foundation of America
	Alzheimer Research Forum
	Alzheimer's Resource Room
	Alzheimer's Society
	Alzheimer's Society of Canada
	Association for Frontotemporal Dementias
	Creutzfeldt–Jakob Foundation
	Lewy Body Dementia Association
	National Institute of Aging
	National Institute of Neurological Disease and Stroke
Health insurance	AARP
	Centers for Medicare and Medicaid
	Children of Aging Parents
Legal assistance	AARP
	National Academy of Elder Law Attorneys
Medication assistance programs	Aricept—Pfizer
	Exelon—Novartis
	Namenda—Forest
Professional organizations	American Academy of Neurology
	American Association for Geriatric Psychiatry
	American Geriatric Society

	American Medical Directors Association
	American Neuropsychiatric Association
	Gerontological Advanced Practice Nurses Association
	National Adult Day Services Association
	National Association of Geriatric Care Managers
Publications	ADEAR
	Agency for Healthcare Research and Quality
	Alzheimer's Association
	Alzheimer's Foundation of America
	Foundation for Health in Aging
	National Institute of Aging
	National Institute of Health
Research—clinical trials and funding information	ADEAR
	Agency for Healthcare Research and Quality
	Alzheimer's Association
	Alzheimer's Disease Cooperative Study
	Alzheimer's Disease Neuroimaging Initiative
	Alzheimer Research Forum
	Alzheimer's Resource Room
	Alzheimer's Society
	Alzheimer's Society of Canada
	Association for Frontotemporal Dementias
	Lewy Body Dementia Association
	National Institute of Aging
	National Institute of Health
	National Institute of Health (clinical trials link)
Safety	Alzheimer's Association
	Alzheimer's Foundation of America
	ParentGiving

AARP
American Association of Retired Persons, 601 E Street NW, Washington, DC 20049, 1–888-678—2277, www.aarp.org

ADEAR
Alzheimer's Disease Education and Referral Center, PO Box 8250, Silver Spring, MD 20907–8250, 1–800-438–4380, http://www.nia.nih.gov/alzheimers

Administration on Aging
Washington, DC 20201, 1–202-619–0724, www.aoa.gov

Agency for Healthcare Research and Quality
540 Gaither Road, Rockville, MD 20850, 1–301-427–1364, www.ahrq.gov

Alzheimer's Association National Office
225 N. Michigan Avenue, Floor 17
Chicago, IL 60601, 1–800-272–3900, www.alz.org

Alzheimer's Disease Cooperative Study
9500 Gilman Drive # 0853, La Jolla, CA 92093–0853, 1–858-822–1030, www.adcs.org

Alzheimer's Disease International
64 Great Suffolk Street, London SE1 OBL, UK, www.alz.co.uk

Alzheimer's Disease Neuroimaging Initiative
4150 Clement St., San Francisco, CA 94121, www.adni-info.org

Alzheimer's Foundation of America
322 8th Ave, 6th Fl, New York, NY 10001, 1–866-232–8484, www.alzfdn.org

Alzheimer Research Forum
www.alzforum.org

The Alzheimer's Resource Room
Administration on Aging, Washington, DC 20201, 1–202-619–0724, www.aoa.gov/alz

Alzheimer's Society
Devon House, 58 St Katherine's Way London E1W 1JX, 011–44-20–7423-3500,
www.alzheimers.org.uk

Alzheimer's Society of Canada, 20 Eglinton Ave. W., Ste. 1600, Toronto, ON M4R 1K8,
1–416-488–8772, www.alzheimer.ca

The Alzheimer's Store by Ageless Design
12633 159th Court North, Jupiter, FL 33478–6669, 1–800-752–3238, www.alzstore.com

Alzonline
Alzheimer's Online, 1–866-260–2466, www.alzonline.net

American Academy of Neurology
1080 Montreal Avenue, Saint Paul, MN 55116, 1–800-879–1960, www.aan.com

American Association for Geriatric Psychiatry
7910 Woodmont Ave., Suite 1050, Bethesda, MD 20814–3004, 1–301-654–7850,
www.aagponline.org

American Geriatrics Society
The Empire State Building, 350 Fifth Ave, Ste 801, New York, NY 10118, 1–212-308–1414,
www.americangeriatrics.org

American Geriatrics Society (education link)
www.healthinaging.org/aging

American Health Assistance Foundation
22512 Gateway Center Drive, Clarksburg, MD 20871, 1–800-437–2423, www.ahaf.org

American Health Care Association
1201 L Street NW, Washington, DC 20005, 1–202-842–4444, www.ahca.org

American Medical Directors Association
10480 Little Patuxent Parkway, Ste 760, Columbia, MD 21044, 1–800-876–2632,
www.amda.org

American Neuropsychiatric Association
700 Ackerman Road, Suite 625, Columbus, OH 43202, 1–614-447–2077,
www.anpaonline.org

Aricept Patient Assistance Program—Pfizer
PO Box 679, Sommerville, NJ 08876, www.aricept.com

Assisted Living Federation of America
1650 King St, Ste 602, Alexandria, VA 22314–2747, 1–703-894–1805, www.alfa.org

Association for Frontotemporal Dementias
Radnor Station Building #2, Suite 200
290 King of Prussia Road, Radnor, PA 19087, 1–866-507–7222, www.ftd-picks.org

Caregivers World
Lakeside Road, RR #1, Box 1442, Hop Bottom, PA 18824, 1–800-239–4116,
www.caregiversworld.com

Centers for Medicare & Medicaid
7500 Security Boulevard, Baltimore MD 21244–1850, 1–800-633–4227, www.medicare.gov,
www.cms.gov

Children of Aging Parents
PO Box 167, Richboro, PA 18954, 1–800-227-7294, www.caps4caregivers.org

Creutzfeldt-Jakob Foundation
P.O. Box 5312, Akron, OH 44334, 1–800-659–1991, www.cjdfoundation.org

Eldercare Locator
1–800-677–1116, www.eldercare.gov

ElderCare Online
Prism Innovations, Inc., 50 Amuxen Court, Islip, N.Y. 11751, www.ec-online.net

Ethnic Elders Care
Department of Psychiatry, University of California, Davis, 1–925-372–2105,
    www.ethnicelderscare.net

Exelon—Novartis Patient Assistance Program
PO Box 66556, St. Louis, MO 63166–6556, 1–800-277–2254, www.exelon.com

Family Caregiver Alliance
180 Montgomery St, Ste 1100, San Francisco, CA 94104, 1–415-434–3388,
    www.caregiver.org

Financial Planning Association
4100 E. Mississippi Ave., Suite 400, Denver, Colorado 80246–3053, www.fpanet.org

Foundation for Health in Aging
The Empire State Building, 350 Fifth Avenue, Ste 801, New York, NY 10118,
    1–800-563–4916, www.healthinaging.org

Geriatric Resources, Inc.
www.geriatric-resources.com

Gerontological Advanced Practice Nurses Association
East Holly Ave., Box 56, Pittman, NJ 08071, 1–866-355-1392, www.gapna.org

Healing Well
www.healingwell.com

Lewy Body Dementia Association, 912 Killian Hill Road, S.W., Lilburn, GA 30047, Caregiver
    Helpline: 1–800-539–9767, National Office (Atlanta, GA): 1–404-935—6444,
    www.lbda.org

Namenda—Forest Pharmaceuticals Patient Assistance Program
13600 Shoreline Drive, St. Louis, MO 63045, 1–80-851–0758, www.namenda.com

National Academy of Elder Law Attorneys
1604 N. Country Club Road, Tucson, AZ 85716, 1–520-881–4005, www.naela.com

National Adult Day Services Association
www.nadsa.org

National Association of Area Agencies on Aging
1730 Rhode Island Ave NW, Ste 1200, Washington, DC 20036, 1–202-872–0888,
    www.n4a.org

National Association of Geriatric Care Managers
1604 N. Country Club Road, Tucson, AZ 85716, 1–520-881–8008, www.caremanager.org

National Family Caregivers Association
10400 Connecticut Avenue, Suite 500, Kensington, MD 20895–3944, 1–800-896–3650,
    www.thefamilycaregiver.org

National Hospice and Palliative Care Organization
1700 Diagonal Road, Ste 625, Alexandria, VA 22314, 1–703-837–1500, www.nhpco.org

National Institute of Aging
Building 31, 5C27, 31 Center Drive, MSC 2292, Bethesda, MD 20892, www.nia.nih.gov

National Institute of Health
9000 Rockville Pike, Bethesda, MD 20892, www.nih.gov

National Institute of Health (clinical trials link)
www.clinicaltrials.gov

National Institute of Neurological Disease and Stroke
PO Box 5801, Bethesda, MD 20824, 1–800-352–9424, www.ninds.nih.gov

Parentgiving, Inc.
105 Grove Street Suite 5, Montclair, NJ 07042, 1–888-746–2107, www.parentgiving.com

Index

AAN guideline, 175
Aberrant motor behaviors, 109
  treatment, 109–112
Acetyl cholinesterase inhibitor agents, 58
AChEI drugs
  dosing, 60
  duration of benefit, 63
  efficacy, 59
  frequency of response, 61
  magnitude of response, 62–63
  proportion of, 61
  timing of response, 62
  tolerability, 63–64
Adaptation theory, 225
ADAS-cog scores, 59
  graphical presentation, 62
Agency for Healthcare Research and Quality, 241
Alzheimer's disease, 1, 5, 8, 169, 178, 225–226
  behavioral symptoms, 72
  demographics, 27
  diagnosis, 27–29, 173–174
  drugs, 177–178
  efficacy of AChEI drugs, 59
  evaluation of, 30–31, 175
  genetics of, 32
  imaging techniques, 30
  informed decision making, 219–220
  issue, 226–227
  living arrangements, 180–181
  management, 175–176
  pathology of, 26–27
  protective factors, 32
  recognition of, 173
    risk factors, 173
    warning signs, 173
  stress, 225
Alzheimer's Disease Assessment Scale
  (ADAS), 31

Alzheimer's Disease and Related Disorders
  Association (ADRDA), 28
Alzheimer's Foundation of America, 240, 244
Alzheimer Research Forum, 240
Alzheimer's Resource Room, 240
Alzheimer's Society of Canada, 240
APOE allele, 31
APOE genotype, 31
Association for Frontotemporal Dementias,
  240
American Academy of Neurology, 30, 240
American Association for Geriatric
  Psychiatry, 174, 40
American Medical Association, 29
American Medical Directors Association, 241
American Neuropsychiatric Association, 241
Amyloid angiopathy, 45
Amyotrophic lateral sclerosis (ALS), 33
Anticonvulsants, 83, 98, 101
Antioxidants, 14–15
Apraxia, 147–148
Aphasia, nonfluent, 37
Ataxia, 33, 44–45, 49, 77
  hereditary, 33

Baltimore Longitudinal Study of Aging, 182
Basic activities of daily living (ADLs), 141
  bathing, 142
  dressing, 142
Benzodiazepines, 72, 94, 97, 102, 105, 114,
  177
Blood pressure, 9, 89, 202
Body mass index, 10
Buspirone, 77–78, 94–95, 97–99, 101

Caregiver stress
  challenges, 227–228
  health outcomes of, 230–231
  interventions, 231

Caregiver stress (*Continued*)
   issues, 226–227
   role of relationships, gender and ethnicity,
      228–230
Cerebrovascular disease/stroke, 9
Cerebrospinal fluid, 49
Cholinesterase inhibitor, 178
CERAD battery, 31
Consortium to Establish a Registry for
      Alzheimer's Disease (CERAD), 31
Creutzfeldt-Jacob disease (CJD), 48

Degenerative Parkinsonian syndromes
      disorders, 38–39
Dementia, 1, 226
   age-specific incidence rates, 2
   aggressive and agitated behaviors, 78–79
   aggressive and agitated studies, 79–82
   air travel tips, 133–134
   apathy behaviors treatment, 92–96
   apathy, 92
   behavior management, 71–74
   behavior modification approaches, 73–76
   corticobasal degeneration (CBD), 38–39,
      42–43
   culture, 205–206
   depression, 88–89
   differential diagnosis of, 32
     alcoholism, 32, 49
     Alzheimer's disease, 32
     drug/medication intoxication, 32
     Parkinson's disease, 32
     vascular dementia, 32
   driving, 129–132
   ecology of, 171
   economic impact, 5
   epidemiology of, 1–2
   environmental/experiential factors, 8–9
     age, 8
     female sex, 8
     race/ethnicity, 8–9
   ethical issues, 188
     diagnosis, 188
     diagnostic disclosure, 188–192
   genetic factors, 7
     promoting, 7
     protective, 7–8
   head trauma, 11–12
   history of, 1
   household management, 137
   incidence, 2

   legal issues, 210
     advance health care planning, 212–213
     decisional capacity, 211–212
     informed consent, 210
   management of finances, 134–135
   management of function, 141
     dressing, 142–143
     grooming, 143–144
     oral hygiene, 144–145
   meal preparation, 137–138
   medication administration, 135–137
   mild cognitive impairment (MCI), 25
   mortality of, 3–4
   nutritional issues, 145–148
     apraxia, 147–148
     home safety, 148–149
     toileting/sphincter issues, 146–147
     weight loss, 145–146
   obesity/metabolic syndrome, 10
   prevalence, 4
   psychotic behaviors, 83–84
   psychotic studies, 85–88
   recognition, 170—172
   risk factor, 6–7
   senile dementia, 27
   smoking, 12
   technology, 139–140
   terminal condition, 200
   traveling, 132–133
   vascular risk factors, 9
   yard maintenance, 138–139
Dementia of depression, 50–51
Dementia/amnestic syndrome, 49
Dementia Rating Scale (DRS), 31
Department of Health and Human Services
      Administration, 5
Depressive symptoms and loneliness, 11
Depression, 88–89
   treatments, 89–92
Diagnostic and Statistical Manual of Mental
      Disorders, 27, 50
Diurnal rhythm disturbance, 101
Drugs
   behavioral disturbance, 179
   depression, 179
   use for dementia syndrome, 77–78
Durable powers of attorney, 213–214
   living wills, 214–215

Eating disturbances, 105–106
   treatment, 106–107

Electronic medication dispensers, 136
Eosin histologic staining, 42
Estrogen therapy, 15–16
Ethical issues
  autonomy versus beneficence, 195–196
  decision-making capacity, 193
  dementia caregiver, 192–193
  disclosure process, 189–190
  genetic testing, 191–192
  management of, 196–198
  mild cognitive impairment, 192
  nondementia illnesses, 198–199
  palliative care, 201
    restraints, 196–197
  societal level, 203–204
  terminal condition, 200

18-F-FDDNP, 30
Fluoxetine, 77–78, 89, 90, 92, 99, 113
Folic acid, 15
Frontotemporal dementia (FTD)
  diagnosis, 33
  features of, 35
  imaging of, 34–35
  neurochemistry, 35
  pathology, 37–38
  symptoms of, 35
FTD-motor neuron disease (FTD-MND), 33
FvFTD, 36

Genetic counseling, 190–191
Genetic testing, 191–192
GRN mutations, 38

Hachinski Ischemic Scale, 47
HDL, *See* High-density lipoprotein
Hematoxylin staining, 42
High-density lipoprotein (HDL), 9
Hypersexual disturbances, 107–109
  treatment, 107–109

Inflammatory markers, 13
Initial Assessment of Alzheimer's Disease and Related Dementias, 29
Institutional review board (IRB), 220
Instrumental activities of daily living (IADLs), 127
  driving, 129–132
  occupation/life role, 128–129
  management of function, 127
  traveling, 132–133

Intermittent emotional expression disorder (IEED), 97–98
Intrasynaptic enzyme, acetylcholinesterase, 58

KISSES Mnemonic, 183
Korsakoff's psychosis, 49

LDL, *See* Low-density lipoprotein
Lewy body dementia, 40–41
  features, 40–41
  pathology, 41–42
Low-density lipoprotein (LDL), 9

Major depressive disorder (MDD), 175
Magnetic resonance imaging (MRI), 30
MAPT mutations, 38
MDD, *See* Major depressive disorder
Metabolic syndrome, 10
Mild cognitive impairment (MCI), 192
  diagnosis, 26
  pathology, 25–26
Mini-Mental State Examination (MMSE), 172
Mood lability, 97
  treatment, 98–100
Moral agnosia, 35
MRI, *See* Magnetic resonance imaging (MRI)
Multi-infarct dementia, 45, 48
Multisystem atrophies, 39, 44–45

National Academy of Elder Law Attorneys, 240
National guideline clearinghouse, 174
National Hospice and Palliative Care Organization, 240
National Institute of Aging, 241
National Institute of Health, 241
Neurodegenerative disorder, *See* Alzheimer's disease
Neurological and Communicative Disorders and Strokes (NINCDS), 28
Neurological signs, 35–36
Neurotransmitter acetylcholine, 57
New England Journal of Medicine, 170
NINCDS, *See* Neurological and Communicative Disorders and Strokes
N-methyl-D-aspartate modulation, 65
  dosing, 66
  duration of benefit, 67
  frequency of response, 66
  mechanism of action, 65

N-methyl-D-aspartate modulation
(*Continued*)
receptor, 177
studies, 65–66
timing of response, 66
tolerability, 67
N-methyl-D-aspartate receptor, 177
Normal pressure hydrocephalus (NPH), 48

Obsessive-compulsive traits, 113
treatment, 114
Orthostatic hypotension, 44

Palliative care
definition, 201
special issue, 201–202
Parkinson's disease, 12
PET, *See* Positron emission tomography
Pharmacotherapy approaches
aggression and agitation behaviors, 76–77
Pharmacotherapy of cognition, 56
cholinesterase inhibitors, 57–58
therapeutics outcomes, 56–57
Pittsburgh Compound B (PIB), 30
Positron emission tomography (PET), 30
Progressive nonfluent aphasia (PNFA)
disorder, 37
Progressive supranuclear palsy, 42
Prototypical cortical dementia, 39

Screening tests
mental status questionnaire, 31
short probable mental status questionnaire,
31
Self-determination Act, 212
Semantic dementia (SD), 36–37
Severe Impairment Battery (SIB), 59
Short Kurtz test (SKT), 31

Single photon emission tomography (SPECT),
30
Sleep disturbances, 101–102
treatment, 102–104
Steele-Richardson-Olszewski syndrome, 42
Subcortical dementia, 39
Surrogate decision making, 216
involuntary commitment, 218–219
planned, 216
unplanned, 216

Thyroid function test, 175
Toxic disorders, 32
Tolerability, 58, 63–64, 67, 92

Ubiquitin-associated TAR, 37
Uniform Health Care Decisions Act, 213
Ubiquitin inclusions, 37
Ubiquitin-positive inclusions, 38
Ubiquitin immunohistochemistry, 38
Ubiquitin-proteasome system, 42

Valproate, 78, 81, 92–94, 97–98, 102, 105–107,
107, 110
Vascular dementia, 45–46
diagnosis, 46–47
evaluation for, 47–48
treatment of, 48
VCP mutation, 38
Verbal agitation, 111
Vitamin E and nutriceuticals, 67
Vomiting, 63–64, 77–78

Warning signs, 130, 172, 180, 183
Wear-and-tear hypothesis, 225
Wernicke's encephalopathy, 32

Ziprasidone, 77–78, 81, 84, 86, 88

Milton Keynes UK
Ingram Content Group UK Ltd.
UKHW020026071024
449327UK00032B/2949

9 780367 383398